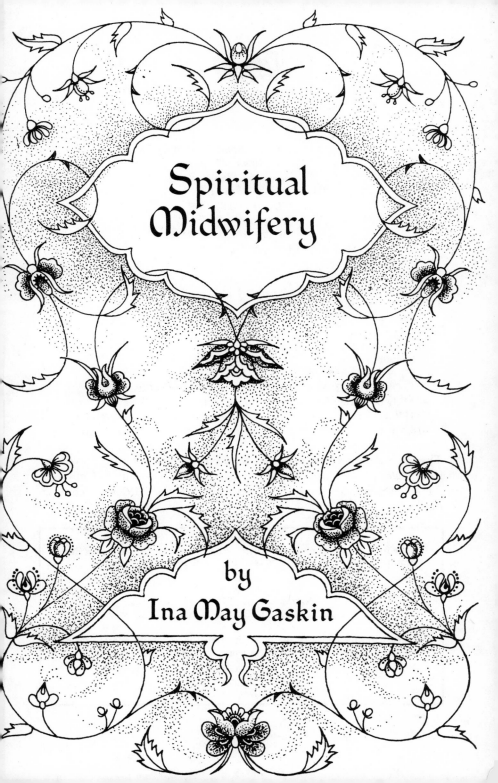

Spiritual Midwifery

by
Ina May Gaskin

© 1977, 1980, 1990 The Book Publishing Company
Summertown, TN 38483
All Rights Reserved
Printed in the USA
ISBN 0-913990-63-9

Library of Congress
Card Catalog Number
89-31060

Gaskin, Ina May.
    Spiritual Midwifery / by Ina May Gaskin. --3rd ed.
        p.   cm.
    Bibiography: p.
    Includes index.
    ISBN 0-913990-63-9
    1. Obstetrics. 2. Midwives. 3. Natural childbirth--Case studies.
    4. Midwives--Tennessee--Biography. I. Title.
RG526.G37 1989   89-31060
618.4'5--dc19   CIP

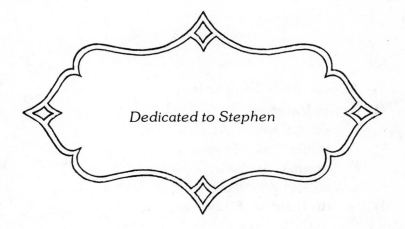

Dedicated to Stephen

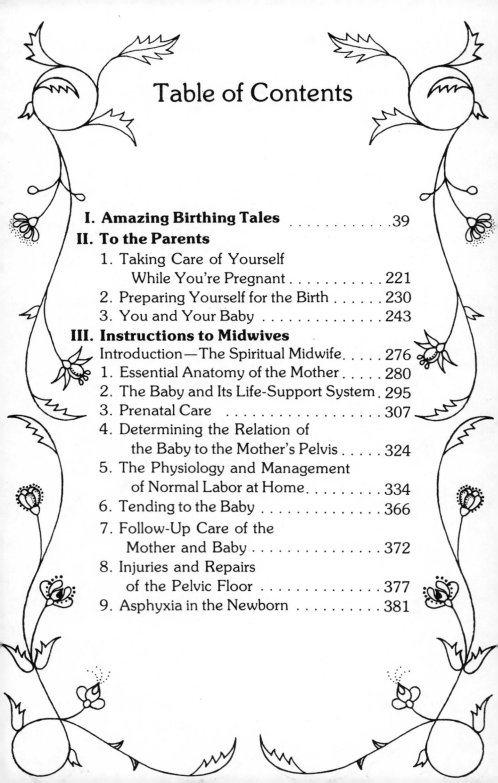

Table of Contents

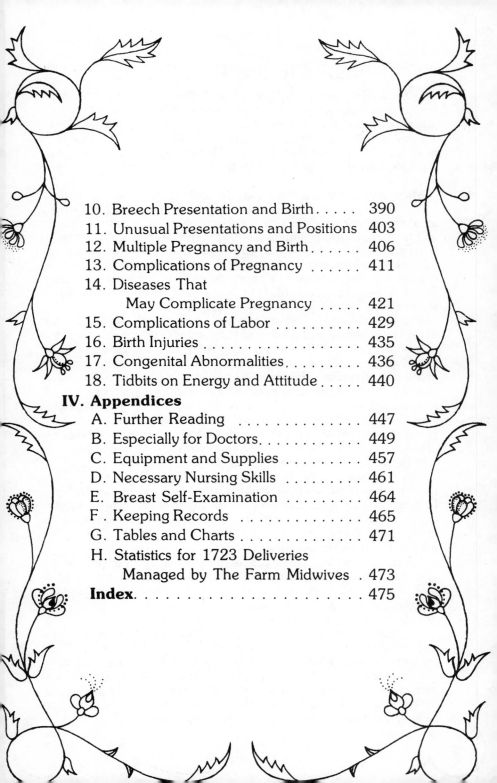

Preface to the Third Edition

In the fifteen years since **Spiritual Midwifery** was first published, it has become even more evident than before that the return of the birthing process to women is important to society at large, not just to the women and children directly involved. The way babies are treated at birth is likely to affect them forever. The way women are treated during childbirth affects them in all their relationships for the rest of their lives.

Many seeds for later actions and relationships are planted in the birth room. Marriages may be made or broken here, mothers form lasting ideas about their strengths or weaknesses, about their mates' strengths and frailties and lasting impressions about the "personality" of the newborn are created. The woman who is gently mothered by a midwife or nurse through her labor learns by absorption some of the most important skills she will need as a parent. When she is showered with sweetness and love, she is more likely to have a fund of generosity on which she can later draw when her patience is tested.

The United States, the industrialized country with the highest rate of teenage mothers giving birth, needs to provide these young mothers (many of whom will be keeping their babies) with the most sensitive care that can be organized. Machines and high tech equipment cannot provide sensitive care; only human beings can carry out this important task. Once we are able to provide our young mothers with really excellent and appropriate care, whether or not they give up their babies for adoption, we may be smart enough to dissuade people who are too young and uneducated for the responsibility of parenthood from beginning pregnancies. At the time of this writing, we, as a society, are very far from knowing the answers to the problems of teen pregnancy.

The information in this book is almost exclusively derived from women by women. This fact alone makes this information rare and unique. In today's world, particularly the industrialized portions of it, we have almost no data available to us that come exclusively from women, even in areas such as pregnancy and childbirth, where we are discussing behavior that is solely feminine.

For this and other reasons, the childbirth experiences of people who gave birth within The Farm community are relevant to the world at large. Here, the culture surrounding pregnancy and childbirth was put together by the women who were still having babies. The care system was designed by those who were using it.

The men of The Farm community provided technological assistance and moral support to the midwives and birthing women, but they did not interfere with the ideas, the organization, the customs and ways, and culture that developed among the women. This behavior on the part of the men was not random or accidental, but part of a philosophical decision to give the women the kind of chance they weren't able to have in much of the rest of the Western world.

Spiritual Midwifery is a book primarily written by women about women's experiences, expressed in women's terms. Because women tend to form their deepest attitudes about childbirth by listening to the stories of others, I included a lot of the women's own stories of their pregnancies, their births, their miscarriages. What makes these stories rise above the usual value given information that is anecdotal is that these come from a community of women who knew one another intimately. Many of them lived in the same house for a period of time, they exchanged babysitting from the time their babies were very young, they ate the same food, knew the same people, shared the same values — in short, they established a culture that was unique to The Farm. Within this culture, certain patterns may be discerned that may shed light on little-understood or little-investigated areas of human experience.

I believe that the origins of compassionate behavior in humans come from the female side of experience. It is difficult for any human to express compassion who has not been on the receiving end of it. Being compassionate to the pregnant or birthing mother is not just an insignificant nicety of our practice — it lies at the very heart of our success. Kindness begets kindness that is passed on to nursing babies and to proud fathers, to brothers and sisters, cousins, aunts and uncles.

It is possible to reach, in meditation, a level of consciousness which gives deep insight into oneself. Impulses and motivations that may not ordinarily be apparent may become crystal clear. In an even deeper level of meditation, it is possible to reach a level of insight that goes beyond the inner personal wellsprings of thought, worlds and behavior into a consciousness of what is universal in humanity. Such insight and power is available to birthing women under the right circumstances. We think our community was able to discover the qualities of favorable, even ideal, circumstances for giving birth and raising children.

This complex of values that attends each birth is so profound and universal that I use the term "spiritual" when I talk about midwifery. What is caused in the birth (or delivery) room does not end there.

My hope is that the collection of information that follows will aid women in attaining the insight that can lead to power that equals that of men. Only in this way, I believe, can we reach a real balance in our society.

The creation of this book began in 1975, with the innocent cultural expectation that the language and values in it would continue. This third edition has been revised with the intent of keeping these important ideas and concepts fresh and available to a new generation of women who need some form of cultural stability behind their own birthing efforts.

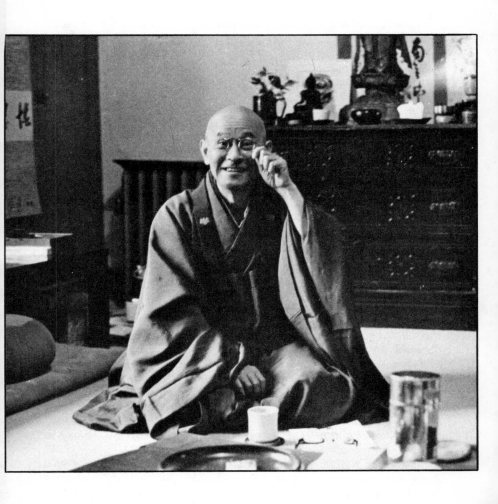

Once at a Zen Center picnic in Golden Gate Park, I saw Suzuki do what I felt was a silent teaching on the nature of Enlightenment.

When he arrived at the gathering he saw a baby blanket on the ground and he lay down on it and rolled up in it and just lay there a while in his black robes, rolled up in a lacy pink baby blanket.

—Stephen
Gaskin

In the Zen tradition, a line of succession of Zen Masters is supposed to be linked together by transmission of mind—pure thought transferred from mind to mind with no words. I think that with midwives there is a similar kind of transmission that can take place and link them together and that is a transmission of touch.

Touch is the most basic, the most non-conceptual form of communication that we have. In touch there are no language barriers; anything that can walk, fly, creep, crawl, or swim already speaks it.

I first experienced a transmission of this kind, not with another midwife, but with a lady Capuchin monkey, a couple of years before I ever thought of being a midwife. I learned something from her in touch language that has stayed with me, and this is part of what I have felt I must pass on to any midwife that I teach. A young man who knew my husband, Stephen, stopped by one day to show us his monkey. She was a pretty little thing with delicate features and a very expressive face, and she was trusting and friendly. Stephen motioned for the monkey to come over to him, and she came over and climbed into his lap. She chattered at him a little, examined his shirt and then spied his cowhorn, which was hanging on the wall over his shoulder. He saw how interested she was in the horn so he took it down from the wall, put it to his lips and blew a long, clear note. The monkey lady was thrilled and wanted to try to blow it herself. Stephen handed her the horn and she tried to blow, but she didn't know how to purse her lips and direct the stream of air into the horn. Stephen tapped her to get her attention, pointed to his mouth and demonstrated how to blow by doing it himself so she could see it. She watched him very closely and tried it herself a couple of times and then suddenly dropped the horn, threw her arms around his head because she was so glad that he had treated her like an equal and volunteered to teach her something. It really got me high to see her do that and I slid over to her and offered her my finger to hold because I wanted to be her friend, too.

She took hold of my finger in her hand—it was a slender, long-fingered hand, hairy on the back with a smooth black palm—and I had never been touched like that before. Her touch was incredibly alive and electric. There was so much concentrated feeliness in her hand that I felt this warm glow travel from her hand to mine, on up my arm, and then I felt a nice electric rush spread over my whole body. I had a flash of realization then that my hand wasn't made any different than hers— same musculature, same bony structure, same nervous system. I knew that my hand, and everyone else's too, was potentially that powerful and sensitive, but that most people think so much and are so unconscious of their whole range of sensory perceptors and receptors that their touch feels blank compared to what it would feel like if their awareness was one hundred percent. I call this "original touch" because it's something that everybody has as a brand new baby, it's part of the kit. A baby born blind doesn't lose his original touch because he can't afford to pull his attention out of his skin and out of his hands when he gets so much of his information about the Universe this way. Many of us lose our "original touch" as we interact with our fellow beings in a fast or shallow manner. As I transmit the knowledge of spiritual midwifery to other women, I feel that compassion and true touch are of foremost importance.

—Ina May

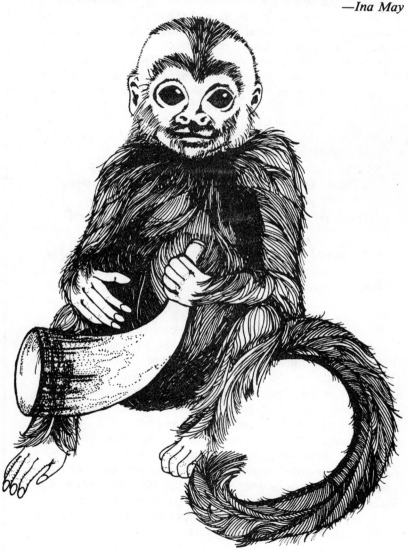

This is a spiritual book, and at the same time, it's a revolutionary book. It is spiritual because it is concerned with the sacrament of birth—the passage of a new soul into this plane of existence. The knowledge that each and every childbirth is a spiritual experience has been forgotten by too many people in the world today, especially in countries with high levels of technology. This book is revolutionary because it is our basic belief that the sacrament of birth belongs to the people and that it should not be usurped by a profit-oriented hospital system. The authors of *The Constitution of the United States* included an amendment to protect any basic human rights which might not have been covered in the rest of the Constitution—the Ninth Amendment:

The enumeration in the Constitution, of certain rights, shall not be construed to deny or disparage others retained by the people.

The midwives represented by this book feel that the rights of women, the newborn, and the family during the passage of childbirth are among those unenumerated rights which are to be retained by the people. We feel that returning the major responsibility for normal childbirth to an abundance of well-trained midwives rather than have it rest with a predominantly male and profit-oriented medical establishment would lower rates of premature birth, infant mortality, and cesarean section, not to mention skyrocketing costs. Mothers, babies and fathers need midwives to nurture them through the very impressionable and vulnerable period of pregnancy, labor and birth, and the time following birth. The wisdom and compassion a woman can intuitively experience in childbirth can make her a source of healing and understanding for other women.

When a child is born, the entire Universe has to shift and make room. Another entity capable of free will, and therefore capable of becoming God, has been born. In that way, every child's birth is exactly like the birth of a world teacher. Every child born is a living Buddha. Some of them only get to be a living Buddha for a moment, because nobody believes it. Nobody knows it, and they get treated like they're dumb. Babies are not dumb. Just because they don't speak English doesn't mean they're dumb. A newborn infant is just as intelligent as you are. When you're relating with him, you should consider that you are relating with a very intelligent being who just doesn't speak your language yet. And you shouldn't do anything gross to him before he learns to speak with you.

—Stephen

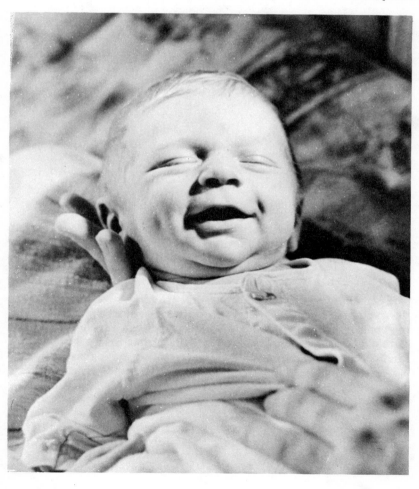

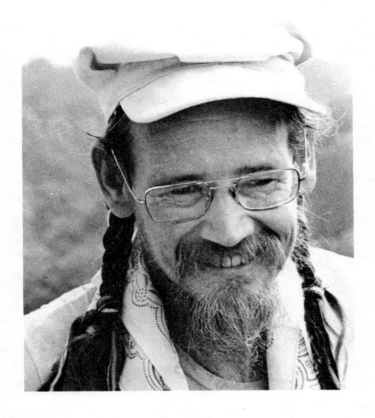

Stephen is my husband. I had been with Stephen for four years before I had anything to do with midwifery. He was always saying in the early days of our community that if we had a platform, it was clean air, sane people, and healthy babies. That sounded right to me. When I decided to learn about midwifery and was attending those first births, I applied the principles I had learned from him. He taught me respect for life force and truth and holiness, how to manage spiritual energy, how to be compassionate even when it's hard to be that way, how not to be afraid, and how to help people relax. These principles worked then and they continue to work so well that we felt that we would make this book so we could tell you about it. The rest of what I know, I learned from some compassionate doctors; from the women whose births I have attended; from studying medical textbooks; from my mother, who taught me that childbirth was not something to be scared of; from my father, whose common sense about pregnancy and birth gave me strength; from the five children I have given birth to; and from all the children whose births I have attended. I'm still studying.

We are a group of midwives who provide prenatal care and attend births for our community of three hundred people. The community, which came to be known as The Farm, was founded in 1971, when the first three hundred of us settled on a large piece of land near Summertown, Tennessee. The group of original settlers had come together in San Francisco during the late 1960's, attending open meetings held by my husband.

We are not just a community. We are a church. We hold our land and its assets in common. The community has gone through many changes since its founding, not the least of which has been its economic organization. For the first twelve years of its existence, the years during which the midwifery system was developed, we in the community shared fortunes in a way unknown to most Americans. We organized ourselves according to the Book of Acts in the *Bible* (2:44-45): "And all who believed were together and had all things in common: and they sold their possessions and goods and distributed them to all, as any had need." No money was exchanged for goods or services among the people of the community during those first twelve years.

The passage of time brings many changes to any community. Ours was no exception. We grew from three hundred to twelve hundred and shrank back to three hundred. This number includes quite a few original settlers, among them three of the four midwives who still work together. When the community revised its economic organization so that individual families became responsible for their own welfare, we midwives, like most other midwives in North America, began to charge money for our services.

It was even before we settled in Tennessee that we knew we were going to have to learn how to attend our own births. The original three hundred settlers spent several months accompanying Stephen on a national lecture tour, traveling in a caravan of remodeled schoolbuses and vans which were both our homes and our transportation. Several of us were pregnant when we left San Francisco, including myself. No one on the Caravan had ever attended a birth before. One woman had had her own baby at home, but her knowledge was limited. Our funds were primarily what savings we had among us and what we could earn on the way, so it seemed beyond our reach financially for each woman to give birth in a hospital. We were a transient population with no desire to leave a trail of debts behind us and we had an ethic that did not allow us to accept welfare. We were aware that many of our contemporaries were accepting the benefits of the larger society at the same time they were loudly criticizing it, and we had no wish to be associated with this position. Besides this, several of us had given birth in hospitals previous to the Caravan and had been unsatisfied with the way we and our babies were treated. We wanted our men to be with us during the whole process of childbirth, an option that was not available in American hospitals at the time, we didn't want to be anesthetized against our will, and we didn't want to be separated from our babies after their births. We were already looking for a better way.

Current Staff

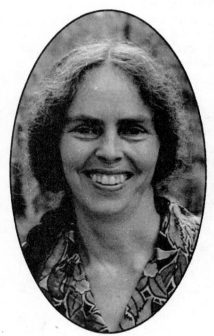

Ina May Gaskin

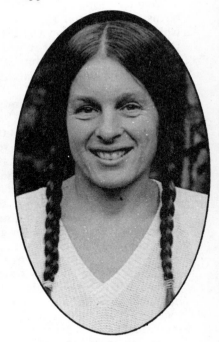

Pamela Hunt

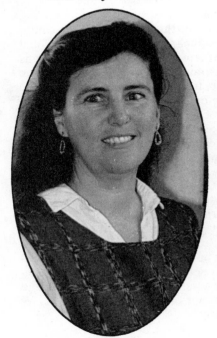

Joanne Santana

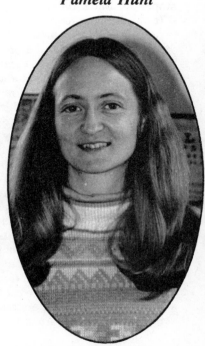

Deborah Flowers

Former Colleagues

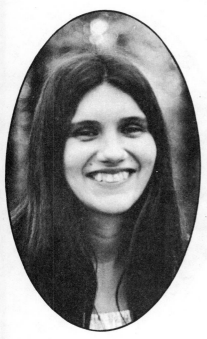

Kathryn McClure

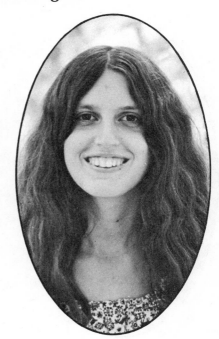

Leslie Luna

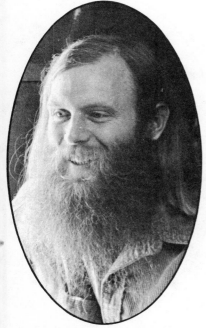

Jeffery Hergenrather

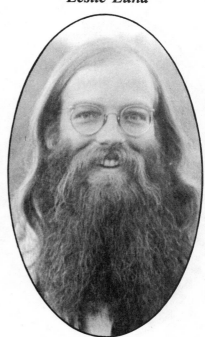

Gary Hlady

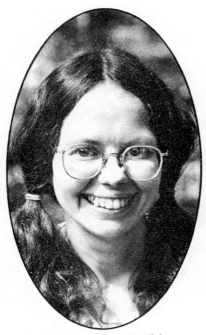

Mary Louise Perkins

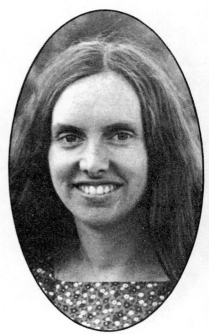

Cara O'Gorman

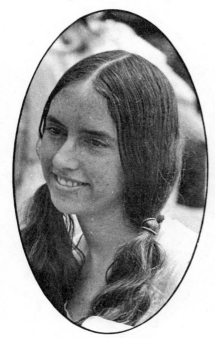

Mary Fjerstad

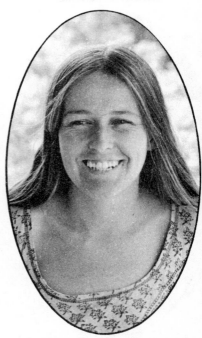

Kay Marie Schweitzer

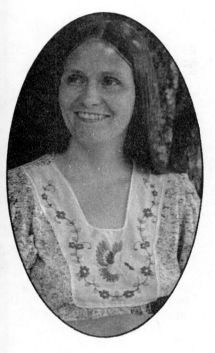

Tina Moon

Ruth Thomas

Elizabeth Maxen

Gladys Leininger

Gerri Sue Chappell

Diane Hoffman

Susan Rabideau

Isabel Serrano Perez

Carol Nelson

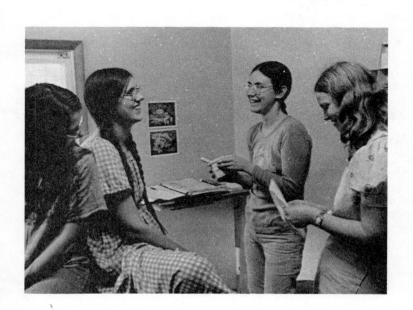

How We Started

Our first baby was a fine boy, born in his parent's schoolbus-camper in the parking lot at Northwestern University — the first birth I had ever seen. Just as Stephen was preparing to go into the lecture hall at Northwestern to address an audience of several hundred people, the baby's father came over to our bus to ask for Stephen's assistance at the birth. (Stephen had had combat experience with the Marines in Korea, where he received first-aid training and dealt with some life and death situations as a result. Because of this he was regarded as the most qualified person among us to attend a birth.) Knowing that he had to go ahead with his lecture, I volunteered to help at the birth.

The entire labor and birth lasted only three hours or so. I was no midwife at the time, but I was able to help the mother stay relaxed during this quick labor. I was struck by how beautiful this woman looked while she was laboring. The father actually "caught" the baby, who came out easily and started breathing by himself. There were no complications of any kind with mother or baby. I was in a state of amazement for several days. I had never seen a newborn baby before (my baby was almost a day old before I was allowed to see her), and I was struck with how perfect this baby looked, right from the time he took his first breath.

I felt a definite calling to be a midwife, but my Master's degree in English had not prepared me for anything so real life as a birth. It was during the second birth on the Caravan that I began to realize more fully the responsibility that goes with being a midwife. (See page 40, "Amazing Birthing Tales....") I saw that if I made any mistakes, or if I let any mistakes happen in my presence, I was going to have to live with them for the rest of my life. I began to study whatever I could find about pregnancy and childbirth.

My first real training in the essentials of midwifery was given to me and one of my first assistants, Margaret,* following the birth of the third Caravan baby, my first actual delivery. Dr. Louis La Pere, a Rhode Island obstetrician who had read in the newspapers about the Caravan and its births when we passed through there, took the trouble to come and visit us where we were parked. He gave Margaret and me a hands-on seminar on how to recognize any complications we were likely to encounter, and what to do if we did, demonstrating how to stimulate a baby to breathe, what to do if the umbilical cord was wrapped tightly around the baby's neck, what to do if the mother hemorrhaged. He taught us sterile technique and provided us with some necessary medications and instruments, my first obstetrics textbook and gave us instructions on how to provide good prenatal care. It was a great blessing to have met such an understanding obstetrician when we did, because what he taught Margaret and me enabled us to safely deal with the complications that

*Margaret Nofziger, Farm nutritionist and author of *A Cooperative Method of Natural Birth Control.*

came up in the very next birth on the Caravan. The cord was tightly wrapped around this baby's neck, the baby didn't breathe spontaneously and needed suctioning and stimulation to get him going, and the mother hemorrhaged following the expulsion of the placenta. We got the baby breathing, and stopped the mother's bleeding, immensely grateful for the training and courage we had absorbed from our friend.

The excitement generated by each Caravan birth was contagious. Each mother who gave birth became an inspiring and encouraging example to the other women. We came to look at birth as a sort of initiation or rite of passage—something for which you could gather up your courage with the help of your friends and contemporaries. (Even though more than half of the women during the first seven or eight years of our midwifery experience were having their first babies, they were able to give birth with the same help and encouragement that the others had.) Those who had given birth in hospitals were unanimous about how much easier and how much less painful it seemed to give birth in one's own bed than in the hospital.

As we travelled, we had common experiences and began to know each other better. When each birth took place, we all parked in a sort of protective formation around the bus in which the birth would take place, and everyone waited for the baby's first cry.

It wasn't until the two Wyoming births that we really had to deal with extreme weather while a labor was happening. It was early March, and the temperature was below zero every day, twenty degrees below at night. The differential on our schoolbus shattered when we tried to push start it on the first bitter cold morning. Another bus towed ours to Buck's Garage in Rock Springs so we could have a new rear end installed. It was relatively cozy inside the garage, but outside, where everyone else was parked, the winter winds whipped across the high plains, making it nearly impossible to keep warm in the schoolbuses, which were heated only by tiny woodstoves.

Two women went into labor at once; one who had given birth before and my current partner, Pamela, who was having her first baby. Up to then, we hadn't had any really long, drawn out labors, and Pamela seemed so strong, healthy and eager for the birth that I expected her to give birth quickly. She didn't. A full twenty-four hours passed, with very little dilation. She ate and drank as usual, as did all the laboring mothers who didn't give birth within five or six hours. Still, the baby's heart rate sounded fine, and Pamela looked healthy, though tired. By the end of the second day I was getting worried. Stephen and I began to wonder if Pamela had anything on her mind that was bothering her. I asked her, and she said that one thought had kept coming up. She wondered if her husband was going to stay with her for life. When they had married, they had had one of those new age ceremonies in which they had written their own vows. Neither Pamela nor her husband had wanted to mention "death" in their marriage vows, as in the phrase "till death do you part." Their pastor at that ceremony had thought this omission was a little strange, but he didn't argue with the young couple. When

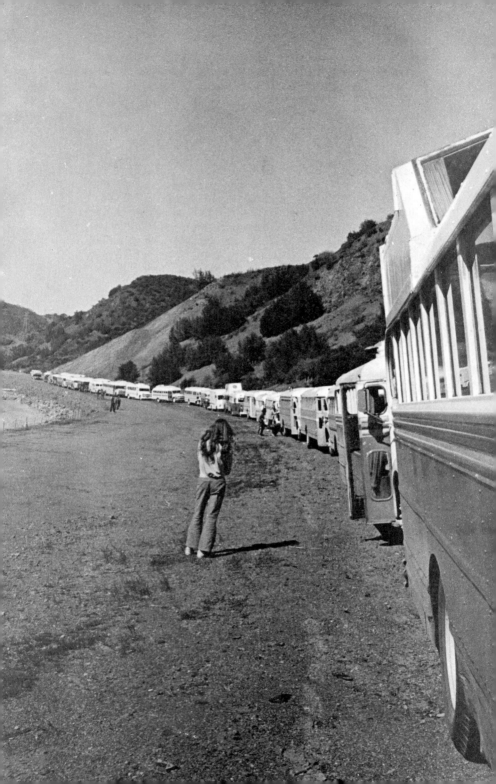

I heard about Pamela's concern, it felt significant, and I went inside the garage to our bus and mentioned it to Stephen. He had already been functioning as pastor of our group, and he volunteered to marry them on the spot. He said the vows, and Pamela and her husband repeated them after him, including "as long as we both shall live." She then labored on for three or four hours, but it was immediately obvious after the impromptu ceremony that she was making real progress now. When her son was born, Pamela and I talked about how he hadn't wanted to come out until his parents were properly married. The second Rock Springs baby was born very easily just a few hours after Pamela's son arrived.

My next strong lesson in midwifery came on the tenth birth on the Caravan— that of my own baby. Just before we reached Nebraska on our way to Tennessee to buy land, I started labor two months before my due date. My rushes** were light, so we decided to drive on across Nebraska. As it turned out, we had to stop in North Platte for a couple of days because of a blizzard. I'll never forget how kind the people there were; they brought us boxes and boxes of bread, milk and eggs. All this time I was trying to keep the rushes at a minimum, but by the third day it became obvious that I was going to give birth pretty soon. We had driven on from North Platte, and we found a place to park the buses for one night in Grand Island, and Stephen, with Margaret's assistance, caught my boy a few hours later. He was tiny—three pounds or less—and had extreme difficulty breathing right from the first. He lived for twelve hours, enough to see the light of day, and then he died in my arms, probably of hyaline membrane disease, the most common cause of death in premature babies in those days. I was filled with grief. At the same time, I knew he had taught me something I was never going to forget. I was also relieved that if we had to lose a baby that it was mine and not somebody else's. But it still took me several months—in fact, until the birth of my next child—to heal from the grief I felt at his death.

I learned a lot from those first few births I attended on the Caravan. Altogether, there were eleven babies born while we were on the road: one in Illinois, one in Michigan, one in New York, one in Nashville, one in Kansas City, Missouri, two at rest stops in California, two in Rock Springs, Wyoming, one in Grand Island, Nebraska, and one at Percy Priest Park near Nashville. All are indelibly engraved in my memory.

It wasn't until we started delivering babies in Tennessee and filling out birth certificates for them that we realized we hadn't gotten birth certificates for the Caravan babies. We ran into unexpected problems doing this, since it was so unusual to have a baby out of the hospital; the public health authorities in many places weren't sure how to go about certifying the birth of a baby who had arrived in a schoolbus. We had to get a few people together to remember what California counties we

---

**I like to use the term "rush" in place of "contraction" because I think it describes better how to flow with the birthing energy.

had been in for the babies born at the rest stops. Most of the parents managed to get all the proper papers on their babies within a few days, months or years after the child's birth, but our Kansas City baby only got his birth certificate at the age of 18, when he was preparing to enter college.

We finally settled in Tennessee, in the middle of a thousand acres of oak trees. A few days after our arrival, we were visited by our county public health nurse, and we asked what was the procedure for getting further training as a midwife in Tennessee. This was 1971, sixteen years after the formation of the American College of Nurse-Midwives, but there were still so few nurse-midwives that no one among us had any knowledge of officially-sanctioned, modern day midwives. We were told that Tennessee had no provision for the licensing of midwives to attend home births. She said that Kentucky had some kind of training program for midwives, but let me know that it was necessary to be a registered nurse and that once graduated, I would be violating the rules to attend home births. As I listened to her, my mind was full of the twelve pregnant women who expected me to continue to care for them during pregnancy and birth, my five year old daughter, my husband who was underweight and struggling with sciatica and the six years of university study I had already completed. She left me wondering what I should do.

Two men from the State Bureau of Vital Statistics accompanied the same public health nurse on a second visit with us the next day. She gave me a box of ampules of silver nitrate, and the men gave me a stack of birth certificates and death certificates and wished me good luck. I was glad we had picked a state to live in where enough people had been safely born at home in recent memory that the public health authorities were not afraid of the idea.

We set about to learn everything we could about safe practices and standards of providing midwifery care for all the people we served. Ever since Pamela's birthing, I had thought I would like her to be my midwife the next time I gave birth. I became pregnant again about six months after the death of my little son. I knew I needed a midwife to nurture me during my pregnancy and birthing, and I couldn't think of anyone I felt safer with than Pamela. She was the calmest, kindest, most patient person I knew. Margaret had already let me know that while she had been my very competent assistant at a few births, she knew she didn't want to be a midwife. So I asked Pamela to begin studying with me and attending births with me. Now I had someone to measure my belly and fuss over me as my baby grew.

While I had some fears during my pregnancy, especially before I got to my seventh month, I knew that I was being well cared for and that my chances to give birth to a full term baby this time were good. Dr. Williams was very reassuring, and so were Pamela and Stephen. I was reasonably sure that my previous birth had been premature because I had been anemic, as well as exhausted. During this pregnancy, although I still had births to attend, I managed to catch up on lost sleep by napping whenever I felt sleepy.

Not only did I reach my due date before going into labor this time, I went past it by ten days. When labor began, I phoned Pamela, who was nearly eight months pregnant with her second baby. By this time we lived in an army tent, and it was June of our second summer on The Farm. As I was always a slow baby-haver, and not many hours into my labor, Pamela was called over to Cara's to catch her second baby, another girl. Pamela returned to our tent, smiling and glowing. I suggested that she sleep until I got more dilated. It was a warm June night, so warm that the sides of the tent were rolled up and June bugs and moths were divebombing the kerosene lamps. The woods were alive with crickets, frogs, exchanges between whippoorwills and the soft hoot of an occasional owl. A few hours after sunup, our daughter, Eva Marie, was born easily after a few good pushes, obviously a well done, healthy girl. She weighed eight pounds, ten and a half ounces. The next day I was presented with a beautiful quilt for Eva, which had been made by most of the women who then lived on The Farm. Each of them had embroidered a beautiful square for the quilt, as a way of wishing me well with this baby. I was so grateful for the strength I received from this sisterhood and for my beautiful, healthy baby.

Six weeks later I brought Eva along with me to Pamela's next birthing. This time it was July in Tennessee, and instead of huddling inside a schoolbus in below zero weather, Pamela and her husband had chosen to give birth outside on a platform under the oak trees. It was a lovely place for Stephanie to be born at dawn.

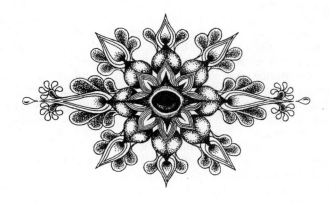

Pamela's Story

Being a midwife is not what I thought I'd do when I grew up. I didn't even know what a midwife was until we came across the word "midwife" in the Bible in my high school church youth group. Our minister told us that midwives were women who delivered babies in the old days before doctors began doing it. I put it out of my mind.

My mother had all her babies in the hospital, and she loved us very much, so I supposed it was a good experience for her. I remember her looking beautiful each time when my father brought her and my new baby brother home from the hospital.

In college I studied interior decorating and fine art, and my studies brought me to the University of Guadalajara in Mexico for two years. Here, one of my art classes was a class in anatomy. One of the field trips for this class was to one of their state-run hospitals. While there, I observed two "natural" births and one cesarean birth. In all three births, when the doctor pulled the baby out, which he had to do because the women were given epidural anesthesia, he slapped the baby on the butt, swung it in the air and gave it to a nurse. Then he walked out of the room. All three mothers looked tired and forlorn after the births. Their husbands had not even been allowed in the room to comfort them. No one else did this either, and here was this class of anatomy students observing, a group of total strangers who didn't know the first thing about birth. Why they arranged for us to be at these births and put these poor women up as models at this most vulnerable time in their lives, I'll never know. We certainly didn't learn any anatomy or compassion for the mother or baby.

I was shocked. Is this what my mother went through? She, too, had an epidural with her babies. I didn't really think she got this treatment when she had her babies, because she always looked so pretty when she came home from the hospital, but seeing that this could happen convinced me that I would find another way to have my babies.

I started to notice when my Mexican school friends talked about their aunts or mothers having their babies at home. About that time, I read a novel about how the peasants in China just squatted in the field to give birth and then went on with their work. That was enough for me. I didn't want to give birth in the field, but I was sure if the peasants could do it that way, that I could do it at home in my own bed with my husband at my side. Actually, the whole idea of becoming a peasant myself was intriguing to me. I saw peasants as honest, hard-working people who loved each other, had big families, believed in God, and knew how to have babies. I had put value in these things for many years already.

During the next two years, I moved back to the United States to finish my education. My parents sent me to San Francisco in 1965 to attend my senior year at San Francisco State College.

There were hippies with flowers in their hair everywhere. They looked pretty and had fun and seemed to share a lot of the same ideals that were strong in my mind, so I became a hippy, too. I hitchhiked to school, figuring God would provide me with the safety I needed. I wasn't afraid of work and worked hard at whatever I did at school or at my jobs.

Around this time I met Stephen Gaskin, a teacher at San Francisco State College. He said, "Helping man is a good place to start your search for God." I was depending on God's help a lot and wanted to be close to him. San Francisco in those days was pretty wild, and I was single and young. I knew I would need His help to get through. Stephen provided me with the spiritual guidance I needed to be close to God at that time.

My mother had also given me a good spiritual background, which kept me in touch with God. I became part of a church that was ministered by Stephen Gaskin. We travelled in 1970-71 around the country, stopping at churches and universities to talk. There were about three hundred of us on the trip, living and travelling in old school buses that we had painted very neatly in pretty colors. They were fixed up like homes inside with rugs on the floor and ceiling, beds, easy chairs, and kitchens. We had about fifty busses among us. There were six or seven families who were expecting their first or second babies. My husband and I were one of these families.

Our first woman went into labor in the parking lot of Northwestern University while most of the group were inside the university meeting hall. Three of us stayed out in her small bus lit by kerosene lamps and helped her through her labor. She had a fairly short labor and a healthy boy. I remember her looking beautiful all through her labor, kind of rosey and glowing.

The second birth took place in a park in Michigan. Cara, later one of our midwives, went into labor. Everyone wanted to see the birth, and as many people crowded into her tiny bus as could squeeze in. The vibes felt strained. One woman who was there was superstitious about any conventional information and criticized Ina May when she began looking through the Mexican midwifery manual we had. This person also thought the husband should be the one to deliver the baby and that no one person should be in charge. The situation felt shaky. Ina May was backed off, even though she was the best qualified person in our group to help the mother.

Cara was young and brave. Her baby was born blue and not breathing and weighing just a bit over five pounds. The father was in the catching position, wondering what to do. A woman went over to Stephen's bus and told him the baby had been born, and he knew by the tone of her voice that something was wrong. He ran over, took up the baby and breathed into her. She took a breath immediately and turned pink; our first miracle and our first heavy lesson. After this birth we didn't allow random people to attend a birthing, and Ina May was established as our main midwife in charge.

One of our women, pregnant with her third baby, went into labor as we were entering a small town in upper New York State. She, too, had a short labor. As her labor came on stronger, we realized we would have to stop the Caravan. We ended up in front of an old church. When the baby was born, the minister rang the church bells, and the townspeople of Ripley came out and brought food and good wishes.

The rest of our deliveries went smoothly. By the time my turn came to have a baby, I had complete confidence in the natural birthing process and in Ina May as my midwife.

The birthing of my first child tested every bit of faith I had. It was a forty-eight hour labor in the middle of Wyoming, with the temperature ranging from zero Fahrenheit to twenty-three degrees below zero, and with the draft board hot on my husband's trail. Every time we crossed a state line, we had to call his draft board. They threatened to come and take him at any time.

I was so grateful for Ina May, Margaret and Mary Louise, who helped me through the long hours of my labor. I never doubted that the baby would come out and that the outcome would be good. I did wonder when it would happen, and I asked often. I learned a lot from Ina May at Christopher's birth about how a midwife is really a wife to the mother. She stays with you through all your changes in labor.

When Christopher was born in the early morning, it felt like a miracle. He was healthy, and I felt tired but good. When he was two days old, we took him to a supermarket in Rock Springs and weighed him on the produce scale in the vegetable section of the store. He weighed 7 pounds and 2 ounces. Then we took him to the local hospital because we wanted a birth certificate for him. We told the lady in the records office that we wanted a birth certificate for our newly born baby, and she looked at us and said that they usually only made birth certificates for babies who were born in their hospital. After all, how could we prove the fact of the birthing, she wanted to know. There I was, with my baby in my arms, milk leaking through my sweatshirt. I was amazed that she doubted me. It was kind of funny, really, so I smiled and so did she. She did fill out the certificate and wished us luck.

My husband and I traveled back to California after Christopher's birth to figure out what to do about the draft board. At the time we turned back, a week after Christopher's birth, we didn't know that Ina May and the Caravan were headed toward some of their hardest times. We didn't hear that Ina May had lost her eight weeks premature baby until we reached The Farm in July. When I arrived in Tennessee, I found Ina May, Margaret and Stephen and many other friends yellow with hepatitis. They had eaten watercress picked from a local creek that was contaminated.

Ina May was skinny, yellow and still sad because she had lost her baby, but she continued to be strong in her convictions to make the community work. She was a real inspiration to me, as well as a good friend.

The day after we arrived, everyone got a gamma globulin shot from the Tennessee Health Department, so those of us who weren't already infected didn't get sick. We healthy ones helped care for those who were sick. We were already in touch with the health department about the hepatitis, and our local doctor, Dr. Williams, was aware of us. Ina May asked me if I would watch out for the health of the thirteen or fourteen children we had with us. These included some new babies and toddlers on up to a twelve year old. She gave me Dr. Williams' phone number.

This was a turning point in my life. I was not only responsible for my baby and husband, but also for a handful of kids who were running barefooted in the summer heat. The woods were full of poison ivy and chiggers, little larvae of mites that burrow under the skin and cause an irritation. The kids, especially the young ones, would scratch and their bites would get infected, which happens easily in Tennessee's sub-tropical climate. I gathered the group together every day in the morning and the evening and took them to the open air shower house the construction crew had built just up from a spring. I would get them nice and clean and then put antibiotic ointment on their infected scratches. I tried to teach them to take care of the bites instead of scratching. Most of the scratches healed right up, but there was one child whose didn't. His skin kept breaking out in little red swollen-looking blisters. I took him to Dr. Williams' office, and he told me how to care for the child and what antibiotic to give him. Dr. Williams was always a help to us.

Around the same time, a local pharmacist gave me a Physician's Desk Reference and Stephen gave me a Merck Manual to use. (See the appendix on "Further Reading", pg 447.) I started to read medical books. A young nurse name Kathryn joined our community, and she taught me how to give injections. We worked with the health department and started immunizing our children against infectious diseases. The health department was interested in us and befriended us. They gave us enough prenatal vitamins, iron and vitamin B12 (an essential vitamin for complete vegetarians) for all our nursing and pregnant women.

My husband built a lean-to next to our bus and hammered an orange crate onto a tree. This was our first clinic. In the orange crate were bandages, tape, alcohol, disinfectant and a bottle of antibiotics that Dr. Williams had given us with instructions on when and how to give them.

At the same time that I started helping with the kids, Ina May asked if I could help her with some of the pregnant women we had. I wanted to help her in any way I could, being grateful to her for helping get Christopher out and I wanted to help her do more of that. She showed me how to do prenatal checks, how to check the position of the baby and how to measure a woman's pelvis. We read everything we could find on pregnancy, birth and obstetrics. We made friends with our local doctors and called them whenever we had a question.

After helping Ina May with twenty-three birthings, I was left on The Farm to deliver several babies while Ina May and Stephen went on a trip to Ohio. One of these babies had the umbilical cord wrapped very tightly around her neck. I followed the steps Ina May had taught me from what she learned from Dr. La Pere. I clamped and cut the cord, unwound it to free the baby, and the mother pushed out a healthy baby girl, beautiful and pink. It worked so well. Every time we ran into a problem, we would read about it and talk it over with Dr. Williams. This is how we learned.

Our land consisted of a thousand acres, mostly woods, with a few fields, one house and a barn. One of the rooms in the house was given to the clinic crew, which now consisted of four women; Ina May, Margaret, Kathryn and myself. One wall of the room was lined with shelves which soon housed our medical library and medicines. By now we had a collection of antibiotics and cough syrups and a few other specialized medicines that were donated to our clinic. Once every couple of weeks we would go through the medicines and read about each one in the Physician's Desk Reference, when and how to use them, as well as the side effects of each medicine. When we had a question, we would call Dr. Williams or a pharmacist friend.

The house had a telephone, so we no longer had to go to the local bar to call our doctor. Meanwhile, The Farm grew in population. Not only were we having babies (about fifty the first year we settled), but new people had heard about our community and wanted to join us. Dr. Williams helped us a lot. Once when one of our mothers had been pushing for four hours with little progress, I called him and he came out. He examined her and said she had a small anterior lip of cervix caught between her pubic bone and the baby's head. He reached in and held the cervix back for one contraction and said, "You'll have the baby in an hour, honey" and then he left. He always made you feel good — and the mother did have her baby in an hour. When Dr. Williams got a citizen's band radio for his pickup truck so we could talk to him while he was away from a phone, his radio handle (nickname) was "Dr. Feelgood".

A few months after we settled in Tennessee, Ina May got pregnant again. This time we took very good care of her. Ina May wanted to come to the prenatal clinic we had for all our women by this time, so we put a big, comfortable chair in the clinic room so she could sit if she got tired. She came to birthings, but that was about all we'd let her do. Cara and Kathryn were helping with birthings, too, so I wasn't alone. Actually, all of us were pregnant, and all due between June and August. We had enough pregnant women that we were delivering between four to six babies a month. Starting families was one of our goals when we left San Francisco to find a place where we could live; we wanted to raise our families in the healthy environment of the country.

In early June, Cara went into labor. She lived in a small bus down a dirt path in the woods. Kay Marie, who was also helping with birthings now, and I had to walk the last 200 yards to her bus. Cara was beautiful in the lamplight and gave birth after an eight hour labor to a healthy, full term, chubby girl. As soon as we had Cara cleaned up, the call came that Ina May was starting labor. Kay Marie was three months pregnant and feeling nauseous, so she went home and I went on to Ina May's.

Ina May was on a bed in the corner of their big army tent with a lamp lit next to her when I arrived. She looked pink and golden as we exchanged smiles. This baby was full term and a good size. She was five centimeters dilated and having good rushes when I got there. I lay down to sleep for a while and dreamt about her baby and Cara's new girl and my baby. My baby was very active that night and kept turning and kicking in my belly, which was very comforting. It felt like there were babies everywhere that night.

I woke up two hours later hearing Ina May, and by the sounds I knew she would have the baby soon. I went to her and about half an hour later, she had a healthy, pink, beautiful baby girl. After Eva was born, my baby settled down inside me and I went home to catch up on my sleep.

A month later on a hot July night, Ina May delivered my baby, Stephanie, outside our bus on a large wooden platform that we had built under the trees for a cool place to rest in the summer. I remember feeling very well cared for pushing Stephanie out with Ina May, Cara and Kay Marie all helping. As the sun came up, a dewdrop fell from a tree and hit Stephanie's forehead. I felt she had been baptized.

Stephanie and Eva, both seventeen now are still good friends.

Carol was a young woman due to have her first baby. We had been on The Farm for a year and a half, and two small A-frame houses had been built from wood we had cut and milled at our own sawmill. Carol and her husband didn't have a place to live and have their baby, so the community gave them a loft in one of these houses. It was very rustic but warm, and Carol had it neatly fixed up with curtains on the window and a covered stand to hold a kerosene lamp.

The loft was only eight feet by ten feet, and you had to climb up a ladder to get to it, but it did have a skylight and was open to the rest of the house at one end, so it was bright and didn't feel that little. Carol felt very grateful to live here. There were two other young couples in the house who helped her with cooking and laundry. She was a quiet woman with long, straight brown hair, and when she smiled, I knew she was glad to be pregnant.

Ina May was off The Farm when Carol went into labor, so I was to deliver the baby with Cara's help. We went right out when we got the call and hoisted the birthing kit up over the edge of the loft, because it wouldn't fit through the hole for the ladder. We got everything ready and Carol proceeded right along with her labor.

After about six hours, she pushed out a healthy boy. As soon as the placenta came out, I noticed something else was out of her and realized immediately that it was her uterus inside out. I put on a sterile glove, made my hand into a fist and gently pushed the uterus back up inside her where it belonged. I massaged her uterus for a few minutes to stop the bleeding.

Carol was a little dizzy for about five minutes after all this happened. She started to nurse her baby and felt better so we fed her some warm soup. She was tired, but her color was greatly improved.

I had read about inverted uteruses and what to do about them a few weeks before this birth, but I didn't really think I would ever see one. When it happened my reaction was instinctual. I didn't think about it; I just did what was obviously necessary. I found out from a doctor years later that had I waited, the cervix would have closed and it would have meant an operation to get Carol's uterus back up in her pelvic cavity. We asked Carol to do shoulder stands against the wall and Kegel exercises* for a couple of months following this birthing.

I always say a prayer as I'm going to a birthing or sometime during the birthing. Sometimes I ask for God's help and sometimes I tell God exactly what I need and ask that He help with that specific thing. He has never let me down.

I sort of feel that I have a working agreement with God, that I promise Him I will do the work He puts in front of me. I haven't put any limits on this work. He can give me anything he wants. In return, I ask that He help me when I need help. I feel He is always there for me and I always feel His presence, especially at birthings. (Somehow I think He likes midwives.)

*Kegels are exercises of the muscles of the perineum and the pelvic floor. The woman alternately tightens and relaxes the anal and vaginal sphincters.

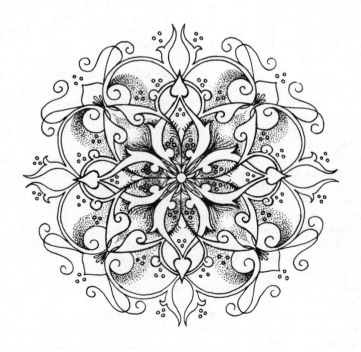

Back-up

During our first summer in Tennessee, we had the good fortune to meet a doctor who would help us in our struggle to take care of ourselves. Dr. John O. Williams Jr. was already used to births at home. In the early days of his practice, he used to go with an old doctor who was his mentor to the homes in the nearby Old Order Amish community. This group of Amish families had come to Tennessee in the 1940's from Pennsylvania, when their elders had decided that the Pennsylvania group was becoming too worldly. The Tennessee group to this date uses only horse and buggy for transportation (unless they are travelling

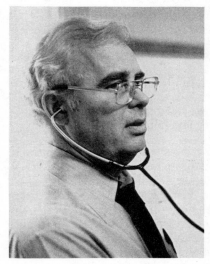

Dr. John O. Williams, Jr.

to other states or to Canada), light their homes with kerosene lamps, grow their own food, have no running water in their homes, and use no form of contraception. They give birth at home unless there is a life-threatening situation.

Dr. Williams' mentor had been attending Amish births when the community settled nearby. The women insisted on covering themselves with a blanket and having him catch the baby under the blanket without looking. When the old man died and Dr. Williams took over this part of the practice, he kept attending the home births but insisted the blanket had to go — so it did. He noticed that the Amish women and their babies ran a significantly lower rate of infection than the mothers and babies he saw in the hospital in the rest of his practice. His theory was that the lower rate of infection in the home births was due to the resistance the mothers built up to disease-causing organisms in their own environment. Also, since hospitals are places were sick people go, they are apt to have more dangerous microorganisms than a carefully kept home has. Dr. Williams let us know right away that he was interested to see if his theory would be borne out by the statistics of our home births. (It was.) We were told to call him any time of night or day if we had questions about the pregnant or birthing women and their babies.

An interesting note about Dr. Williams and the obstetrician who gave me my first seminar on emergency midwifery techniques is that both men are skilled at helping certain animals give birth when they have difficulties. Dr. Williams raised horses at the time we arrived in Tennessee, and the obstetrician often assisted his goats in birthing their young. I once told Dr. Williams that I thought he was good at attending human births because he treated women as well as he did his mares. (You have to be telepathic with mares to help them, or they'll give you a swift kick.)

Facilities and Communications

The Farm Midwifery Center has always been a mainstay of The Farm's primary health clinic. The clinic started as an orange crate containing bandages and antibiotic salve and has grown over the years to include examining rooms, laboratory, pharmacy and the equipment necessary for the primary health care of a community.

Those women who come from outside of our community to give birth here usually do so in Tower Road House, our birth house. It is equipped with oxygen tanks (we take portable tanks to other home births) and bilirubin lights, in the rare event that we have to deal with a baby with a high bilirubin count. We can provide around-the-clock nursing care if that is necessary.

In the early days of our settlement, when Margaret, Pamela and I were the only ones attending births, we had no communications other than how loud we could shout from hill to hill to relay a message. If we needed to make a phone call, we had to drive out three miles to a local bar to use the phone. When we did get a phone, we were on a party line with eight of our neighbors, and "we" amounted to three hundred people.

Of course, when we city folks moved out onto 1,000 acres that were mostly covered with oak trees, many of us headed for the borders. At first, not too many people wanted to live next door to one other. If we were called to a birth in one of the outlying areas, we'd have to stay at the couple's home from the beginning of the labor until the baby was born because we were still learning what constituted labor. Sometimes we'd spend two or three days sleeping out under the oak trees in our sleeping bags; or if it was cold, sleeping on the floor of the couple's house or bus, waiting to get the baby out. They always came out, we observed. That became an article of faith.

Sometime during the late winter of our first year, The Farm acquired its own telephone system as well as an outside phone line. We started getting telephones in our homes. Each pregnant woman had priority in having a phone installed. This meant that we no longer had to drive a few miles to the nearest public phone in order to consult with Dr. Williams. We could call him from the home of the birthing mother, patched into the outside phone system by our Farm switchboard.

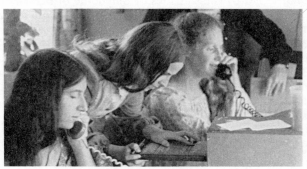

Communication is Intelligence

Later our community acquired a lot of citizen's band radios, making our communications instantaneous. Each midwife was provided by our community with her own pick-up truck or four-wheel-drive jeep, kept in twenty-four hour running condition by the men in the motor pool and each equipped with its own citizen's band radio.

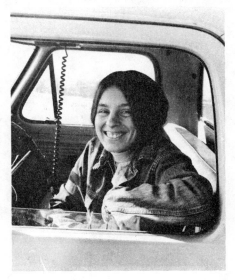

During the years of peak population of our community (1974-1982), our motor pool kept two state-certified ambulances running. We also had a crew of more than forty state-certified emergency medical technicians, including a state approved emergency medical training instructor.

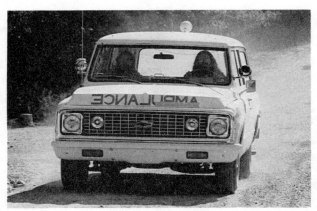

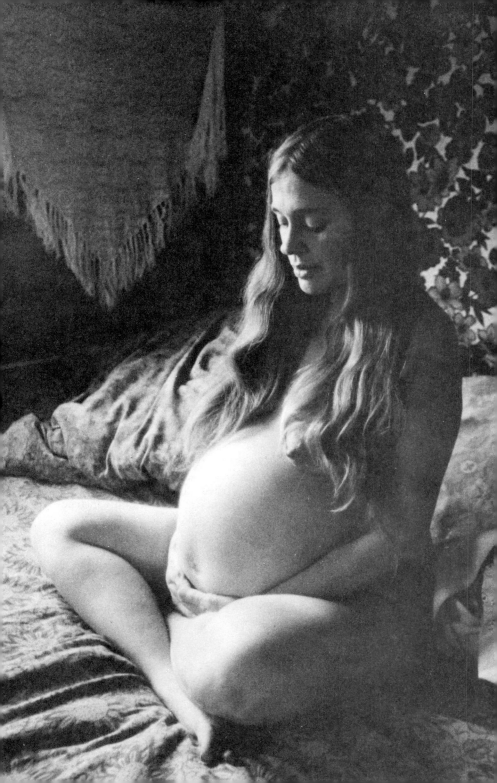

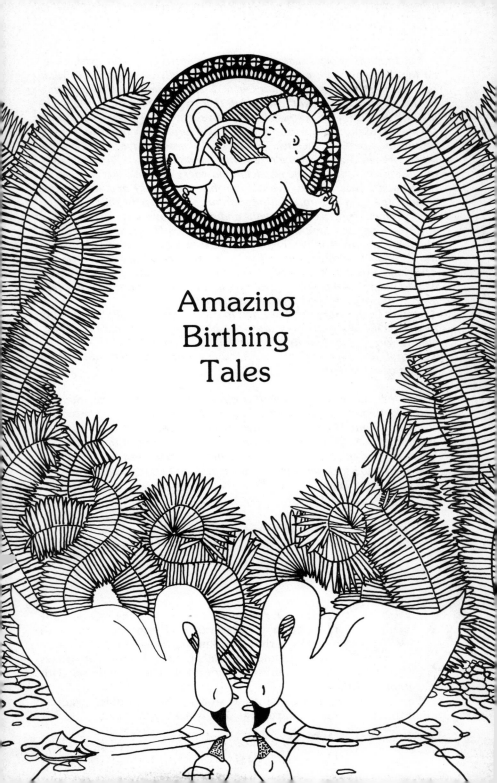

Amazing
Birthing
Tales

I include this story because I learned so much from this experience. At the time I was not a midwife and didn't really understand yet what one was, what the responsibilities were. I tried to help Cara relax during her labor. Michael "caught" Anne, but there was no midwife at the birthing. We had a rather confused committee instead. Pamela and I both felt there was not good reason for the tiny schoolbus to be crowded with several men besides Michael, so we asked them to leave. Two or three other women besides Pamela and me remained in the bus. My next impulse was to pick up the Mexican midwifery manual (this was before my Rhode Island friend gave me an obstetrics book) and study what to do if the baby did not breathe spontaneously after birth. One of the other women there became nervous and superstitious when she saw what I was reading, and took the book out of my hands, afraid that if I read about something negative, I would cause it to happen. Instead of taking the book back, I allowed myself to be intimidated by the other woman. The result was that neither of us knew what to do when Anne did need help to breathe. An interesting note is that the woman who took the book away from me has since become a physician.

Anne's birth taught me that I had to accept the responsibility of being a midwife if I was going to be attending births. A midwife has the responsibility for at least two lives in her hands at every birth.

Cara joined the midwife crew after a few years and attended the birth of one of my children.

Another interesting note to this birth: during Cara's labor, Stephen had been in our schoolbus, which was parked thirty or forty yards away from Cara and Michael's bus. Seconds after Anne was born and was lying there, one of the women who had been at the birth ran over to Stephen's and my bus to tell him that the baby had been born. She said that everything was fine, but Stephen could tell that it wasn't by the way she said it and came fast to check for himself.

Anne's Birth

ara: Our daughter, Anne, was the second baby born on the Caravan.* I went into labor five weeks early. Not knowing what to do, Michael went and told Stephen's family. It was after Anne's birthing that Ina May decided to be the midwife, with Margaret assisting her.

We were concerned because it was so early, and we didn't want to admit that it was really happening. But when Stephen came into our

*Stephen's national speaking tour in 1970.

truck to see us, it started coming on and we had to accept it and let it happen.

We had the birthing in the schoolbus next door because our truck was too small to fit enough people in to help us. It seemed like the word got out that there was a baby-having, because as soon as I laid down on the bed about twenty-five people filed into the bus to watch. It got so uptight that my rushes stopped, until Ina May told the menfolks to leave. We still allowed all the ladies to stay. We learned from Anne's birthing that only family and midwives should be there. Most of the folks there weren't directly involved and mainly just added subconscious to the situation. The birthing was surprisingly easy, though. It felt ecstatic. Everything that happened in my body felt really natural. I just had to keep paying attention to what was happening. After six hours, Anne was born. She was small, about five pounds. She gave a small cry and then turned blue and just lay there. It was a heavy place and no one knew what to do. During the labor when we read the midwife manual, we didn't read what to do if your baby comes out blue, because some ladies got superstitious. So Anne turned blue and Michael and I and Ina May just prayed. At that moment, Stephen walked in and went right to the baby and picked her up. He said, "In cases like this . . ." and breathed into her and got her going. She turned pink and cried. Stephen looked ancient, and Anne was the newest being on Earth. We all knew it was a miracle. Stephen looked out of the window at the trees and birds and said to Anne, "Welcome to the planet."

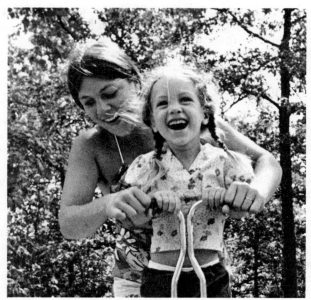

Anne and her teacher

41

Our First Hospital Birth

*T*he first time I had to take a laboring mother to the hospital was in the summer of 1972, our fifty-sixth birth. When I learned that Carolyn was in labor, I went to her bus to check the dilation of her cervix. To my surprise, I discovered that her baby was coming bottom first. I headed out to the neighborhood bar to phone my obstetrician friend in Rhode Island. I was pretty sure that I should take this mother into the hospital, but I wanted his advice on how to go about dealing with the hospital staff. He was glad to know that I had diagnosed the breech before the baby started being born and encouraged me to stay with the mother during her labor, once she was admitted to the hospital. Stephen drove me and the laboring couple the thirty miles to the county hospital in Columbia. As we entered the emergency room, I recognized Dr. Hargrove, the obstetrician who had checked one of the women in our community for a gynecological problem. I pointed him out to Stephen, who went over to him, following him to the stairwell and engaging him in a conversation on the stairs. He talked the doctor into letting me accompany Carolyn into the labor room, as well as to the delivery room, once she was ready for that. It was a great bit of persuasion, I thought. Stephen later said it was like selling a set of encyclopedias. Actually, it was the only one he ever sold.

The odd thing in those days was that Harlan, her husband, would not be allowed in either the labor or delivery room. The general feeling seemed to be that husbands would only be in the way, that they were likely to faint and that they could do their laboring wives no good. As I got dressed for the first time in a scrub suit (I noticed that I was wearing clothes more like the doctors' than the nurses'), I decided that we had to go along with the rules in order to have a good relationship with the hospital. Since Carolyn wanted to be with Harlan as long as possible during her labor, we decided to sit in the visitors' lounge with the families of the other women in labor after her initial checkup.

Fortunately for everyone, Carolyn was a student of yoga, and I really didn't have to do anything to help her relax with this first baby. She sat cross-legged on the plastic covered couch, next to Harlan, with Stephen and me on another couch across the small, smoke-filled room. There were five or six nervous family members waiting for news of the other women in labor. Occasionally we could hear their screams and curses when a nurse or doctor would come through the double swinging doors to the labor rooms. The relatives would cringe and chainsmoke.

Between rushes we read magazines. When we would hear Carolyn's breathing deepen, we would put down our magazines and pace our breathing with hers as she relaxed her way through another rush. We helped by relaxing, too, and smiling at her now and then.

I'm sure that we were the weirdest sight those relatives had seen in recent years, but after the experience of the Caravan, we were pretty used to going about our business, even if the onlookers thought we were strange. Carolyn looked vibrant and beautiful; everyone there had to be impressed with her courage as well as her beauty. It wasn't long before she began to feel that she could have to push. She and I got up, she holding the back of her hospital gown together, and walked through the swinging doors of the labor rooms. I felt blessed to be going with her.

The obstetrician was impressed with Carolyn's ability to relax and was obviously pleased that she had dilated so quickly. Carolyn reminded him that she wanted me with her in the delivery room. Once Carolyn was on the delivery table, it took only a few pushes before we began to see Matthew's pink little bottom emerging. A few more pushes and the rest of him was out, all five pounds and twelve ounces of him. Dr. Hargrove seemed as excited about the birth as Carolyn and I did. Later on, he told me that I was welcome in the maternity ward whenever I came in with a woman. He was very happy to see a woman have her baby without anesthesia, especially since he had spent most of the night worrying about a young woman who had come very close to dying from aspiration under anesthesia the week before. It was very satisfying to be able to know that we could accompany a laboring mother into the delivery room when she needed hospital care.

Here's Carolyn's description of what happened:

Carolyn: My baby's birth was the most incredible experience I had ever had. Stephen drove us to the hospital. The hospital looked surreal and weird to me at first, as I hadn't been away from the dirt roads and woods of the Farm for a long time. Then I looked closer and saw it was just a hospital with some nice Tennessee folks in it. It must have been interesting for them, too, to see these four hippies, one of them about to have a baby, her midwife at her side. Folks there were kind of formal and stiff with us at first, didn't want us bending any rules but the longer we were there, the more compassionate they became. Stephen got an okay from a doctor for Ina May to come in with me so I could have help during labor. It was wonderful that they let her be there, because it made it like a Farm birth, even though it was actually in the hospital. From that point on we just relaxed and tripped; each rush would get us more stoned, the vision got better, and folks got prettier.

When it started getting super intense for me, I had to adjust my attitude to the sensations. Part of me wanted to complain, "Hey, nobody told me it was gonna hurt," to "Eeoww, I can't stand it!" And part of me said, "Where's that at?" I asked Ina May what about it, and she said, "Don't think of it as pain. Think of it as an interesting sensation that requires all of your attention." That stoned me. It was still kind of rocky, but I could let go of the pleasure-pain sensation continuum by thinking of it as one thing and then letting it go, and I was glad I knew how to do that. Then I started getting it on, helping it out some and not resisting like before.

My head was really tripping. I could feel so much life force on each rush I couldn't believe it. I wondered, *Is it this heavy for everyone?* I guessed so and that blew my mind. Learning where folks come from, not in the textbook biological sense so much as what heavy tripping woman in birth do each time, showed me some of where it's at. I felt like I had to give up some of my personal ego. It was neat. I couldn't do anything but lie there and let it happen. Something more powerful than me was at work. I knew it was going to happen and that it wouldn't help to complain, so I just hung out and paid attention to see what I could learn. I thought, *Far out, generations of women have been doing this. That's how we all got here. The trip seemed very precious, very spiritual, sacred, in fact. I can understand that we want to do it at home when we can, but it doesn't make much difference really—anywhere can be stoned. Just to get to is a blessing.*

I also learned a lot of textbook stuff about how the body gives birth, involving parts of my body I had never used that way before, and I was just amazed each step of the way. Far out automatic birthing mechanisms we have that contract and open and push out a new soul. It's beautiful how it happens. It took some hard work, too, and some skillful maneuverings on the doctor's, nurse's and midwife's part. I couldn't tell from my end what they were doing, but I could tell they were delighted about how it was going. The doctor was showing Ina May just how to do it, and she was picking it all up. Everyone felt awestruck there in the delivery room—it felt like one intelligent consciousness, brought together and unified on the energy of the birthing. When the baby was out, Ina May brought him around where I could see him, and I realized I'd forgotten I was going to get a kid out of it. I was amazed to see this perfect little newborn babe. I felt a big rush of love for him and felt really blessed. I still do.

Ina May: From that point on, we have enjoyed an excellent relationship with the staff of our local hospital. It wasn't long before they revised their policy about husbands in the labor and delivery rooms, and when the hospital went through expansion and remodeling, a birthing room was installed.

Not long ago I attended a mother who developed pre-eclamptic symptoms just as labor began and had to be transported to our hospital in Columbia. She asked for the woman obstetrician who had begun her prenatal care before she decided to have a home birth. This mother had been so disappointed when I told her I thought she needed to have her baby in the hospital that tears streamed down her face. Even though she had told me earlier that she liked this obstetrician, when the doctor entered the hospital room after we arrived, she asked, "Is it all right if Ina May delivers the baby?" The obstetrician had to refuse, because of hospital rules, but she let the mother know that I could be with her throughout the labor and proceeded to treat the mother the way a midwife should. The women in that room became sisters, and everyone cooperated as totally as they possibly could to help the baby come easily. The baby was born in the same bed her mother labored in, with no episiotomy or tear; the obstetrician sat on the bed like a midwife, her gloved hands supporting the perineum as the baby's head emerged. Everyone seemed proud that we had been able to have such a lovely birth there.

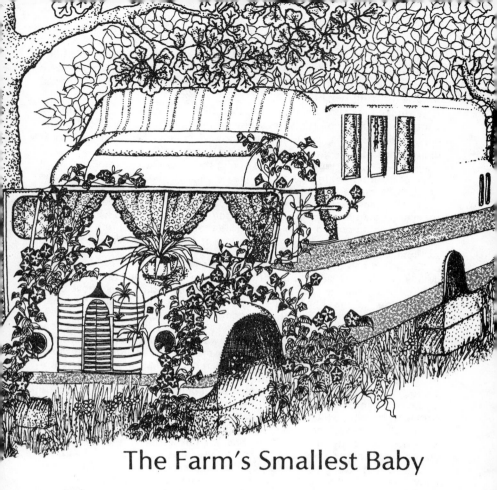

The Farm's Smallest Baby

Ellen: Having a baby was the most impressive thing that ever happened to me. I didn't want to believe at first that it was happening because I was two and a half months early, but I noticed right away that it felt Holy and visionary. I tried not to think so I could feel what it felt like. It didn't hurt; it was a spiritual high and I enjoyed it. At times I forgot about me and felt one thing with everything around me. I felt God creating life through me and I felt that I was God.

She came out very quickly. She started moving right away and she opened her eyes. She was two and a half months premature because I had been sick. She weighed only two pounds and ten ounces. We took her to the local hospital right away and they put her in an incubator. She never needed oxygen, all her body was together, but she needed to be kept warm. She went down to one pound and fifteen ounces during the first two weeks. They had to feed her with a tube. We didn't know if she would make it, but we prayed. She was always strong and she started gaining weight soon after that. When she got up to three pounds, we thought she was fat, and at four pounds, fourteen ounces, we got to bring her home.

It amazed me that a monkey that small could make it. It taught me a lot about life force. It always seems to me that it is a miracle that she gets to be here. I saw real clear how it is not the meat part that determines life, because she hardly had any.

Ina May: This birthing happened during the early days of the Farm when most of us still lived in the schoolbuses we had arrived in and the Farm had no phone system. Having heard that Ellen was having rushes five minutes apart, I hurried over to her bus to see how far along she was. She was dilated four centimeters and was obviously not going to stop until she had her baby. I wanted to find out from the doctor if he thought I should bring her to the hospital to deliver, so I drove out a couple of miles to the nearest phone to call him.

"Go ahead and deliver her there," he said after I had given him all the details. "Bring the baby to my office if it's under five pounds."

I agreed and hurried back to Ellen's as quickly as I could. As I drove up to park beside the bus, I heard Ellen's husband, Neal, call, "I can see something purple and shining starting to come out."

I jumped out of the car, bounded up the bus steps and went over to Ellen. She was about to deliver. I could see the water bag right there. I wanted to break it before the baby's head came so the membranes wouldn't be covering the face if I should need to help the baby start breathing. I showed Ellen how to pant to slow down her contractions and looked around me for something sharp. On the table behind me, I saw a small plate with a piece of raspberry pie and a fork on it. I grabbed the fork and carefully punctured the water bag with it. By this time Ellen couldn't wait anymore. Her uterus contracted and the smallest baby I had ever seen spurted out into my hands: head, shoulders, and body all in one rush. She was tiny but perfect and right away she opened her eyes and looked at me. I fell in love with her. Her heartbeat was good and strong and her breathing remarkably clear for such a small baby. Margaret, who had come in the same time I had, suctioned her throat and nose and I bundled Naomi in several blankets to keep her as warm as possible.

We sent a message for someone to get a vehicle and we drove the ten miles to our doctor's office. I had asked someone from the Farm to call and let him know we were coming, so he was there to meet us when we arrived. I got out of the little bus holding Naomi close against me. Dr. Williams was in the parking lot next to his car. "Oh, she's a good one!" he said. "She's a little doll." I thought so too, and was glad he had noticed. He felt big and strong and I was glad to turn Naomi over to him.

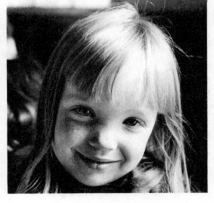

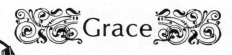
Matthew: I came home from work around six o'clock and Kathryn's water bag broke as I was coming in the door. I went and got one of the midwife crew, and we relaxed and had dinner. Then Kathryn said she had to go to the outhouse, and one of the midwives told her to wait and make sure it wasn't the kid she was feeling. It turned out that it was the kid. Kathryn's rushes started coming on stronger, so she got in the birthing position. I was holding Kathryn's hands and helping her, and one the midwives was telling her what to do. It started feeling really high—all of us were loving Kathryn a lot and helping her deliver the kid. Actually we wanted to wait a little bit until Ina May got there. But the rushes started coming on stronger, and one of the midwives told Kathryn she could push some if she felt like it.

Kathryn told me I could help out by breathing with her. We looked in each other's eyes and breathed together and panted together throughout the rest of the birthing. I found I could help her keep relaxed just by paying attention to her. She would start to tighten up and I'd just look at her and she'd realize what she was doing and relax—or she'd look at me and I could tell where she needed to be rubbed and I'd rub it.

Pamela asked Kathryn how she was doing, and Kathryn said she felt tired. Pamela said that was silly—she'd only been doing it less than an hour, and Kathryn had helped at birthings that had taken a day or so. Kathryn said she knew, and didn't be tired anymore.

The rushes started coming closer together and it started feeling really Holy. Ina May and the other ladies came in, and somehow Ina May was in the catching position, cleaned up and all, by the next rush. She felt very slow and loving. Ina May told one of the ladies to slow down some—they'd just been driving down the Farm in a jeep, and they had to slow down a bunch to match speeds with the birthing.

All during the birthing, Pamela and Ina May kept a running commentary on what was happening—how much they could see, what they thought was happening and stuff like that. "One more rush," Ina May

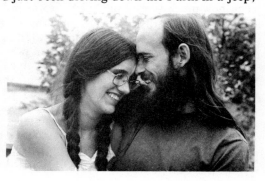

said, and then one more and the baby's head came out. "Oh, it's face up!" Margaret started syringing the baby's nose and mouth, and the rest of her body came out on the next rush. Ina May looked at her and saw her nose was crooked, so she pushed it back in place.

I got to hold the baby, and the whole bus lit up with a golden light as I looked at her. She was really pure and beautiful. I felt amazing rushes of gratitude to all the folks who'd helped with the birthing. The midwives cleaned everything up, thanked us for a nice birthing, and left. Kathryn and I lay down with the kid between us and just loved each other and the baby for a long time. We'd keep waking up to check her out, and every time we'd see that she was okay, we'd look at each other and feel really grateful. We named her Grace that night, because it felt like that was how she got to us, through Grace.

Rose

athryn: Friday night we borrowed a truck to go and take a bath, hoping the bumpy ride might get the baby coming. Sure enough, I woke up at three o'clock with a rush and my water bag breaking. We called Pamela after I'd had a couple of good rushes and she came over. It felt like a slumber party, everyone laughing and having a good time. I remember going out to pee and the moon was full and it was starting to get light and all the birds were singing and everything was so clear and it felt like Heaven.

When I got to be about eight centimeters, it started feeling different than my first one. At Grace's birthing I sincerely and truly was glad when a rush would start coming. This time I had to remind myself that it was fine and that that was what was going to get the baby out and I knew how much I loved the baby. It was just like a short feeling in the beginning of the rush, like, uh-oh, and then I'd get myself together. It made me more compassionate with ladies who have a hard time in labor. It was like I could see the root of it and could see how there was a place where you could not like it and you could just freak on out if you wanted to do that. And that was a good thing to learn. I think the reason for that was that Matthew and I weren't as connected as we could be. At Grace's birthing it was like we were one body and Matthew would do stuff like rub exactly where I needed it most right at the same time I'd think of it. At Rose's birthing, we felt high and loved each other a bunch, but didn't quite connect a hundred per cent. We had a great time, but it wasn't quite as easy.

It was a lot different than Grace because with her I pushed and pushed, and with Rose I never felt any compelling urge to push. I would just bear down a little bit for about five rushes and I looked down and saw her head halfway out. I was amazed that she was almost out. She started crying when just her nose was out, and when the rest of her came out she was the pinkest baby I ever saw. Mary Louise put her on my belly and I could hardly believe she was our baby, she looked so different from how Grace had. She was real fat and had a huge nose that was mashed over to the side and dark hair and she was so soft and pink and golden and beautiful and new.

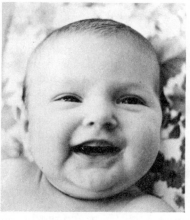

Then my placenta wouldn't come out. We tried everything but it didn't come out for forty minutes. During that time I thought, now, the baby's out and okay, and it's this third stage that's hard on the mother sometimes. When the placenta did come out I bled a lot. After the midwives worked on me some and gave me a shot, the bleeding slowed down. I was grateful that we had a phone. We called the ambulance and it came down to get me. I was really conscious and all for a long time, and then all of a sudden I got hot and felt my whole body go to "sleep" and my head swim and I felt really crummy. They gave me oxygen and I immediately felt better. In the middle of this, Grace woke up and came to see what was going on. Mary Louise showed her her new sister and I gave her a kiss and she went off with Mary Louise next door. I knew I was going into shock because I'd lost a lot of blood. By the time the ambulance got there I'd pretty much stopped bleeding, except for occasional gushes when we'd go over a bump. It was good that we went in to the hospital, because I wound up needing three pints of blood.

It was really good that, if it had to happen to someone, it was us—because Matthew and I had both worked at the hospital and it was neat to get taken care of by our old friends. Everyone was super nice. I even got to have Rose with me. And Matthew. We had a good time. We were there three days. It wasn't until the last day that we had a chance to finally name her. But by then, we were calling her Rose because she was so pink, and the nurses were too, and writing Rose McClure on her papers. So we named her Rose.

And sometimes I think about it, and I think, if I'd lived fifty or a hundred years ago, or if I'd just had some lady or Matthew to deliver my baby, I wouldn't have made it. I'm grateful to be alive.

I Learn About Fathers

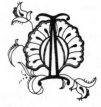

I started my career as a midwife with a pretty sure feeling of what a woman needed to do during labor. I knew less about how the baby's father should conduct himself during labor, especially those fathers who were so nervous that they made their mates more uncomfortable and nervous with their presence than with their absence. I had already seen how much comfort and encouragement a man could give his mate while she labored. Most of the first couples whose births I attended were very physically affectionate with each other during labor. They would kiss and hug between rushes, there would be soft sighs, and I could feel in my own body the relaxation that such loving communication brought. These women did not seem to experience severe pain during labor; they knew that relaxation was the key, and they appreciated their men for being able to help in such a practical way.

But there were a few labors in which the man clearly didn't know how to behave. He would put his hand on his mate's belly, and she would snap at him about how bad that felt. Sometimes he would rub her back, and she would get angry because he was pushing in the wrong spot or pushing too hard or not hard enough. On these occasions, I would feel my insides twist into a cramp and wonder what I ought to do next. The problem was how to get a couple out of a snarl when angry words had already passed.

I soon learned that prevention was the best answer. Realizing that the men who were clumsy and awkward during labor were usually the ones who were scared, I tried to relieve what fears I could before the birth and to provide some advice about communication. The nervous man needed to know that his main role was not in telling his mate what to do but rather to follow her directions about how best to help her. I learned to watch the body language of a couple to know if they were comfortable in how they touched each other.

Some men were so concerned with their mates' comfort that they forgot their own. I remember one man, whose wife needed the assistance of forceps to get the first baby out. I knew that her pelvic measurements were generous enough that cephalo-pelvic disproportion (the baby's head being too big for her pelvis) couldn't have been the reason why the forceps were needed, but when I heard their birth story, I thought I understood at least part of the reason she hadn't been able to push the baby out without assistance. He was a huge bear of a man, very strong, and she had labored for several hours sitting nearly upright in bed, leaning against him. Labor was intense for her, and she was comfortable only when he was there, so much so that when he needed to get up to pee, she wouldn't permit it. He had sat there for several hours of labor, having to pee and not doing so. I am certain that his inability

50

to relax his pelvic muscles and sphincters affected her ability to relax in the same area. The next baby was a pound and a half larger, she allowed him to relieve himself and no forceps were necessary.

Some men will feel guilty about eating during labor unless the midwife gives permission. In such cases, I made sure the man knows that he must also keep up his strength so he can be there for his mate when she needs him.

I remember a birth, the couple's third, when more than half an hour had passed since her cervix was fully open. Still she had no urge to push, and we were beginning to wonder what was going on. Knowing that stimulation of the breasts can encourage the flow of oxytocin into the woman's bloodstream, thereby stimulating uterine contractions, I asked the husband if he would squeeze his wife's breasts. He was somewhat self-conscious about doing this in front of us, I suspect, and used only one hand. After one rush in this lopsided condition, his wife leaned over and whispered in his ear, "Squeeze the other one, too." Not more than five seconds after he had both of her breasts in his hands, she had an enormous urge to push, and the baby's head was visible!

I remember an early birth: the couple's second baby. Their first child had been born after what I consider a perfect labor, one of those in which the cervix was more open each time I checked and the baby moved right down the birth canal after cervical dilation was full. During the second labor, the mother's cervix opened as nicely as it had during the first, but when it was fully open, nothing much happened. Regular rushes continued, but they weren't strong enough to start moving the baby down the birth canal. I remember being struck by how pinched this mother looked around her mouth and chin. On an impulse, I asked if she ever told her husband that she loved him. I could tell I had touched upon a nerve in their relationship, when he quietly said she had never told him that. Surprised, I suggested that she try it. A few moments passed. Her features softened, she looked at her husband and said, "I love you."

At that moment a powerful rush rolled through her, and she began to push her baby out. It was impossible not to make the connection between the mother's expression of love and the uterine action that followed it. I don't mean to say that declarations of love will always be followed by such dramatic results, but if such sentiments are missing in the relationship, there is apt to be a powerful release of energy, which may greatly enhance labor.

Pain and Endorphins

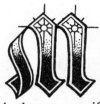uch of the art of midwifery, the kind that is comfortable with the baby's father helping with the birth, lies in creating an atmosphere that is easy, humorous and sensual. Not everybody is comfortable with necking and petting during labor, especially with the midwife in the room, so if the woman was in early labor and I would sense that her man's touch would be relaxing to her, I would withdraw to another room, coming in periodically to check the baby's heartbeat or the dilation of her cervix, so as to let them experiment with the kind of touch that would best enable her labor to progress.

I believe that much of the reason why the women whose births we attended were able to get through labor without anesthesia or tranquilizers had to do with the atmosphere we learned to create at a birth. There is a sound physiological explanation for why some women experience more pain in labor than others. A woman who is the center of positive attention, feeling grateful, amused, loved and appreciated, has a higher level of the class of neurohormones called endorphins. Endorphins actually block the perception of pain.

On the other hand, there are also adrenalin-like substances which may be secreted by the body during labor, especially when the woman is afraid, cold, angry, humiliated or experiencing any other disagreeable emotion. Adrenalin is part of the body's protective mechanism when it is presented with danger; the heart rate quickens, the muscles tense, labor contractions may be inhibited, and the perception of pain is intensified. The mother is made ready to fight or to flee when adrenalin levels are high, not to have her baby.

Much of the midwife's responsibility during early labor is to give the mother so much positive, loving attention (and to encourage the baby's father, if present, to do likewise) that the mother's endorphin levels are as high as possible. I learned humor could be a great help, in that it seemed impossible for a woman to be amused and afraid at the same time. The challenge then became (and still is) how to amuse a woman in labor. Naturally, this is a much easier task if you and she know each other well. It's not easy to know what will be amusing to a stranger during the intensity of labor. Some women simply won't think anything is funny, in which case, the main rule is to be soothing, sympathetic and encouraging.

Karen: Wilbur and I spent the day together and that got me real relaxed. That's the thing that was missing at my other birthings. Being in your own home with your old man lets you get real relaxed. My rushes hardly felt heavy at all, but I knew they must be because I was opening up. We just kept making out and rubbing each other. We got to places that we had forgotten we could get to. Since that day we have been remembering to really get it on. Going through the birthing I felt his love very strong. It was like getting married all over again.

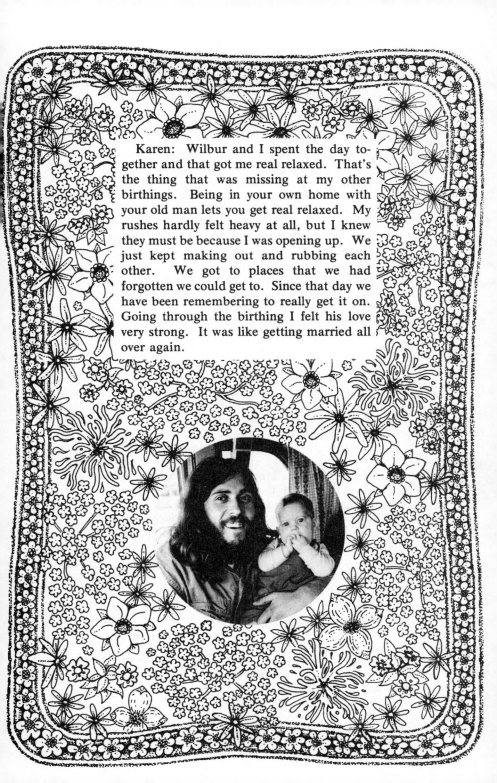

A Husband's Story

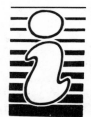

—Rudolph

was being self-conscious and uptight and was unable to change at the time so Ina May told me to go away for a while. I started for the showers on a bicycle and on my way there I saw a friend of mine and asked him to lend me a towel. After talking with him a while I was afraid I was going to miss the birthing so I told him I decided not to take a shower and went back to our van. Ina May let me in saying that Marilyn had waited for me and wanted me to be there when she had the baby, and that made me feel really good.

The ladies told me to eat something, so I ate a little bit but I didn't feel like eating much. I thought I wasn't supposed to be hungry because Marilyn wasn't hungry. I wanted to cuddle up with Marilyn but when I touched her it didn't feel like she wanted me to. I was being very clumsy and Ina May had to warn me a couple of times when I was about to back up into the kerosene lamp. I didn't feel very telepathic. I was self-conscious all the time the midwives were there, until the baby started to come out.

Marilyn's contractions stayed about the same for a long time, because I wasn't putting out any energy. She wasn't putting out too much energy either, until Stephen came, and then she started to get high. She'd have a contraction and get amazing mind-expanding rushes and everyone in the room except me would be rushing too. I knew I wasn't being telepathic and I was nervous about it. Stephen said I wasn't being telepathic with my body, and I asked how was that? He said that for example when I had passed him a jar of soymilk that I passed it as if his hand were six inches farther from me than it actually was, so there was six inches of shove in there. He was on one side of Marilyn and I was on the other side, and I was jealous of him because he was getting connected with Marilyn and I wasn't.

Someone suggested that I squeeze Marilyn's leg on the inside of her thigh when she was having a contraction, and I did. They told me to hold it longer and to let go when I felt a rush of energy, but I held it too long that time, and I kept trying to do it but I didn't really feel what I was doing. Stephen or Ina May said I thought I was a crane operator up in my head telling my hand what to do instead of me being my hand and the leg being squeezed, and feeling what was really happening. I still didn't change. I understood mentally what was happening, but I was still holding on to my ego. I was afraid I was going to faint at the sight of blood but I didn't tell anyone.

So Ina May said that we needed something to be like a waiting room, and Marilyn suggested the outdoor kitchen, which was several yards away from the van. I went out there and felt sick, so I laid down on the ground and tried to vomit for a while and kind of wallowed around in self-pity and felt pretty rotten. After a while I started to notice the ground I was lying on and the trees and the wind and things like that. It was a really nice night. I decided to get myself together and to try to help out. I went to the kitchen and nibbled a little bit of food. Stephen and Ina May came in and they were hungry and ate a bunch. I really liked that because I had had the idea that it was a bring-down to eat when it's really high. Thinking that had really tightened up my stomach, along with the rest of the stuff I had been thinking.

When I went back into the van Marilyn told me to leave. Then Pamela came out and told me to go back in, that Marilyn was in there by herself. She said that Stephen and Ina May had gone into the other van to take a nap and that they would get up when the baby was closer to happening. So we lay there and I gave Marilyn sort of a pep talk after a while and told her that she could do it and that she was going to have to try really hard, harder than she had probably ever tried before. Then she fell asleep and I might have fallen asleep too, and when she woke up she was dilated wide and she was having strong ones. Ina May and Stephen and Pamela and Mary all came in. The contractions felt like rushes that happen making love, and it got more and more intense. Marilyn looked like I'd never seen her before. Her face was bulging with energy and she was really working. She was intensely powerful and looked like a deity I've seen in pictures of Hindu temple carvings. I was amazed at how much energy she was putting out. It got to a place where her puss was bulging out from the head being right underneath it and then really soon after that we could see the top of the baby's head through the opening and then with one big push the head came out. Ina May made sure the cord was like it was supposed to be and then she pulled Luther's arm out by the hand and he came surfing out, peeing as he came out along with all the water and some blood that was in the womb. The second he was out he looked so familiar to me that it was as if I'd already known him; he looked just like himself. I really loved seeing him; he was beautiful. Pretty soon he was lying by Marilyn's side sucking her tit. *It felt like there was no space or time barrier to anything, and we were in Holy times in Holy land.*

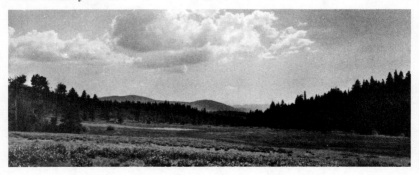

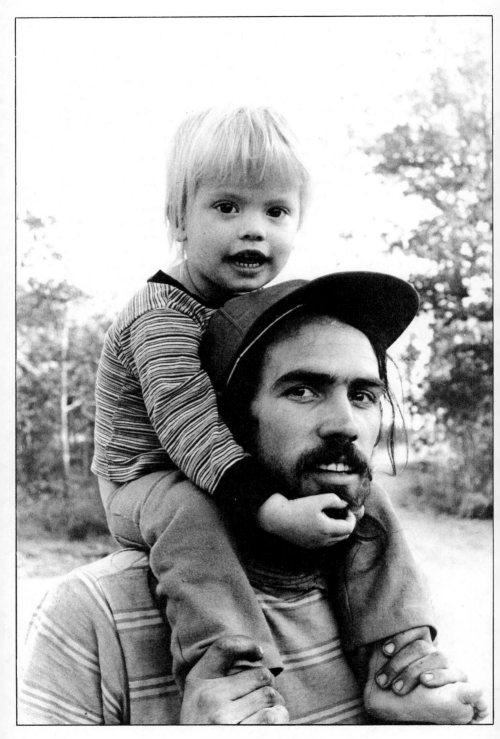

Luther and Rudolph

George's Birth

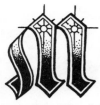

arilyn: It was pretty late at night and I was making a sterile pack, because that was my job, and there was a possibility that both me and another lady could have our babies that night. I was sort of half asleep doing that, and then I started feeling something in my lower back. I thought I might as well wake up and pay attention to what I was doing, because I thought I might be going into labor. I went to bed and lay down there feeling what the rushes felt like. They started out feeling like a little ache in my lower back that turned into a bunch of energy, and went up my backbone. Rudolph and I decided we'd go to sleep and see whether the rushes would wake us up later or else go away. The next morning I got up and made breakfast, and after some of the folks we lived with went to work, I started having rushes again. I kept on cleaning the house and such, and every once in a while I laid down and paid attention to what it felt like. I remember from when I had my first kid that at one point Ina May told me I'd have to want the rushes to get heavier. When she told me that, I couldn't imagine wanting it to get heavier, or at least I wasn't into it at that time. So this time I decided that I would want it to get heavier from the start. Every time I had a rush, I relaxed and thought that it was fine and that I dug it, and that I wanted it to get heavier. After a while I quit trying to do anything in the kitchen, and Rudolph and I went to our bus and lay down and made out a lot, especially while I was rushing. We were having a good time.

Then Ina May and Cara and Denise came down the path, and things seemed to pick up speed after they came. Ina May blew my mind. She was stretching my cervix out with her fingers. [*I had a sterile glove on. I noticed while checking Marilyn's dilation that if I pulled out a little bit on her cervix that it would open up a bunch more, so I stayed in there and did that for a while. —I.M.*] Rudolph was kissing me and the rushes felt more connected. Sometimes I couldn't tell who was rubbing me. The rushes felt a lot smoother than they did before. I started pushing a little bit too soon, and Ina May figured that out and told me not to. It felt like she knew exactly what was going on in my body. When I was pushing the baby out, every once in a while, she'd tell me to stop pushing so that I'd stretch out a little bit. The baby came out and I was glad to see him. He was nice and fat. They asked us if we had a name for him. I thought of George, and it turned out Rudolph was thinking the same thing. Then we both considered a middle name, and it turned out we both thought of the same middle name, too.

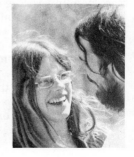

An Account of a Miscarriage, Another Miscarriage, and Then a Baby

Mary: A miscarriage is when you lose the baby before the fourth month of pregnancy. I had two miscarriages before I had my first baby, and I learned a lot about the changes you go through when it happens, and why it happens.

I got pregnant right after Stephen married Paul and me, the summer that we first settled on the Farm. When I was about three months along, I started spotting like a very light period. I wasn't quite sure if that was normal or not, so Paul and I went and told Stephen and Ina May and they told us to take it easy and be good to each other. Ina May called our doctor and he said some doctors say you might as well get up and be doing your regular thing, because if you're going to miscarry, lying down won't prevent it, but he himself felt it was better to lie down. I continued spotting for eight more days. I've found out since then that your hormones are going through tremendous changes and this can make you feel very emotional. I kept thinking about anything wrong I'd done in the past that was the reason for all this. Later a doctor told me that a miscarriage happens usually because the baby is not viable. He said if the baby is healthy, you don't have to worry because you won't make it come out by working or getting around.

On about the tenth day of spotting, things felt heavier and I was having wave-like cramps. Ina May came down to check me at my place, a small, temporary shelter. She, Stephen and Paul took me up to a house that had a phone and electricity in case I bled too much. I rode up sitting next to Stephen sort of cuddling and feeling good that it was all covered and enjoying seeing everything that was happening on the Farm as we went by, including the shocks of sorghum cane that were standing getting ready to be made into syrup. Almost immediately when I laid down on the bed at the house I could feel a soft ball come out. I saw the white and pink umbilical cord. It looked real clean and pretty. There was a part of me that was really upset that I'd lost the baby, but I read some of Stephen's transcripts and other spiritual teachings and they helped me remember where it was at. I also walked out to a field behind the house and looked at a big purple cabbage with dewdrops on it. It was so beautiful and full of life force that I started crying. I felt a lot of love and a little sad but I basically knew that everything was all right.

Paul and I still wanted to have a baby. He was very accepting of what had happened and completely confident that we would have a kid. I really had to struggle with my emotions for a while, and he made it easy for me because he'd let me talk out what was in my head, no matter how silly or paranoid it was. It felt necessary to clean out my head as I went along to keep from feeling real emotional.

I got pregnant about nine months later. I felt pretty healthy, but I was worried about how everything would go. At about three months along, I started spotting again. After three days, I had a miscarriage. I think that baby wasn't a together one. I remember seeing a lot of light. Everything looked golden and full of energy. I saw if I could cut loose gracefully that there would be a lot of life force happening, because there always is a lot of it, it just moves on. After the first miscarriage, I got back together right away, although Ina May told me to lay down for a day. After the second one, I still had strong cramps for a while. About a month after that, I started a period that kept on for three weeks and occasionally I would gush some blood and I'd lie down because it felt heavy. I hadn't wanted to tell anybody because I had something in my head about thinking a D & C* could make it harder to get pregnant. I finally confessed this to Ina May and she chewed me out in a nice way and said there was probably stuff in there that was rotting and it would be better to have it out. The doctor did a suction D & C in his office and it worked out good and got me back together.

I still really wondered whether I would ever have a baby, but I got to the place where I knew I had to strive for the good of mankind and enlightenment, and not be so attached to whether I was going to have a baby. It taught me some about patience. Paul was still sure that we could have a kid, and wasn't worried at all. I got pregnant again about eight months later and whenever I'd tell him I was scared I was going to lose this one too, he'd never have any doubt that we were going to have a baby. It did feel like a healthy one and we had a seven pound, two ounce boy, Ernest. It was a miracle. I really know in my heart of hearts that choosing to be spiritual instead of depressed was what got me together enough to have a baby.

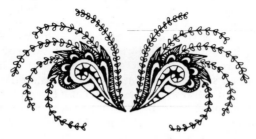

*D & C—dilation and curettage. A minor surgical procedure in which the cervix is dilated and the inside of the uterus is gently scraped to remove any material that was not expelled by the miscarriage.

After Mary's two miscarriages, she started helping out at birthings and training to be a midwife.

Mary: At the first birthing I went to, Stephen was stitching the lady up. He asked me to hand him a sterile gauze pad. I had no real definition for sterile, so I touched it instead of pulling back the wrapping and letting him take out the sterile pad. He said, "Don't touch that!" Then, he told me to hand him the suture and I goofed by touching it, too. He had another lady assist in doing the stitching. I felt like I'd been dumb not to have any idea what sterile really meant, but at the same time at least I know now for real what being sterile is all about.

Another time, Pamela told me that I didn't have to try to do anything that I didn't know how to do, that I would be told specifically what to do as we went along, and to not get ahead of myself wondering what to do next.

Ernest's Birth

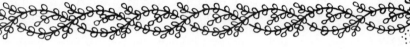

ary: My water bag broke about seven at night and I went to the phone to call Pamela and kept giggling because it was dripping down my legs and it was all so exciting. The water bag broke during a rush and the rushes kept on steadily, very light at first and getting stronger. We called Paul home from his ambulance course and he got home as I was getting an enema. Cara and Pamela came over right away. All night long I rushed. They got very strong and it was heavy, but I was really grateful to be doing it. As each rush came on I told myself, "Keep your sense of humor," or a thing Ina May had said, "It's an interesting sensation that requires all my attention." In between rushes Paul and I would doze off in a blissful meditative state. I really liked the way he rubbed me out—he grabbed me strong enough that it kept my muscles loose. Cara, my twin sister, held my hand and we looked at each other a lot while I was rushing. It felt like we were one person. She had had two babies and knew what I was feeling. I knew she had given me energy to have a baby for a long time and helped me out a lot while I was pregnant, so I was glad that she was helping me have the baby. I had a deep, loving relationship with Pamela too. The midwives sat around while I was rushing talking about their kids, how they were toilet training them, the latest news on the Farm, and I really liked listening to them talk and talking with them. It grounded me because it was the same kind of stuff we always talked about when we got together and now we were having lots of time to talk and enjoy each other's company. I really loved everyone a bunch. We felt like old buddies, life-time friends enjoying the occasion.

As I started to get fully dilated I was using my whole mind and body to integrate the rushes. Pamela asked how I was doing and a whole continuum flashed through my head ranging from, "It hurts!" to "Great!" I said, "Great!" and everybody laughed. *I saw how it's really free will whether you have fun or not having a baby and at each point along the way when the rushes got heavier I deliberately decided to have a good time because I really was grateful to be having a baby after having had a couple of miscarriages.*

Paul: Around dawn Mary was dilating more and more. Then it seemed like we clicked into something. It got very psychedelic and we could see the head and then it would go in again. Mary was pushing so hard the veins in her tits stood out. We all cheered and she would push and the head came out. It was beautiful. He was sky blue and streaked white. The cord was around his neck so Mary panted and Kathryn took the cord and put it over his head. It was tight and felt like a rubber band stretching over. Then the next push he came out. He felt like a spirit while he was blue and then he started breathing and getting more and more body as he got redder and redder. He got red all around his body and his legs and arms were still blue. You could see his heart pumping good red blood to his whole body and soon he was red all over. It's the most incredible thing I'd ever seen. It let me see that if every man could see his kid being born it would be a much more pleasant culture or world to live in.

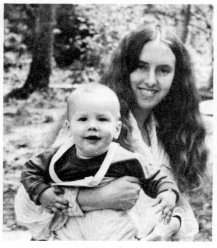

Mary: Later that evening we were going to put Ernest in his crib for the night. He opened his eyes and looked at me and he knew we were his folks and that we all really loved each other and that we would all be involved in a deep relationship that would last the rest of our lives. The three of us felt the miracle together.

Mary and Ernest

61

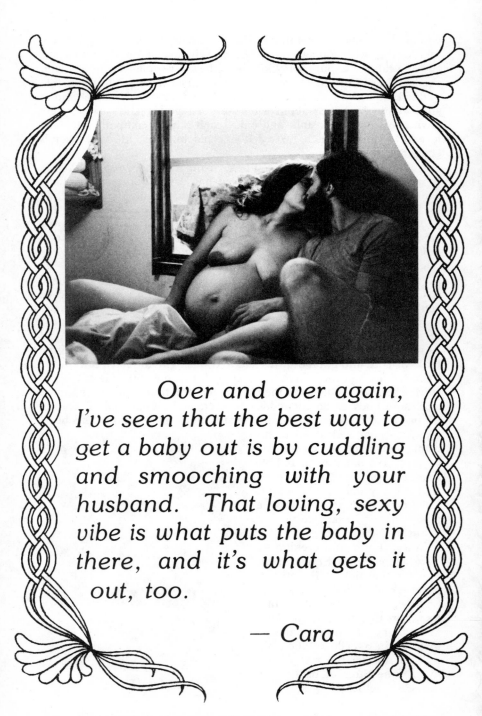

Over and over again, I've seen that the best way to get a baby out is by cuddling and smooching with your husband. That loving, sexy vibe is what puts the baby in there, and it's what gets it out, too.

— Cara

Hazrat Inayat Khan once said, "With love, even the rocks will open."

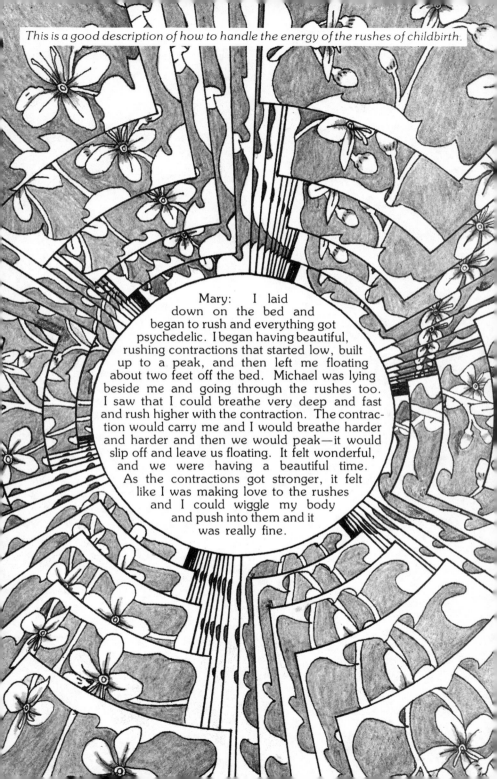

This is a good description of how to handle the energy of the rushes of childbirth.

Mary: I laid down on the bed and began to rush and everything got psychedelic. I began having beautiful, rushing contractions that started low, built up to a peak, and then left me floating about two feet off the bed. Michael was lying beside me and going through the rushes too. I saw that I could breathe very deep and fast and rush higher with the contraction. The contraction would carry me and I would breathe harder and harder and then we would peak—it would slip off and leave us floating. It felt wonderful, and we were having a beautiful time. As the contractions got stronger, it felt like I was making love to the rushes and I could wiggle my body and push into them and it was really fine.

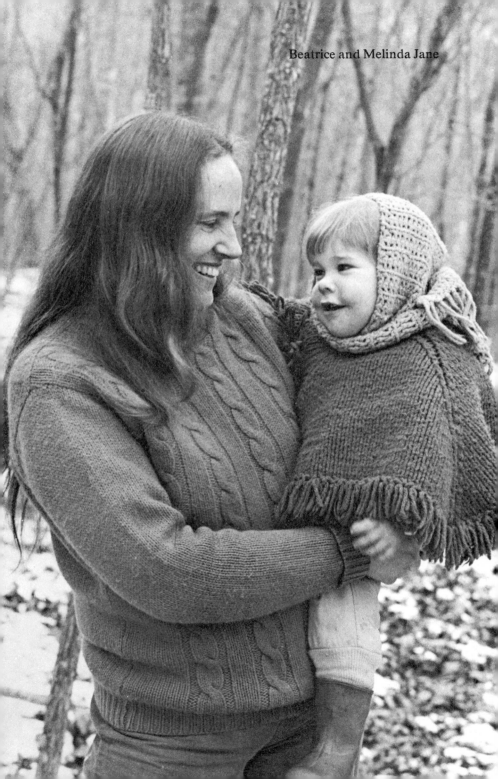
Beatrice and Melinda Jane

Melinda Jane

Beatrice: I had had four other children, and one before with a midwife, but never was it like this. I was feeling so psychedelic I couldn't stand up or even think about what I'd do next. I thought I was just getting started because I mostly remembered it being uncomfortable and having pain when my other children were born. Ina May sat me in her lap and said, "Okay, let's see who this baby is."

I went over and lay down on the bed again. She started messing with my breasts and my rushes came on very strong. My head was feeling so far out I couldn't understand some of the stuff folks were saying, but I knew what was happening and I felt great. James was sitting there watching Ina May, and looked amazed. Ina May asked him what was up and he said, "She'd never let me do that." Ina May laughed and talked to me about how I had James intimidated and said I was going to have to let him come out. It was one of those times when the truth was so real that the sun came out and shone through the windows and lit up everything—kind of saying, Yes, yes, for everyone to know. It changed our relationship with each other and made us more together. We talked a while about our relationship and the sun kept coming on like the fair witness for the truth.

My head was clearer with the subconscious sorted out, and the talk was understandable. James was on the bed with me and rubbing my back. The midwives were rubbing my legs and I was rushing heavy. I could see a silver pink shimmering throughout the room. It was really pretty so I told everyone and one of the midwives said that she had seen that the night before. She later also said she knew I was going to have a girl. The midwives started to scrub up and one for some reason turned and looked in my puss. Just then my water bag broke and the head started to crown. She said, "Here she comes." The midwives were hurrying to get a sterile sheet under me. I felt good and kept thinking it was going to hurt now, but when I'd think that, I'd look in Ina May's eyes and feel good again because I could relax and know everything was all right.

I always thought painless childbirth was just something folks said so you wouldn't be afraid, but it's really true. It astonished me how good it felt to have Melinda. She came out all purplish-blue and wiggling like a fish. She was so slippery Ina May had to keep getting a hold of her. She asked me if I'd like to watch her turn pink. I never knew babies went through that change. It was wonderful to watch the life energy come into her. James and I were both so happy, we just kept on feeling what a miracle it is to have a baby. We just hung out with her for a couple of days. I had visions of Buddhas and Bodhisattvas, birth, death and life while looking at her. You could see her aura, and even flies and August bugs didn't go beyond that Holy light.

My Training

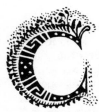

ara: After I had my first baby, I felt like what I wanted most in life was to help deliver babies. But I needed to make friends with my daughter Anne and have another baby, Emma, before I had grown up enough to actually help. After I had Emma, I felt like I went through a heavy change in consciousness where I felt more compassionate with the human race and, for the first time, made a decision to work hard. My sister, Mary, started to help on the midwife crew, and I thought that was great. She had been really brave·during her two miscarriages. After attending birthings for several months, Mary got pregnant, and it really felt like she would have a real live baby this time. When she was around six months pregnant she needed to take it easy because of some early labor. This left the midwife crew short, and Ina May was soon to leave on tour with Stephen and the Farm Band.

The first few birthings I went to I mainly watched. I felt like I mostly learned from Pamela, who was my midwife for my second baby. I felt complete love and trust in her. When I was pregnant with Emma, I had recurrent dreams about Pamela swimming out into deep water and saving souls.

One night I got a call "Would you like to help at birthings? David and Kathleen are having their baby—could you go over?" It felt like my dream come true. After saying I'd love to help, I hung up, fell into Michael's lap for a minute and hugged him, and quickly set off to go.

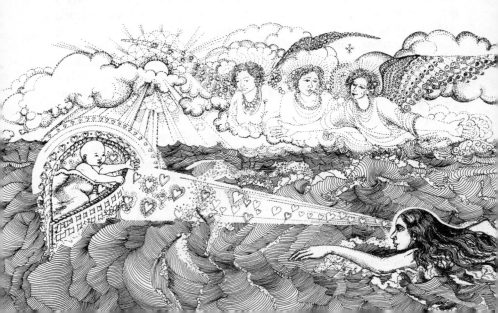

I got to do a few birthings with Ina May, and it was an incredible experience. Seeing Beatrice have Melinda taught me a lot about how loose and joyful you can be having a baby.

As I attended a few birthings, the other midwives would tell me to do something, like hand them a gauze pad, peeling down the wrapper from the corner so as not to contaminate the sterile gauze pad, which took my full attention. There was no such thing as practicing; it's always real life and matters that you do it right here and now. At the same time, I realized that just having a good time and being grateful to be there was also a help.

Each birthing, I was expected to do something more complex and of heavier responsibility than the last birthing. In a way I felt like I was barely able to keep stretching with such non-linear speed, but it kept me amazingly high to do it, and besides that, I had to—I was really counted on.

Then, around my tenth birthing, I was posted by myself to check Sara's dilation. To be the only lady present with a lady in labor felt like a tremendous responsibility.

I was at twenty-three birthings before I delivered my first baby. Ina May was with me, and it was really fun. I loved it. For the next birthing, too, Ina May was there. And then Ina May told me to deliver the next one solo! There I was! But I was ready to jump right in. I couldn't imagine anything I'd rather do.

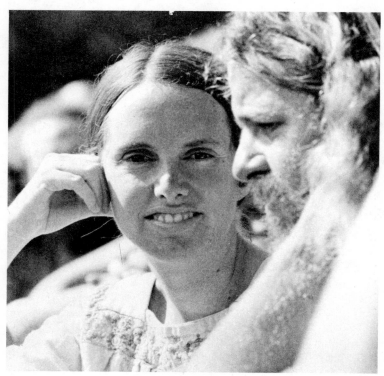

Cara and Michael

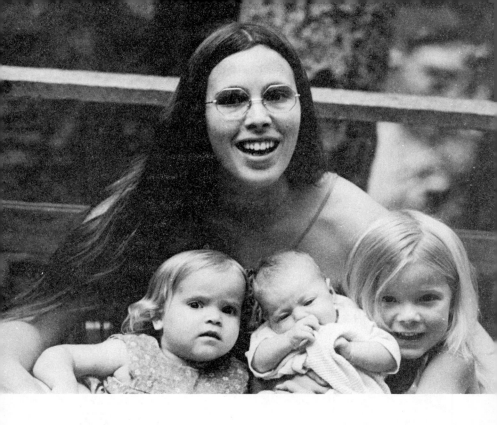

When Donna began labor on her third baby, her son Abraham asked, "Is it going to hurt, Donna?" She said, "No, Abraham, it's going to be **strong.**"

A Close One

ara: This birthing was one of the most unforgettable things that ever happened to me. Diane's labor was fairly smooth, even though the midwives had to encourage her to be good to her husband. She was dilating easily. When the baby's head moved through the cervix, though, it was a different story. Diane started screaming. I told her to shut up and keep herself together, but the baby was moving so fast that she wasn't going to listen. It was storming out and the lightning and thunder were so loud it was hard to hear much. The baby's head came out and I had to cut the cord right then because it was so tight around her neck. Her body came out and it looked healthy, but she just didn't have any muscle tension. I couldn't get anything happening from clearing her airway or stimulating her body. It felt like she was so scared that she just went way back and didn't want to come out. I started doing mouth-to-mouth resuscitation and heart compression. As I was doing mouth-to-mouth, I felt like this baby had to make it, and it was up to me. As I would bend down and put my mouth on hers, her eyes looked kind of glassy with no recognition. I made a decision in my heart that this baby was going to make it, and I didn't care if it cost my life. On a spiritual level, I felt a miracle happen. I really understood why they call it "the kiss of life." Her eyes brightened and she recognized me and started to breathe. All this time I had been hauling ass at working on her, but I really believe that it was that soul telepathy that got her started. I loved her so much for coming through and making it.

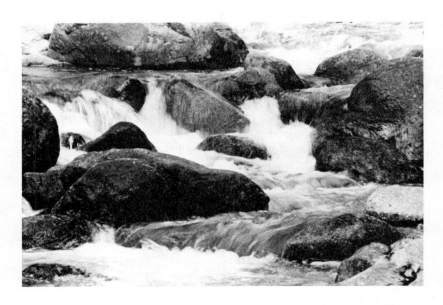

Mary Louise Becomes a Midwife

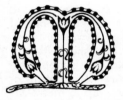ary Louise: I grew up the eldest of six children and always had a good time taking care of the babies. Then I got into a place where I thought I wanted to be a famous artist, travel around the world, and not get married. But it was obvious that I really wanted to be around babies, because it wasn't long before I had a fine baby boy. He was born in a hospital where they did everything backwards and I was completely unaware—I loved my baby, but didn't know about doing that trip again. Meanwhile I got married.

Then on the Caravan I got to be at some births and help out some. Seeing babies born in a compassionate, loving way blew my mind. Having a midwife there who was compassionate with the lady in labor really made a difference. It made me feel that I'd like to try it again, so I did.

Ina May delivered my next baby, a girl, here on the Farm. I loved it. It was the most beautiful, fulfilling experience I'd ever had.

I was glad when Ina May asked me if I'd help at birthings. It was something I really wanted to do. I got to be with a lot of ladies during their labor. Later, I got to help take care of the babies when they were born. I learned from each birth and each midwife. I hadn't really thought of becoming a midwife myself, but now I can't think of anything I'd rather do. There's a feeling of being One with the mother and the baby and everyone ever born that comes on strong at each birth. It makes me feel grateful to be there and help in any way I can.

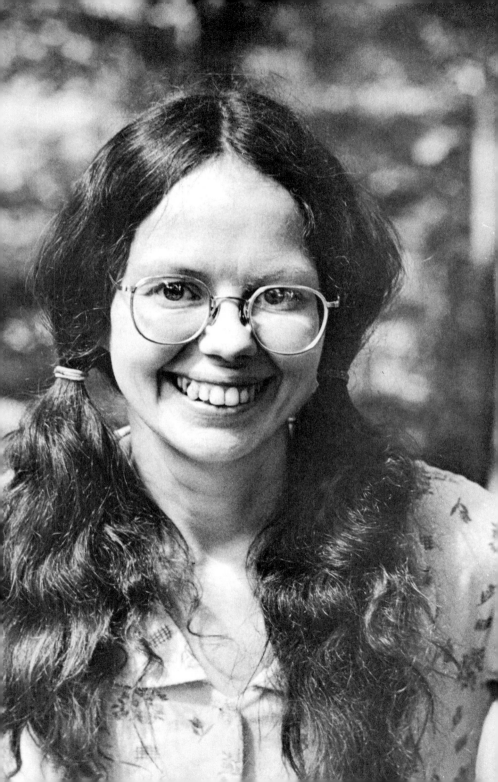

Maureen

Mary Louise describes the birth of her own daughter.

ary Louise: Maureen's birth was a very psychedelic experience for Joseph and me. Each rush
we felt our baby stronger and stronger. She
seemed to be filling us with her consciousness.
I'd look into Joseph's eyes and see a perfectly
clear vision of a new baby's face looking back at me. At one point I
looked at the rug and there was a beautiful newborn baby—looking so
real it amazed me. I could feel her coming closer. It was time to push,
her head was out—Cara said, "There's a cord. Pant." She said, "The
cord's around the neck twice and is pretty tight, I'll have to cut it." I
watched her—everything suspended—she cut the cord and out came a
baby girl. I felt her presence but saw she hadn't come into her body.
She was limp and quiet. *There was a timeless place where we all knew
she needed help.* I felt an urge to get up and start working with her,
and then felt all my trust in Cara. She was putting everything she had
into bringing our baby through. The agreement and love was so strong.
Soon we heard a small sound, she opened her eyes and made noises that
sounded like talking. Cara handed Maureen to me and we connected
through touch in an incredible loving rush. She looked at me and said,
"Hi." I could hardly believe it but Cara said, "Wow, she's talking to
you." She sure was. She was so glad to be here with us. I felt so
grateful. Joseph told me that during the rushes he'd seen exactly
the same visions of a baby's face when he looked into my eyes.

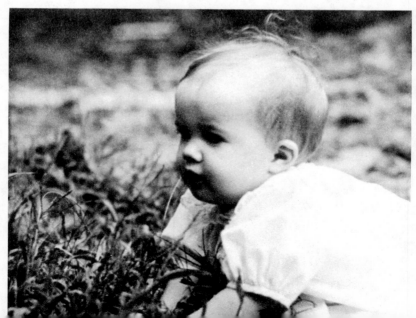

This story dates from the Caravan, long before Mary Louise ever thought of being a midwife. It shows that her heart was really in it, even then. She was already taking responsibility for clearing the minds of any subconscious emotional barriers to the smooth flow of labor.

Jennifer
Born March 2, 1971, 12:20 p.m.
Rest Stop, Sierra Nevada, Calif.

Sheila: On February 28th Andrew and I caught up with the Caravan on the way to Tennessee to buy a farm. The next morning I woke up feeling great. Outside I saw Stephen coming our way so I went out to say hi and give him a hug. At the moment I hugged him I started contracting, but I thought it was just gas or a cramp. Stephen looked at me and asked when I was due and I told him any time. It felt very telepathic that he knew I was going to do it then.

After breakfast the Caravan pulled out and we drove all day. The contractions kept coming on stronger all day, but I still wasn't admitting to it happening yet. It finally got to a place where I couldn't get comfortable. Andrew was pacing the bus asking, "How come it feels like this in here?" At that point I broke over and told him I was in labor. As soon as I said that my contractions came on fast and heavy. At that point I had the option to be graceful and do it or to complain a lot. I complained. At first it looked like I'd do it in a few hours or sooner, but my complaining made my labor last until 12:20 p.m. the next day.

On March 2, I was doing it for real. I could feel her head getting close to popping out. At this point Mary Louise came over. I was still some tight. She walked in the door of the bus and said, "Has Sheila told you all about her mother yet?" There was a lot of energy in that, so we talked about how I thought my mother had died in childbirth. Talking about it released a lot of energy, and the contractions started coming on real fast and heavy.

Mary Louise came over and put her attention totally to me. She and I swapped bodies. It was far out. I felt myself leave and enter Mary Louise's and she came over and did a few contractions for me. I found myself in a beautiful place with a green field and a house. It was a place I'd never seen before. I could still tell my body was contracting, but I was detached from it. Then the head came out. I told Mary Louise what happened and she said she'd been doing that contraction and had been able to feel it all. Then I felt the next contraction coming on and I knew she was going to come out. So I sat up real fast and looked at the head between my legs. What a beautiful sight! Then I laid back and out she came.

She was very blue-purple and didn't cry right off. Stephen had caught her and was working on getting her started. When she did start, we all got ecstatic. As soon as she cried, I wanted to take her and hold her to me. It was such a far-out, heavy, maternal feeling. After Jennifer was cleaned and dressed, they handed her to me and I put her on the tit. They cleaned up, and the Caravan rolled twenty to forty minutes later.

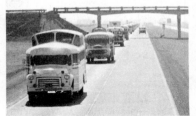

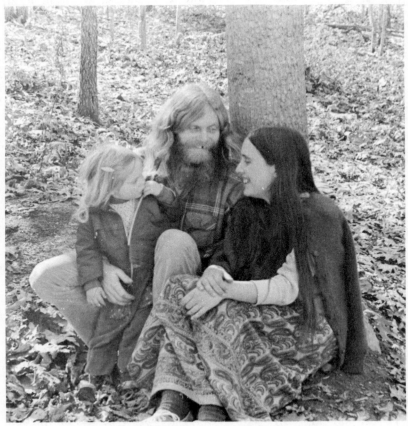

Jennifer, Andrew, and Sheila

Noah's Birthing

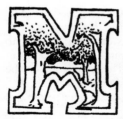y pregnancy with Noah started out in an unusual way. I had been having some pain in my eyes for a couple of weeks, and the two different doctors I went to about it just told me to get my glasses checked. I didn't know that I was pregnant at the time, but I had some suspicions. We'd been trying to get pregnant for four years so I had my doubts too, because I had thought I might be pregnant several times before.

My eyes kept on bothering me, and one of them got fuzzy and hard to see out of, so I went to another doctor who told me I probably had optic neuritis, and come back in a few days for more tests. Two days after that, I woke up in the morning and it was dark, and I went in the bathroom and turned on the light and I thought the bulb had burnt out, so I went back in our room and turned on the light and it was still dark but I could tell the light was on because the darkness was a little brighter. I realized then that I couldn't see much of anything, and I told John. I tried not to get emotional or scared about it, and I felt strongly that since it had come on so quickly that it couldn't be a permanent thing.

It was really something to integrate being blind—I could tell lighter and darker shades of gray, so I didn't bump into large objects very much, but I couldn't see any colors or detail. I really felt reliant on John and my friends—one time that day, John left me standing by a busy street and went to talk to somebody, and I couldn't move at all, I had to wait for him to come back and guide me. I felt helpless, and also amazed at how blind people I had met got around so well. I knew I was going to have to get it together if I was going to be blind for very long.

We went to the hospital for tests the next day. I had a pregnancy test and we were still waiting for the results when it was my turn to see the doctor. He checked out my eyes and I could tell he was worried about me. I told him not to worry. Then another doctor came in and they were talking, and they told us "by the way, your pregnancy test was positive" and we just about went through the ceiling. We were hugging and kissing and I was really amazed. Then they told me that I would have to be admitted to the hospital. I didn't want to go in the hospital, I wanted to go home and celebrate. But John told me to be reasonable and do what they said.

They did a spinal tap, X-rays, and blood tests, and they wanted to put me on medication right away, but we wanted to wait and check it out and make sure that it was safe for the baby. We called Ina May and Jeffrey and they called Paul and Dr. Williams and another doctor, and they all agreed on which medicine would be safe for the baby (Paul told me later that he had just been studying what I had when Ina May called him). I didn't want to do anything that would hurt the baby, but I trusted them. I was so grateful to have folks I could count on like that.

With the medicine, my eyes started getting better day by day. The doctors had told me that it might be months before I could see again, but I didn't really believe them. It took about 3 weeks for the fog to clear altogether. When I got home from the hospital all the colors in my room and the house were so beautiful, and it was so good to be home and to be able to see everyone again that I just cried.

All the tests they did turned out to be normal, and they never did figure out what caused my going blind.

The day after I got home from the hospital I started spotting, and I kept on for a couple of days. I stayed in bed with my feet up and prayed a lot, and it stopped. The rest of my pregnancy was normal.

Noah's birthing started when my waterbag broke as I was carrying a bunch of laundry in off the line. I wasn't having any rushes, so John and I walked to the showers and took a shower and walked home, gushing all the way. It was the middle of July and very hot.

Later that night I started having light rushes and Barbie came and checked me. She couldn't find my cervix at all but she could feel the baby's head so she thought I might be fully dilated. I didn't think so, but she called Kathleen and she and Eleanor raced down from the gate and the ambulance raced over with the sterile pack. Kathleen checked me and I was only 1 cm. dilated—the cervix was tilted back behind his head some. We all had a good laugh.

Faylee came over and stayed most of the night—I was too excited to sleep, and I kept thinking I was getting more dilated, but every time she checked, I'd be the same—1 cm. She left around 3 a.m. and right after that my rushes got a lot stronger. I didn't know what to do to integrate them and John didn't know what to do either.

After a couple of hours of trying different things and feeling scared and tight, I called Kathleen and she said she'd come over. She fell back asleep though, and when she did come over a while later, I was feeling pretty miserable. I wanted to have a good time, but I didn't know how to handle the rushes. Kathleen told us that having a baby was designed to put us through changes that would help us be better parents. I really dug that. She got Lizzy and Janet Sue, and Faylee came back and they would rub my legs and my back when the rushes came on and that helped so much. I could feel the energy stack up there and rubbing would release it. It felt so good. Barbie came to help and I was glad to see her—we had known each other for a long time, and I love her a lot.

Every hour or so I would open up another centimeter, and by the time I was 5 cm., Kathleen checked me and said his head was trying to come through the cervix already, and we'd have to do something to get

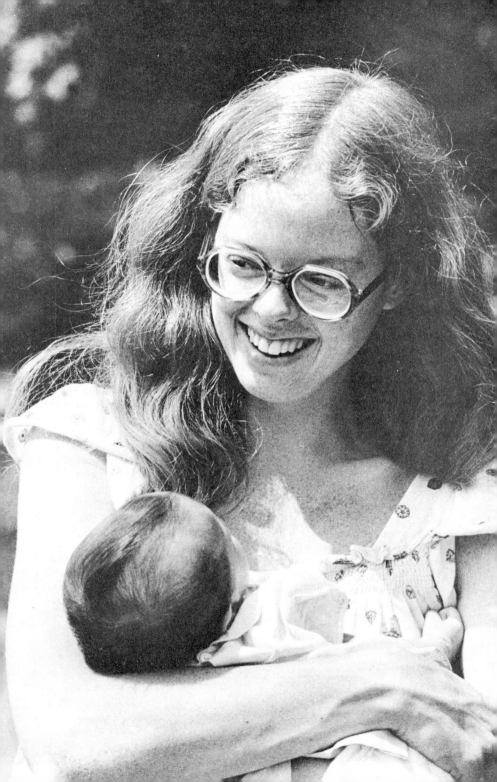

me to open up the rest of the way. We took some walks and I got up on my hands and knees for some rushes and after a couple more hours, I was fully dilated. I remember I could hardly believe it. Learning how to integrate the rushes was like climbing a mountain—just when I'd get to a place where I could integrate them pretty well, they would change and get a lot heavier and I'd have to learn to integrate them again.

When it was time to push, it took me a little while to get the hang of it. Kathryn and Susan Rabs came then, and I was glad to see them. They looked really pretty and clear. Kathryn said "this part is like the Olympics" and that's what it felt like to me, too. It took a long time for his head to get through my bones—I would push and he'd come through a little and then when I stopped pushing he'd slide back. I kept trying to push harder and longer—the ladies were a great cheering section. I'd fall back on John between pushes and try to catch my breath.

I really felt like the Incredible Hulk when I was pushing—the rushes were really strong and I was grunting and making a lot of noise, but it felt good because I knew there was no going back, he was going to come out. I also felt like I had no brains at all, and I was really glad the ladies were there helping me and telling me what to do.

We tried some squatting pushes and finally got through my bones, and after a while I could reach down and feel the top of his head—that was an amazing feeling. I pushed his head halfway out, and they cut me a little, and then his head came out and then his body. What an incredible rush. He looked huge to me—the midwives had said all through the birthing that he was a boy, so I wasn't surprised. I was so glad and relieved that he was all together—they got him going pretty fast and handed him to me. I felt so good and like I had the strength to do anything. While Susan cleaned him up he was crying and we were all guessing how much he weighed and getting the placenta out. It was like a party. When she gave him to me he sucked his thumb and looked so content I could tell he felt right at home. We were so happy.

I flashed on the name Noah when I was looking at him and John liked it too. There was a full moon and Kathleen stitched me up and the ladies all went home. I kept thinking that I never could have done it without their help.

Noah caught on to nursing right away and he was really relaxed and didn't cry much right from the start. *We fell into a deep sleep and I knew that God was watching over us.* I felt so much peace in my heart.

Love,

Marcia

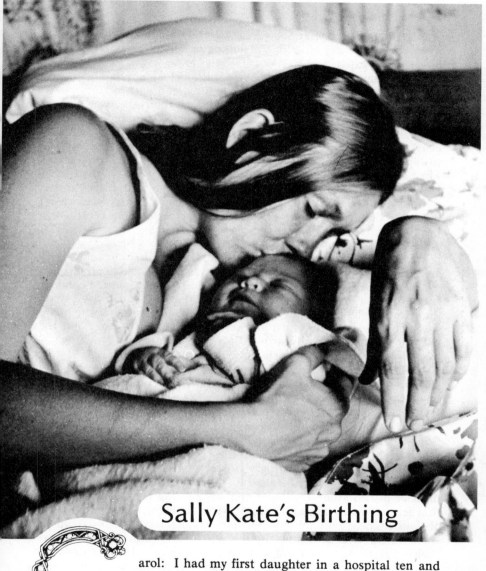

Sally Kate's Birthing

Carol: I had my first daughter in a hospital ten and a half years ago. She was an eight-pound breech, and I was completely knocked out. I nearly died from aspiration pneumonia caused by my vomiting while under anesthesia. My next pregnancy and birthing was very different. It was a lot of fun.

I was really grateful to be pregnant. I had had an operation for endometriosis* four years earlier and was told it would be beneficial but difficult for me to ever get pregnant again.

*Endometriosis: Some endometrial tissue, the lining of the uterus, occurring outside of the uterus in the abdominal cavity, usually on and around the ovaries.

I felt like I had gotten unattached to getting pregnant and that when we made love I wasn't thinking of getting pregnant, I was really trying to get Donald high and was loving him a lot.

When I started labor, I asked Donald for a clock to time the rushes. I couldn't believe it, but they were only three and four minutes apart. I decided I'd better call Ina May even though the rushes weren't very heavy. I got up to call her and the rushes started coming on stronger. I had to pee and when I squatted down to do that, the rushes came on heavier and one right after the other. All of a sudden I was peeing and rushing all at once. I could feel myself opening up—I really felt great. I had a little bloody show then too. I called Ina May. She had Mary Louise come over and check me. Mary Louise said I was almost completely dilated. I tightened up some then because Ina May wasn't there and neither were the sterile packs. The rushes kept coming but I was holding them back some. All of this had only taken about an hour.

When Ina May got there she checked me. I was about nine centimeters dilated then. Ina May broke my water bag. I told her that I had tightened up and I relaxed again and the rushes really started coming.

Donald and I made out and he rubbed my back. It felt good to do that, and it helped me stay relaxed. I loved Donald and everyone there so much; there was so much love all around for each other and the baby. I could feel it really strong. It helped a lot to say, "I love you," to everyone. It made me rush and helped me stay relaxed.

I felt higher than I ever had in my life. It was such a heavy spiritual experience, and so much fun. In between rushes I'd laugh at how telepathic it was. When I was ready to push it was all I could do. It was very compelling and required a hundred per cent of my attention. It felt good to have a direction to put all of that energy. It was some of the hardest work I've ever done. Between rushes I'd relax so much I felt like I was melting into the bed. It all felt good.

Ina May kept giving me progress reports on what was happening; it helped a lot to know what was going on. She also was massaging the muscles in and around my puss and was putting baby oil on. All of that felt good and helped me keep loose. It became more and more obvious that the only thing happening was that a new soul was about to be born. It kept getting prettier and clearer and higher. It was such a rush to look down and see her head coming out from between my legs. Donald was really amazed by that, too. Her head popped out, then her shoulders, then the rest of her body. It was such an amazing rush. It felt really good. She started to cry as soon as she came out. She was really beautiful and very aware of everyone around her. Ina May put her on my belly for a few minutes before Mary Louise cleaned her up. It was so great to have her there.

I was very grateful to have her and to have had the experience of having her at home. It was really Holy. I'm glad to have been able to share it with Donald. It really helped make our relationship solid.

Mary Louise brought Sally back after cleaning her up. Ina May held her for a few minutes, then gave her to me. Ina May said, "Nice cure for endometriosis, huh!" She sure was. Nine pounds, nine ounces of healthy baby girl. Donald and I are really grateful for her.

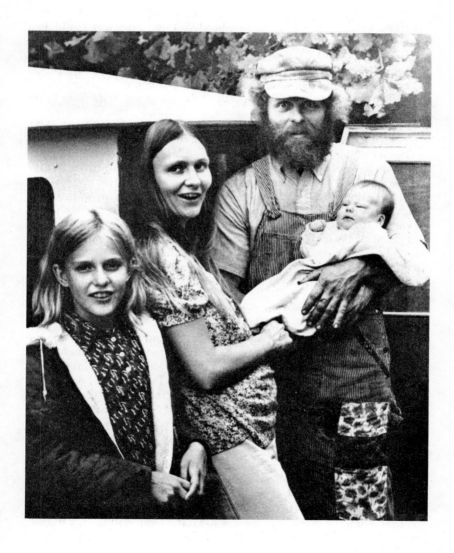

Keif Oliver

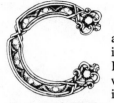

Carol: I was only six months pregnant when I went into labor with Keif. It was a Sunday evening and I started rushing every two or three minutes. It was happening for a while before I really admitted it. I told Donald that I felt like if I could just relax and fall asleep I could get the rushes to stop. Donald rubbed me out really good and I fell asleep while he was doing that.

I woke up the next morning very grateful to have stopped. It was Monday and I had an appointment with Dr. Gene, our local doctor, for him to see a pregnant couple (I was the midwife on our Wisconsin Farm at the time). We all went to the doctor's office and when Dr. Gene was through with the pregnant couple I told him what had happened to me the night before. I had been rushing some that day too, but irregularly.

Dr. Gene checked me and I was one and a half centimeters and over 50% thinned out. Whew! "It's too soon for you to have this baby," Dr. Gene said. We agreed!

What to do now? I knew it was too soon—the chances of the baby making it if he was born now were slim—but there's always a chance. I went through heavy changes in my head. I had to get very unattached and get at peace with the idea that I might just go ahead and have this baby. I prayed a lot. I felt very close with God. I understood what was happening. "If there is anything in my power I can do to keep this baby in, please help me to do it." I knew I had to be grateful for being pregnant and keeping the baby in as long as I did. I felt a great love for Dr. Gene and everyone around me. I knew my friends were going to help me through this, whatever the outcome.

Dr. Gene and I decided I should go home and go right to bed, see what that did and take it from there. I went home and got in bed. The next two days I stayed in bed, but my rushes kept coming on more.

On Wednesday night I called Ina May in Tennessee. I felt like I really needed to get connected with her. She said I should start drinking some booze to see if we could slow me down. Dr. Gene thought so too. So I did. I got drunk and stayed that way for about ten days, rushing on and off regularly and irregularly. Drinking helped keep my body relaxed and made it easier to stay in bed. It also took some of the psychedelic feeling away. My rushes slowed down.

Dr. Gene came and checked me again. I was a little more dilated and more thinned out. I stopped drinking for a few days. Then it got to where all I had to do when I noticed a rush was sip on a drink and that would be enough to mellow me out. I still had to stay in bed, lying flat most of the time, occasionally sitting up. Every time I got up I started to rush.

I had to pay close attention to the energy. If it started feeling really psychedelic and good all over I would drink. I had to be careful to not get into how good I felt, because that would bring the rushes on. Donald and I had to not get too close to each other—we couldn't smooch or cuddle because that would make me rush. Every morning when I woke up I was very grateful to have made it through another day. I felt like I was lying there being an incubator. At times I got impatient and wanted to get up but how could I? I would put those thoughts out of my head and think more of how grateful I was to be able to keep my baby in.

I sewed and read and slept. I had a lot of help from Donald, Kimberly, our twelve-year-old, and our friends we lived with. Everyone was really nice to me and took really good care of me and kept it very mellow around me.

I rushed on and off for ten weeks. I watched the leaves fall and the snow come. Thanksgiving, Christmas, New Year's went by on into January. I was grateful for every day. Dr. Gene said if I kept the baby in until he was 36 weeks (eight months) he would come to the Farm and deliver me. How could I resist that! I really didn't want to have to go to the hospital. As nice as the folks were there I'd still rather do it at home. So I stayed in bed and paid good attention.

I was eight months on January 22nd. I started rushing pretty heavy that night. I knew if I was going to stop this I was going to have to get good and drunk. Sips weren't going to work. I got drunk and fell asleep. I woke up several times in the night to pee. Then on towards dawn I was waking up quite often. I would get up to pee (I had a pot right beside the bed) and just a little would come out. Back to bed and sleep. A few minutes later I'd have to pee again. Then I realized the sensation was rushes coming on. As soon as I realized this I looked at my watch. Three minutes apart and coming on strong. I called Karen, my friend and assistant midwife, to come and check me out. I was about three and a half centimeters.

We called Dr. Gene. He said to try to stop them—it would be good if we could hold off a little longer. I told him I wasn't sure if I could but I would sure try. I went back to my room and drank about three ounces of vodka. It slowed me down some but I could tell they weren't going to stop. Just as I thought that Dr. Gene called to see how I was doing. He said to stop drinking. He'd make the hospital rounds and be right out. He said, "This baby's wanted to come out for a long time. Let's let him out—and have him be sober!"

Whew! What a relief! I really started to come on then. It felt so good to let go and open up. The energy was making my whole body shake. Donald and Lisa, our friend, rubbed on my body. It felt so good and really helped me channel all of that energy. I was really coming on strong. Karen and Susan set up and got things ready for Dr. Gene. They were going to assist him. I asked Karen to check me again. I was about six centimeters. I told her to call Dr. Gene back and tell him to hurry. She did; he was already on his way.

Donald kept rubbing me and we cuddled and smooched—it felt really good to get to do that; it had been so long since we'd been able to. It really helped me. I loved Donald so much and was so glad to get to have him there with me.

When Dr. Gene got there I was really relieved to see him. I'd been rushing pretty strong. It felt really good. I knew I was opening up.

Then my rushes stopped. Dr. Gene got there about the same time as everyone else in the house got up and the three ounces of vodka took effect. It was too much to integrate.

I kept doing what I know works to bring rushes on. Donald and I cuddled and smooched and he rubbed my belly and tits. Finally I sat up and rubbed Donald's back. That brought them on more. My getting up and putting some energy out helped a lot.

Dr. Gene checked me again. Even though I hadn't been rushing I was still opening up. I was eight centimeters. He broke my water bag and I had several nice strong rushes and was ready to push. It felt really good to push. I felt the baby slide under my bones and start up the birth canal. Dr. Gene rubbed baby oil on and massaged my muscles. He felt as tantric and loving as one of the other midwives. He's really a gentle man. I was very grateful to have him help me.

Once I got the baby through the bones I had to slow down a little. Finally out popped his head—I panted, no cord. I pushed again.

It's a boy! A beautiful healthy baby boy. He weighed eight pounds even though he was a month early. Donald and I have big babies. It was nice to have a boy—we already had two girls. Susan took him to clean him up and put drops in his eyes. Dr. Gene delivered my placenta. I hadn't torn. It was the first home birthing Dr. Gene had ever done. He was amazed, really amazed. He was really glad he'd done it—he'd had a really good time. We all did.

We were all grateful for such a fine healthy boy after all that time. We named him Keif Oliver.

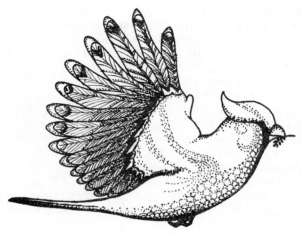

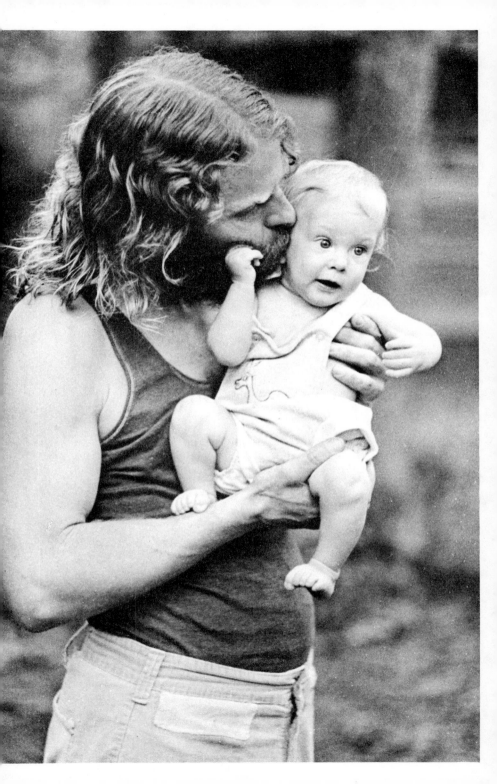

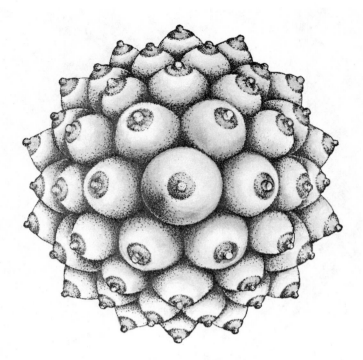

Louisa's Birth

Sometimes a couple is friendly enough but they need a little help in getting their bodies "wired" together so the electricity of the birthing energy flows right. Farm midwives might give a couple some instructions on how to kiss more effectively, which is what we did in the following birthing.

Kathleen: Ina May checked my dilation. She said something about my mouth being tight like it was when we had Samuel, our first baby. A loose mouth makes for a loose puss which makes the baby come out easier. Whatever Ina May said came out funny and everybody laughed but me. I was afraid to laugh because I thought it would make the baby come out. This was true and I realized that if I laughed and loosened up that the pain would go away and Louisa would come out really easy and everything would be psychedelic and Holy. I laughed. Mark and I started smooching a lot to keep my mouth really loose. This made the contractions come on really strong.

Mark: Ina May had Kathleen kiss me with her lips on top and around mine. Kathleen had never kissed me before like that and it was great! I was rubbing Kathleen's breasts and I could feel electricity coming out of her nipples. It was like touching the end of an electrical terminal. [*Mark is an electrician by trade.—Ina May*] The kissing too felt very electrical and I knew that we had gotten to a level of awareness we'd never quite been to before. I realized that what was happening was a fulfillment and what I was feeling was Holy loving energy building up and making the birth of a baby happen.

Holding Louisa for the first time was the most awesome part for me. Her eyes opened right away and it looked like the Universe being unfolded before my eyes. Her face would go through many changes so that she looked like different people that I knew, and I felt telepathic with those folks through her. One time she looked just like my

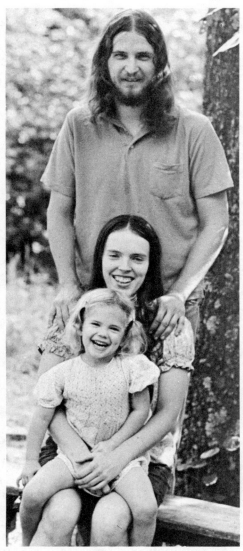

Mark, Kathleen and Louisa

mother, and she felt just like my mother in a peaceful place, and I saw that place in Louisa that was in *all* those people and could feel connected and One with the entire Universe through her. Being with her for her first few hours was the most remarkable thing I had ever experienced. Way after the midwives had left, we were still up, unable to sleep, just feeling wonderful. We had been part of a miracle that had changed our lives and helped us grow.

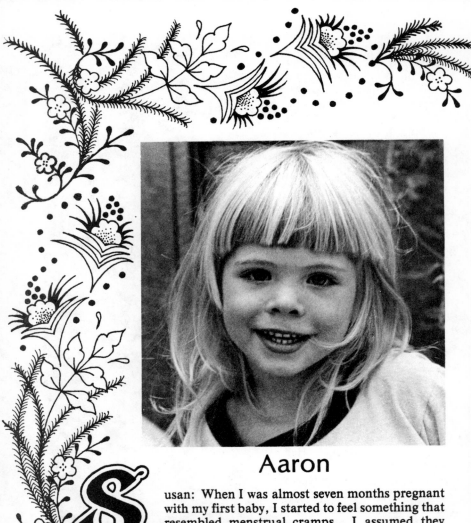

Aaron

Susan: When I was almost seven months pregnant with my first baby, I started to feel something that resembled menstrual cramps. I assumed they were probably gas pains, and didn't give it much further thought. However, they kept increasing in intensity and regularity. Finally, after about two days I realized that these were contractions and that I was probably going to have a baby. My first thoughts were of disbelief and fear. I worried that my baby wouldn't make it, being so early. These feelings soon gave way to a feeling of peace as soon as I decided to enjoy it and have faith that everything would be all right.

My husband called the midwives and they came down to take me to the hospital. It was decided that that would be the best and safest place to have such a premature baby. I had to let go of any attachments to having my baby at home with my husband there.

Ina May got permission to come into the labor room with me. I am really thankful for that. I had some preconceived notions about hospitals and labor rooms. They quickly vanished as I learned to relax and exchange energy with Ina May. She taught me how to relax and breathe right. It didn't matter that we were in a hospital labor room, because we were just being here and now, trying to have a baby.

The baby's head started to come out and the doctor returned with permission for Ina May to come into the delivery room. The delivery room wasn't the weird, scary place I had anticipated. The doctor felt good and I knew the situation was under control. I could tell that the doctor really liked Ina May's presence there and appreciated her techniques. It didn't seem like it took very long to have my baby once we were in the delivery room. I had no anesthesia. Having Ina May there was almost like giving birth on the Farm. We just brought a little Farm energy with us. The baby came out quite small (about three pounds, six ounces), but bright pink and kicking and crying. I knew it would be quite a while before he would be home with us, but he looked so good that it didn't matter. I knew that he would have excellent care until he was big enough to bring home with us and I was very thankful for it.

Ina May: I hardly recognized Aaron when Walter and Susan brought him home from the hospital. It wasn't just that he was bigger and older—almost six pounds at six weeks old by then—he had a whole different look on him than he'd had at birth. He looked like a convict who had been in prison long enough to learn to not move his face. Instead of his face being rounded and soft and babyish, it looked long and lean, and he held the micro-muscles around his mouth and chin so tight that it gave the skin there a greyish cast, making it look like he had a five o'clock shadow. He looked amazingly hard and immobile for someone who wasn't even supposed to be born yet.

I knew that I could get him back looking like a baby, and that he looked the way he did because the nurses who had been taking care of him in the nursery for preemies took care of so many babies that they didn't relate with each one as a unique individual. Nobody had treated Aaron like he was aware and intelligent and capable of communicating. I don't think anyone had looked him in the eyes since he had been born.

I took him in my arms and tried to look in his eyes. He looked away as soon as I got there. I moved with him, caught his glance again and he immediately looked away. Nothing wrong with his synapses, obviously. I chased him for a while in this fashion, trying to get him to hold still and look at me.

After a while I could feel him getting interested, wondering, "Who is this checking me out so close?" Sometimes I would catch his glance for a second and we would get high together—his pupils would dilate noticeably and my head would rush. It was lots of fun. The more I tried to get Aaron's attention, the higher we got; his eyes started looking big and round and alert, and the muscles in his face relaxed, allowing the circulation to improve. He began to look delicious. I nuzzled his cheek and looked at him again and he was even prettier, so I did that a few more times and rushed and rushed. By this time I had achieved good eye contact and *telepathic rapport* with Aaron. I handed him back to Susan so she could get to know him, too.

What I had done with Aaron was a kind of healing that you can give a person just by how purely and cleanly you look at him. The nature of this healing was a communication, which was a two-way transaction and required obtaining his cooperation.

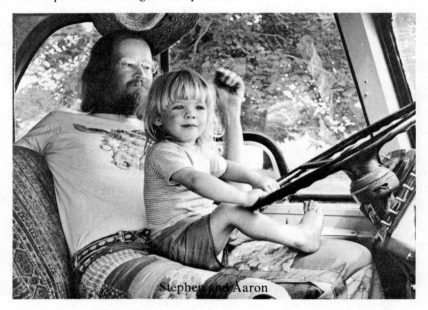

Stephen and Aaron

Ross

Another premature baby for Susan and Walter

Susan: When I was about seven months pregnant with my second child, I lost my mucus plug. I had someone call the midwife, who told me to rest. Shortly after that, I started feeling some light rushes, but I still wasn't really sure I was having my baby then. They got progressively stronger and more regular. One of the midwives checked me and said I was a little dilated, but that I should drink a little booze to try and stop the rushes. I drank quite a bit of vodka, but my rushes continued to get heavier anyway. [*Usually we have very good success with this method of halting premature labor.—I.M.*]

Ina May felt my belly and couldn't tell exactly what position the baby was in. It was definitely not head first. All this time my rushes got heavier and heavier. Since the baby was premature and probably breech as well, we decided to go to the hospital. Kathryn, a midwife trainee, came with me into the labor room. She held my hands as the rushes got heavy and I looked into her eyes. It felt really good to have a Farm midwife there, since my husband was out in the waiting room.

The doctor came in and felt my belly. He, too, wasn't sure of the baby's position, so he sent me up for an X-ray, to figure it out for sure. The X-ray told us that the baby was sideways. The doctor put his hands on my belly and tried to turn the baby around. He kept trying but the baby wouldn't budge. He said that I was too far into labor and it was too late to move him. I really love him for trying, though.

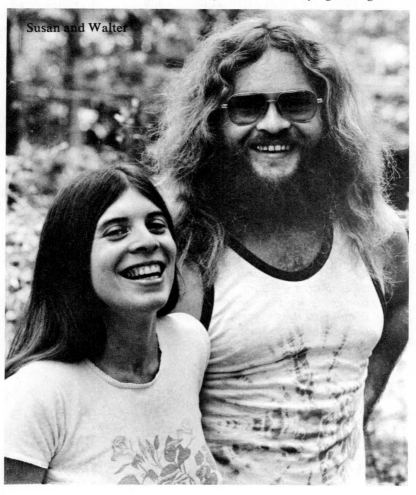

Susan and Walter

He told me he'd have to do a cesarean. He said I could go on for days and days in labor like that and accomplish nothing. The thought of a cesarean blew my mind. I never imagined that I would ever have a baby like that. I knew, though, that it was the only way of getting the baby out alive; so I agreed to it.

They asked Kathryn to leave since I was going into surgery. I didn't really want her to leave but I knew it was their rules. When she left, one of the nurses took my hands and we exchanged energy just like I had been doing with Kathryn. She had been watching us and really liking how we were doing it. She felt good and I was very happy to have her there. She had had a cesarean herself a little while back. Soon after that, I was thinking I'm glad we're going to get this baby out okay, whatever it takes.

When I woke up, my husband was there. I was still a bit groggy, but glad to see him. They had to take my baby to a bigger hospital for more intensive care. (He is now a strong, healthy kid.) For me, it was major surgery, but I healed up fast and was grateful to have my baby alive and well.

Kathryn: The doctor came out of the nursery and said he wanted to send Susan's baby to Nashville because he was starting to have a little trouble with his breathing. The ride in the ambulance felt like a space-ship—it was three in the morning and very still, and we were going about ninety miles an hour and the red light was blinking off and on. It felt very Holy. Felt like those religious pictures of angels flying towards Heaven with a baby in their arms. All the while Ross lay in his incubator, sleeping and breathing softly. When we got to the hospital, there was this big fat nurse in the preemie nursery who picked Ross up and cupped him in her hand and said to the other nurse, "Aw, look what they brought us."

Ross's birth, the 188th of those we attended, was our first cesarean. Looking back on it now in the 1990's, when a 25% cesarean rate is accepted as normal by many people (not the World Health Organization, however), I remember how precious it was for us for so many women to be able to share their strength and knowledge around the time of childbirth. I strongly believe that many of these same 187 women would have had very different outcomes had they given birth in another situation.

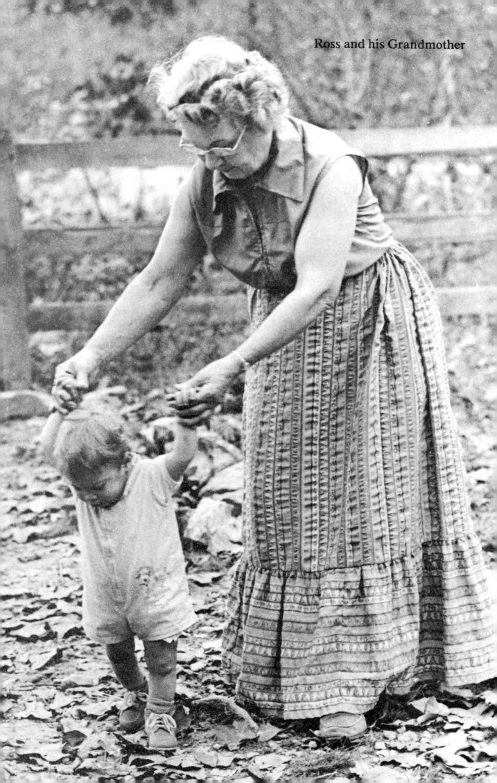

Ross and his Grandmother

Breathing

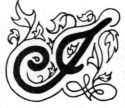na May: We don't practice breathing techniques during pregnancy because we feel that if you practice a lot a certain way, you might tend to be a little rigid when it comes to the actual experience of the childbirth. We work out breathing techniques in the here-and-now at the birthing. If a lady needs to breathe certain ways to help her labor, our midwives will counsel her and demonstrate what's appropriate for the time.

We've also had several instances where the husband gave us invaluable help. One of these was with a lady who was having her first baby. She had assisted at a number of births and thought she knew some techniques. She was having a pretty slow first stage and was only about half dilated after about twenty-four hours of regular, strong rushes. Her dilation had remained the same for many hours. She was not progressing as she had seen many ladies do, and that worried her a little.

Her husband saw this. He also saw that the way she was breathing to deal with the rushes didn't seem to help too much. He told her that to his vision she seemed to gain energy on her in-breaths and scatter it as she exhaled. He suggested that instead of letting her air out right away, she should hold her breath for a bit, then exhale. He was right. As she held her breathe at the top of each rush, she became confident that she could handle the energy of the rushes, and then started to dilate fast. In a few rushes she was completely dilated and starting to push.

The baby was born within about twenty minutes of her tailor-made instructions. It's very good if a couple can figure out how to get the most energy out of the rushes.

Mary of David: Stephen was there looking at a midwives' handbook; he looked at me on the bed and said, "Monkey lady." I didn't like the idea at first. I was brought up with the idea that people had an animal nature and a spiritual one; and that your animal nature was lower. But then I felt One with the monkeys and everything that brings forth new life. It felt very Holy.

Margaret's Birth

ichard: We were over two weeks past the due date when one Thursday morning my wife Marna, feeling herself coming on to labor, asked me to stay home from work. So that day and the next we spent a lot of time together, talking about what was about to happen and just plain old giving each other a bunch. One of the midwives would come by every so often to check Marna out. Marna was slowly dilating (at least slower than some ladies we'd heard tales of), which we were glad for because in those two days all the smooching, cuddling, and back rubbing had really meshed us together.

Towards the end of the second day, the midwives asked us if it was okay to have another couple come have their baby in the room directly below our bedroom loft. For a number of reasons there was only one midwife on the Farm that night who could be there to do the catching, so they wanted both of us couples to be close together. We said sure, and soon William and Joanne were settled in right below us. We could hear each other talking if we spoke up, so sometimes we'd all check in with each other, talk some and compare notes. Cara would check Joanne's dilation, then come up the stairs to check Marna. They were close as far as how fast they were dilating to where we could all feel they were in the same groove. One of the ladies helping said it felt like a close horse race and we all cracked up.

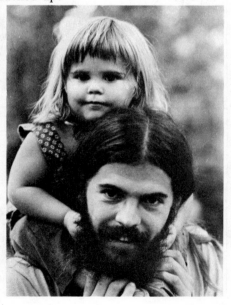

At one point that Friday evening, Marna said maybe she'd not do it tonight, maybe she'd go to sleep and have the baby the next day. That was okay with me—I didn't mind waiting—but something in Marna's voice seemed a little grim. I was sitting there thinking about it when Cara came up to check on Marna. Marna told her what she'd just told me and Cara, picking up on the grim tone right away, told Marna to lighten up, to stop thinking about herself because what she was about to do was for all of mankind. Marna perked up and the next time Cara checked her, Marna was almost fully dilated. You could really feel how Cara's level of truth had opened Marna's heart.

Joanne had fully dilated as well. Cara was downstairs with her as it felt like she might do it first. Mary Louise came upstairs with us. She told us that she was going to catch our baby, with Cara there, as this would be the second time she'd caught. The joy she put out at being there with us lit up the room.

Marna told Mary Louise she felt like pushing and she said go ahead. Marna pushed hard several times. Then Mary Louise told her to stop pushing as she could tell by feeling that Marna hadn't quite fully dilated. She had Marna relax and do short quick breaths while she opened up the rest of the way. It was during that short period of waiting that Joanne had her baby downstairs. The sound of Ida coming into the world, crying, filled the room. The midwives fixed up Joanne and Ida and then came upstairs. It was very soon thereafter that Margaret was born. She was a little hard to start and Cara, helping Mary Louise, got her breathing very soon. I felt so grateful to have these two ladies coming on so heavy with such grace. Margaret squealed a little and I felt a rush of joy come over us, humbled to be there with this new baby and these nice ladies.

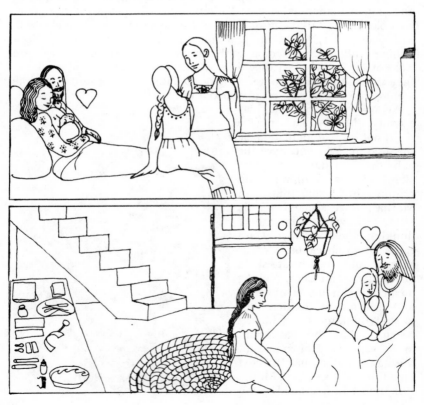

Contractions don't have to hurt. They are energy rushes that enable you to open up your thing so the baby can come out. If you have the attitude that they hurt, then you'll tense up and not be able to completely relax and it will take the baby longer to come through and you won't have any fun either. It is a miracle to be able to create more life force and there is no room for complaining.

—Barbara
Mother of three babies

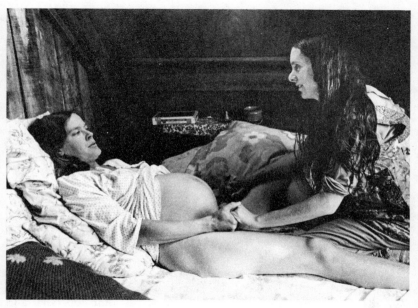

If all your life you never do anything heavy, there's certain passages in life that are heavy. Having a baby, for instance, is one. If you be a total paddy-ass all your life, they're going to have to knock you out when you have your kid, because you're going to be too chicken to have it. And if you do something that builds character ahead of time, you'll have enough character that you can have that kid, and it will be a beautiful and a spiritual experience for you.

—Stephen

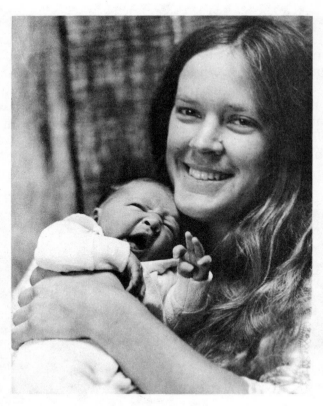

Jenny Rose

When I got pregnant with our third child I knew pretty exactly the day I conceived. I'd felt this strong urge to go lay down. I went upstairs and stretched out on our bed. My body felt good and like it was unwinding. I was laying there feeling stoned when somewhere in the center of me I felt like a flash of energy just spark. It felt like my heart opening. Then it turned into a warm glowy feeling that spread up and down my body. It felt delicious, like falling in love. I lay there and thought, "What is this?" After a while I found myself thinking. "Wow, this feels just like being pregnant." Then I realized what I was saying. Within three weeks or so other signs made it obvious to me, even though I didn't technically know for another three or four weeks that I was pregnant. I feel like I've been knowing this baby right from the start. It settled my mind about the life and soul of a baby being there from the very first.

Love,

Edine

THE BOOK OF LOUEY

Roberta: I woke up around two o'clock Friday morning with light rushes. I felt like I was going to have my baby. I called Mary Louise and she came over to check me. She agreed; my cervix was thinning and I was dilated one centimeter.

The rushes came steady all night. Around sunrise, Ruth checked me. I was still dilated one centimeter and rushing every four to five minutes. Joel and I decided to hang out together. We had a good time; it felt like we were preparing for our new baby.

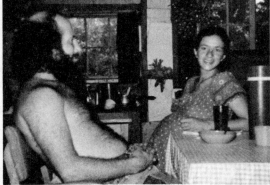

Joel: We had a good time the rest of the morning hours, smooching, joking, and napping. We felt psychedelic, loose, in love.

Roberta: Late in the morning, the rushes were still coming regularly and I was still only dilated one centimeter. I decided I wanted to get up and do something. I felt like working would bring on the rushes. I think what did it was mopping the floors.

By four o'clock Friday afternoon, the rushes were getting so that I had to sit down. I went up to bed and a few hours later, Ruth checked me out. I was dilated two centimeters and the baby's head was pushing up against the cervix. The rushes got more intense and closer together. Joel would rub my back or pull on my belly. He tried to help keep my bottom loose.

Around ten o'clock, Ruth checked me again and I was still only two centimeters dilated. I panicked. The rushes were heavy and very regular. It seemed to be taking a long time to open up. I thought it would take me forever for it to get to ten centimeters. Ruth called Cara because the head was pushing so hard against the cervix. Cara came over and I can remember feeling relieved. Cara told me that it was going to get heavier, and that I had to learn how to let the rushes go through. She taught me how to breathe in a way that would loosen my bottom. She told me that smooching with Joel would get the baby out. It worked really good when Joel and I smooched and cuddled with each other.

99

Cara: I got a call that Roberta was having heavy rushes but wasn't dilating and was having a hard time. I wanted to go see her and help. When I got there, Roberta was writhing with each rush and shaking. She just didn't have any idea how to handle the energy. Joel was sitting beside her looking worried. The whole scene was a bit grim for a baby-having. I got them kissing, hugging, and had Roberta really grab on to Joel and squeeze him. Joel is a big, strong, heavy-duty man. He and I rubbed Roberta continuously and steered in the direction of relaxed. I let her know that she was having good, strong rushes, and that if she'd relax and just experience it and let it happen, her rushes would accomplish a lot and open her up. She gradually accepted the fact that there was no getting out of this, except to let it happen and quit fighting it.

Joel: Cara assured us that everything was going along fine, and when Roberta complained again about how it felt, Cara told her that it was going to get stronger and she should not think of the rushes as being painful, but as an interesting sensation that took all of her attention to stay on top of. Cara told her that when a rush came, she should breathe deep and puff out her stomach as far as she could and to put her attention into smooching with me, or pulling my arms, so that she could keep her bottom loose. Cara also told her not to close her eyes, but keep connecting with the eyes of the rest of us. Cara showed me where and how to rub Roberta to help her out.

Cara: I took a few naps and left Joel and Roberta with Marilyn — she's a close friend and helped a lot. At one point I had some strong thoughts go through my mind that this baby was not going to be an easy one, but I dismissed them because I didn't want to give thought to anything paranoid. His heartbeat was always fine. I decided to get some sleep, though — I wanted to be really fresh and smart when the baby came.

Marilyn: As Roberta's rushes got stronger, I could hear her complaining some and could tell she wasn't handling them too well. Then Cara said I could go and be with her. I was really glad, because we were good friends, and I had had LeRoy six months before. So I went to her room. She was glad to see me. I said, "Well, Roberta, now what do you think about scrubbing all those floors to make your rushes come on?" We laughed. She wanted to know if it had been hard for me. I told her that I had to work at handling the rushes too. She said she thought she was a paddy-ass and couldn't do it. I laughed and told her I'd seen her do hard work in the fields and knew she could do this. We kept connected together. It was so nice. Every time Roberta felt like she was having a hard time, she'd ask me about when I had LeRoy. It was fun sharing the energy with her.

Roberta: As the rushes got more intense, I felt more panic. At first I thought I couldn't go on, maybe I'd even stop. But I knew that thought was ridiculous. What kept me sane was having my family around me. Marilyn had had her baby six months before and I felt like she really understood what I was going through.

Mary: Cara called me to come over to Joel and Roberta's around five o'clock in the morning. Roberta's rushes were obviously very strong, and I could tell she felt a strong bearing down impulse. Cara had been working with Roberta for several hours to help her do her rushes, and she was doing fine when I got there.

Cara: I popped Roberta's water bag at four and a half centimeters. The water came out brown—the baby had discharged his bowels into the amniotic fluid, which is often a sign of fetal distress. Roberta was working hard now—we told her that her sense of humor was a priceless jewel and she knew what we meant. We all knew this was the heaviest thing she had ever done. I took a nap and Mary stayed with Roberta.

Mary: Joel felt real strong and like he wanted to do anything he could to help Roberta out. She hung on to him very tight during rushes and they felt strong together. I sat in a chair and caught eyes with Roberta during the rushes and kept reminding her to relax her bottom. She had a definite tendency to want to push, although she wasn't near fully dilated. One time Roberta got impatient and thought it was going too slow and another time she said it hurt. We told her we knew how it felt, but we could tell when she relaxed during the rushes, that they really opened her up. She listened to us and followed our advice.

Roberta: As morning came on, the rushes got more intense; they came one right after another. I decided to get to work. By then I had learned how to do it and I felt more in control of the rushes.

Mary: When I was sitting in the chair, I saw her push real hard and her face got red. It looked like a real one, so I quickly checked her dilation with a sterile glove. She was almost fully dilated except for a little bit of cervix preceding the baby's head. I told Ruth to wake Cara up right away, and I pushed the cervix back over the baby's head easily. Cara came in and asked me if I wanted to deliver the baby and I said, "Sure."

Cara: When I woke up, Roberta was almost ready to push. Earlier in her labor she had said things like, "This hurts!" and, "I just can't keep doing this." But now we said, "Roberta, you're going to have a baby real soon!" and she held up her hand saying, "That's all right," looking just like Uncle Bill, the eighty-three-year-old man Roberta takes care of. She looked really brave and warm and womanly.

Roberta: Within an hour, my cervix opened up the whole way and the baby was ready to come out. I felt like when I began pushing, I never worked so hard in my life. But it was fun. I knew it was getting my baby out. It felt like everyone in the room and in our house was pushing with me. I remember looking at Cara and she looked so soft and pretty to me. I was really glad to have some folks around me to help me through this one.

Joel: When I would look at Roberta, she looked very beautiful—her cheeks were rosy and her lips were red. Her hair kept making interesting designs against her pillow and always looked neat and pretty.

We could see about three inches of the head. It was wet and wrinkly, and Mary started working to get it out. Marilyn kept squeezing baby oil on Mary's fingers and onto the baby's head. Cara and Mary were coaching Roberta on how to push with each rush. Roberta was working hard and pushing with all her effort, and enjoying it. I found myself pushing along with her. With every push, we could see the head making progress getting out. Mary kept stretching Roberta's puss and moving the baby's head and telling us how everything was going. She said that Roberta's puss was stretching very well and that she didn't think she would tear. I had thought during Roberta's pregnancy that the baby would be a girl, but when the head started coming out, I felt that it was a boy. While Mary was working on getting the head out, I felt heavy waves of energy around my jaws and throat and in my chest, and had to put my total attention into what was happening in order to keep myself together. My eyes were tearing.

Roberta: Suddenly Cara said, "When the head comes out, begin panting." On the next push, the head popped out. I was amazed to see this big head between my legs. It was really beautiful. Cara and Mary checked the cord. The next pushes brought the rest of the body out.

Mary: Roberta looked absolutely beautiful while she was pushing. When the head came out, the cord was loosely around the neck. I didn't cut it because it felt plenty loose enough to slip over his shoulders as he came out. It took four or five pushes to deliver his body, because at first both shoulders were coming out together. I pulled gently on his head in such a way as to coax the upper shoulder to come out first. The baby came out and felt very floppy. His heart was pumping steady and strong but he had by far the most meconium* on him of any baby I've ever seen, and it seemed like he'd swallowed a bunch of it and maybe some water. I picked him up by his feet and stroked his back briskly as Cara was suctioning his mouth and nose. I patted his butt several times, but he hadn't yet responded to anything we'd done. I knew he was in there—he even opened his eyes and looked at us—but his lungs were really full of junk and he wasn't breathing or crying at all.

Joel: The moment the head popped out, it felt like I was zapped with a hundred volts of electricity. I was astonished. The head was purplish-blue and covered with black, sticky meconium. Mary and Cara started working as one thing. Cara started suctioning the baby's mouth and nostrils, while Mary worked to get the rest of the baby out. The head looked larger than I thought it would be when it was coming out. Seeing the head coming out of Roberta, I thought it looked almost as big as her belly, and almost comical, and I wondered how she could have a whole baby in her when the head was so big.

Cara: I took him because I had seen some really hard starters and it felt like this one was going to take all we had. I slapped him on the butt

---

*The brownish-black protective substance in the baby's bowels before birth, sometimes discharged when the baby is under stress during birth.

a couple of times. It sent the meconium flying all over the room, all over everyone. I gave him some mouth-to-mouth and was compressing his heart. It was really intense.

Joel: *It felt like one of those timeless life and death moments where everything is suspended.* I felt helpless, but I knew Mary and Cara were taking care of business, and I felt strongly that they were going to start him.

Marilyn: Mary and Cara said, "We're going to have to help him out." It was amazing tantric touch—as we were giving him mouth-to-mouth and oxygen, it was as if they were one mind completely given to getting him to breathe. Their arms and mouths were so intertwined and moving so fast as they were giving their combined all to the baby, you couldn't tell whose were whose.

Cara: As I squeezed his heart, there was a time where he was grunting very shallow, and I saw this pink aura of light come out from his heart and fill his upper body with energy. At the same time it filled up my heart and all these waves of ecstasy were going from my heart to my head. Then he cried. We knew it was okay then. I looked at Joel—he looked very calm but there were tears in his eyes and I knew how it had been for him. I felt the same way.

Joel: When he finally cried, it was like the top of the pressure cooker blowing off, and we all felt waves of energy. He started breathing, and life came into his body, and his color started changing. He looked a lot fuller and felt strong.

Marilyn: I could feel, so strong, one God-mind reaching out to this baby—breathing for him, praying for him, then, finally breathing with him as he started. We were all crying and laughing, so fulfilled in our hearts that he was doing it, so grateful for this new child.

Roberta: I just watched in amazement. It all happened so fast.
They worked hard and fast together, and they felt like they had it under control. When he started to cry and we knew it was okay, I yelled, "Hey, Louey!" over to him. He looked like he needed a name and he looked like a Louey.

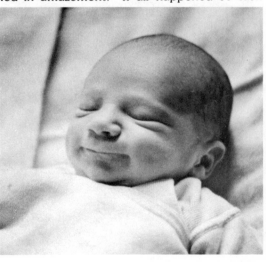

Joel: I had just been wondering if we were going to name him Louey like we had decided, when Roberta yelled his name.

Roberta: Cara wrapped him up and took him downstairs to clean him. His purple coloring turned to pink, but he still had somewhat of a hard time breathing.

Cara: I carried him downstairs to fix him up. My heart was still feeling so much energy it was amazing me. Louey was the most Jewish-looking little baby I ever saw. He looked really wise. He was having some trouble breathing which was causing his chest to retract, so we called Ina May. She came out and we watched him and took his temperature. I held his hand and he was right there, really telepathic. His temperature was 95.4°, so Ina May called our doctor and he told us to bring Louey in to the hospital. Mary wrapped him in a warm quilt and by the time he got to the hospital his temperature was 97.8°. The doctor kept him in overnight and then sent him home.

Mary: It felt like he needed all the mouth-to-mouth breathing, oxygen, and heart massage we gave him to bring him into his body and kick him over. Joel and Roberta were really strong for us and I was so grateful Cara was there to show me how to do it, from having seen Stephen get a slow one going. I also loved Louey because his soul was with us all the time and he was just such a smart, sweet, strong baby.

Cara: I felt a different way since that birthing, and feel so grateful to have Louey here with us and see Roberta so glad to be a mother. I know God helped out with his birth. Louey's one of those babies I''l always be in love with.

Roberta: It's been a month since we've had Louey and I've never been happier. It still overwhelms me that I have a kid.

Louey and Roberta

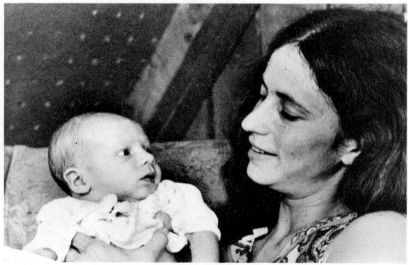

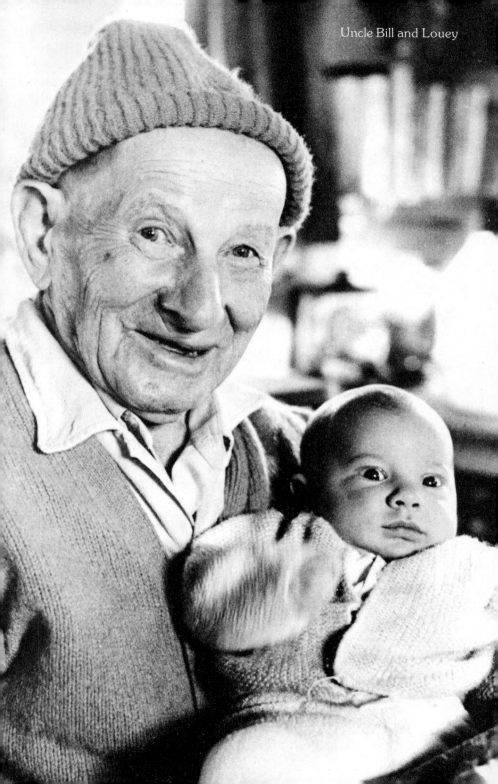
Uncle Bill and Louey

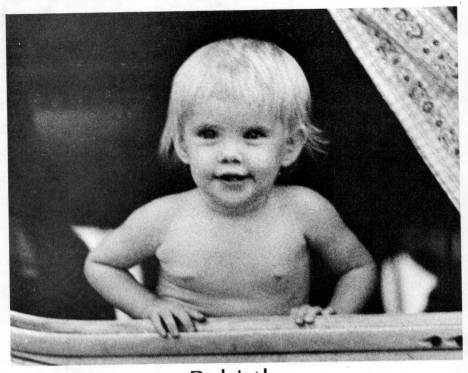

Rebirth

uzanne: I thought maybe we'd spoiled Laura just a little. But after the first few days of a concert and speaking tour with Stephen, the Farm Band, and their families, I started realizing how spoiled she really was.

For her first year, I'd tried to be one step ahead of her all the time, giving her stuff soon, so she wouldn't cry. I had also worried a lot about her, not wanted the other kids to hurt her in their play. Consequently, when we got on the Scenicruiser with other kids, she cried every time anyone said "Hi" to her, looked at her, sat next to her, or another kid walked past her. She spent most of her time in her crib, quietly watching the other kids, hoping they'd be so kind as to leave her alone.

We camped in Texas for close to a week. Laura had me up a tree. She was crying all of her waking moments—I just didn't know what to do. So Ina May began telling me stuff about her. I gave up trying to help the other folks—gave up cooking, cleaning up, and even being with the others. I had to work it out with her first. Ina May told me I got mad at Laura. It was about the heaviest thing anyone had ever told me. Here it had taken us four and a half years to get pregnant and have a baby and now I get mad at her. I felt awful.

Once when Laura was screaming, Ina May told me maybe I'd better take her off to where we could be alone and get it together. So I tucked her under my arm and went to the edge of a gully, the most remote area of the park I could find.

I sat down and wondered what to do next. Laura was crying and carrying on as usual. I yelled at her to be quiet. She kept crying. "Oh, I know what being mad feels like and this feels like I'm mad at her! Well, too bad, the little stinker." My body felt like my insides were pulling and tearing apart. The sun was hot, we were both pouring with sweat. I yelled at her some more; I held her up in the air. She looked terrible, kind of skinny and not much good life force. I put her on the ground. I felt very self-conscious, and hoped none of the other campers would notice me sitting miserably with my daughter.

My body was still aching and she was still crying. I felt like one of those people who have a demon in them—an evil spirit. I realized what I really needed to do was to change my ways, but I didn't know if I could or even wanted to change. I started praying and crying and wishing I could start all over again with her. The more I prayed, the stronger I felt. I had personally seen Stephen help many people change. I could change too. I *had* to. I started feeling like the demon was gone.

I looked at Laura and picked her up and held her. She was finally quiet. I promised her I would never get mad at her again.

As I walked back to camp I realized many things I'd done wrong and thought of things I could change in me that would help—like not worrying when she fell down. And not feeling like I was the only one who could really take good care of her. I realized that she wasn't special but that she just deserved the best I could give her all the time.

Soon after that she started playing with the other kids. My husband quit worrying about her too. Stephen told him that that was how you raise a hypochondriac. It's true.

Jody's Birth

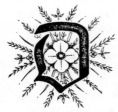

eborah: The first time I was pregnant I miscarried. It was right before we moved to the Farm. I was three and a half months pregnant and I'd been spotting for a few days, which really surprised me—I never thought anything could go wrong.

I knew that sometimes a miscarriage is Nature's way of rejecting a baby that wasn't forming right or something and I should have faith in the Universe that the best thing would happen. Nevertheless, I didn't want to miscarry so I was taking it easy and putting my feet up.

Now that I've had a baby I know that miscarriage was just like having a baby in some ways. I had rushes five minutes apart, for hours, that got stronger and harder to integrate. But the big difference between this and a birthing was I didn't want it to happen and I was fighting it.

When I would try to relax and remember that I should have faith that the best thing was happening, it was much easier to integrate. I kept thinking, "If I can't handle this, how could I have a baby born naturally?"

After several hours of this and the rushes were still getting closer and stronger, we called the doctor. He thought I should come to the hospital for a D & C. That decision was like admitting defeat and I gave up trying. I started complaining and just fell apart. The ride to the hospital was terrible. I learned a lot though. I knew deep down that it didn't have to be that way.

Our first baby was born a year later.

When Cara came she said it looked like I would be an easy baby-haver and she was expecting a good birthing. That really made me feel good and I agreed with her.

My rushes were five minutes apart and I was two and a half centimeters dilated when Cara came. She called two other ladies to come. When they got there they gave me an enema. I was sure glad of it, too.

Cara left. Denise and Carol let Douglas and me be alone and tell each other how much we love each other and get some energy happening. From time to time Carol or Denise would come and check to see how dilated I was. I got to four or four and half centimeters and then didn't seem to change much. I didn't realize it then, but I think I was just waiting for Cara to come back. I was surprised at how fast time was passing. I kept thinking, "I bet I have a baby before dark!" It was a very pretty sunny day and not too hot. It was also very peaceful. For that matter, the whole thing was so relaxed that I could hardly believe it was real. I half expected everyone to get up and leave, saying, "Dress rehearsal is over."

When Cara came she told me to breathe very slowly during rushes, hold it, and exhale slowly. The next rush I went from four to seven centimeters!

Soon I started getting the urge to push. ᾿I was propped up in an almost sitting position with Douglas at my side. When Cara told me to push I was to raise my head up, take a deep breath, pull on the back of my legs and *push*. As soon as pushing really got going, everything else vanished. My back had been hurting a little and my legs were cramped, but that went away.

Pushing was like swimming under water—when you want to come up for air you can usually stay just a little longer. So when I'd feel like giving up during a push, I'd say to myself, "Push a little harder, this may be the one!"

After a while I could see the head. It looked tiny. Once I was crowning, Cara wanted to take it slow so I wouldn't tear. When the head was almost out Cara told me to pant so that I wouldn't push (and she could check to be sure the cord wasn't around the baby's neck). I thought she was crazy, but it worked. Then another push and out came the head. It sure did look big—bigger than the little thing we'd been seeing. I was watching in amazement. Another push (was I still pushing? It seemed so easy now!) and out came a shoulder, then the next shoulder and—wush—a baby!

He had started crying halfway out. Cara said, "It's a boy!" before I'd had time to notice. He peed before the cord was cut!

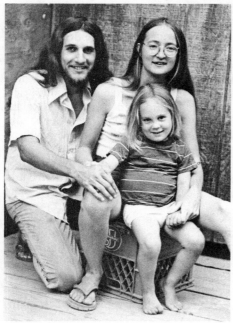

Douglas and I kept looking back and forth from each other to Jody. I felt like I could do anything—I felt so grateful and happy. Carol gave Jody to me after cleaning him up. What a nice baby! He weighed seven pounds, eleven ounces. Cara told me I was a nice lady and thanked me for a good birthing. I thanked the ladies and they gave me a hug and left the three of us together.

He cried a lot at first and wasn't interested in nursing. About eight hours later he stopped crying, and had his eyes open. He looked at me real hard and then started nursing.

Our Second Baby

eborah: I was trying not to be impatient since my due date was past and I seemed so ready. Douglas and I were spending as much time as possible paying attention to each other. Sunday night we went for a walk and the moon looked pretty full so I said to it, "Shine on me, maybe this full moon will bring the baby out." We made love before we went to sleep—that's what put her in there and I think that's what got her out!

At 2:30 I woke up to pee and was so sleepy that all I wanted to do was go back to sleep. Then I had to shit and every time I tried to go back to bed I had to shit again—that's how I started with Jody so I thought hmmm.... I lit a lamp and saw some bloody show. I woke up Douglas and told him to go call Cara.

I was having cramps in my legs that made it hard to squat over the pot. I didn't think they were rushes at first, but they started coming and going so I figured that they must be. I didn't like the cramps; they made it hard to get comfortable. I thought to myself, "No, I don't want it to be like this."

Around 3:00, Cara sent Leslie over to check me out. I wanted an enema so I could stop shitting and get comfortable. Leslie checked me and I was six centimeters dilated so she called Cara. Cara said no enema and she was on her way.

Douglas and I started smooching. My water bag broke during a kiss. I heard it and felt it and told Leslie. Everything was moving right along. I still wasn't having what you'd call strong rushes. I was comfortable now, stopped shitting, legs barely cramping. My whole body was shaking. Douglas had a very tight grip on my hand and it felt like an electrical hookup. I had a rush and said to myself, "Relax, relax, relax." Douglas started shaking all over like I had been, and stopped when my rush stopped! I realized then that feeling everything intensely was good because it put me in control.

Cara came with Cynthia and checked me. I was almost fully dilated and they started setting everything up. I told Cara I thought I could push. She told me to wait because they weren't ready. That was okay with me.

When everybody was ready I tried pushing. I didn't feel like I was rushing any more, but I was in complete control so when I wanted to I'd say in my head "push" and be surprised to find it happening and feeling just as I remembered. Cara said later it looked like "effortless great pure effort." I thought it felt great. I took it slow so I wouldn't tear when her head came out. I looked down and liked being able to see her. On the next push not much seemed to happen and I thought,

"This is going to be a big baby and I'm going to have to push harder to get her out. Can I do it? I have to!"

Out she came on the next push or two, crying a little. Cara told her she was gorgeous. She was lying between my legs getting fixed up and punching me in the puss with her fist! When I could hold her we looked at her and loved her.

Born Monday at 4:19 a.m. weighing nine pounds, four ounces. I didn't have to have stitches.

Nathan

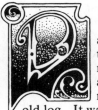aniel: When Nathan was about five days old, a far-out thing happened. I was lying on the bed with him on my stomach. As he started to doze off I could feel his aura opening up, and he kept opening up to where he merged right into me. He was just like a lump on the old log. It was so stoned I just laid there real still for about twenty minutes being one thing with him.

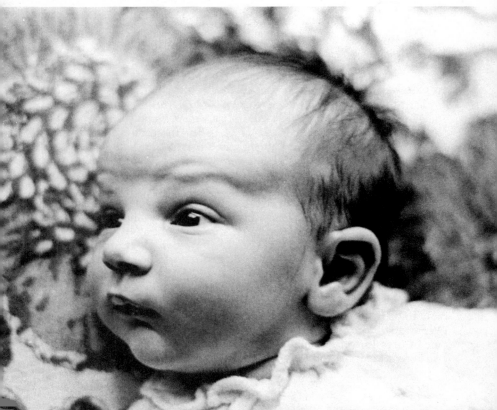

Some Breech Births

The following stories are accounts of breech births, that is, when the baby's bottom or feet come out first rather than the head. Four of these babies were their mother's first child. These stories show how our policy of having breech births evolved from having them all born in the hospital with the midwife but not the husband in attendance (because of hospital rules) to our current way of attending them at home, without anesthesia or routine episiotomy. My training in how to deliver the breech was one that few medical students or residents in the United States have access to, now that virtually all breech babies in our country are delivered by cesarean section. Our record of safety in this department speaks for itself.

—Ina May

Samuel

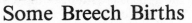

oslyn: Bruce and I made love one morning six weeks before my due date. When we finished, an amazing amount of liquid dripped out of me and it slowly dawned on us that my water bag had broken. The midwives told me to be still because the bag might reseal and fill up again. I was sure it would. [*After the water bag broke, the midwives checked Roslyn's temperature and the baby's heart tones several times each day so we would know if she was developing an intrauterine infection.—I.M.*] But three days later I began to rush, and that evening Pamela came over to check me. She told me I was going to do it. It felt very mellow. When Pamela came over to check me again she could feel that it wasn't the usual presentation. She wasn't sure what it was that was presenting itself first, but it didn't seem to be the head. Barbara didn't know what it was, either. They both rechecked. Then Ina May came. She checked and rechecked and nobody seemed to be sure if the bony little bump they felt was the face, the shoulder, the butt, or what. It turned out to be Samuel's bony little butt. It made me uncomfortable every time one of the ladies felt around, and I had to try not to get uptight. It felt like the midwives brought so much love and humor with them that I wanted to make it as easy for them as I could. Pamela called Dr. Williams and he said to bring me to the hospital when I was dilated to four centimeters. We tripped through the night. As the rushes got stronger Bruce helped me by pressing on the small of my back real hard. We were a team and we kept it together and then it was time to go to the hospital. Walking

112

down the stairs, talking with my family who were waiting in the living room and walking out into the cold stormy night really got my energy up. All the way to the hospital, Pamela had me panting with each rush because she didn't want me to have the baby too soon. A rush would come on. Bruce and I would look into each other's eyes and pant light, fast pants until the rush subsided. It took all of our attention and I don't know if I could have done it without having Bruce to check into. We were having a ball. When we got to the hospital, Bruce couldn't come in with me. I could feel him so strong that it didn't matter that there were about three walls between us. I always knew he was there.

Dr. Williams told us that I would have to have a major episiotomy and be anesthesized for the actual delivery. He said that this being my first baby, there was no way we could convince him to do it naturally because I wouldn't stay relaxed enough for him to do what he had to do unless I was doped up.

But it was happening now. I held Pamela's hand on one side and Barbara's on the other. I was moved from the labor room to the delivery room. Dr. Williams asked the nurse, "Where's the anesthetist?" And then we were delivering the baby. The anesthetist never showed up. I had no anesthesia and no episiotomy. Dr. Williams went inside of me and wiggled out one leg, then the other. I felt his hand go way up inside my belly. It amazed me. He tugged the baby out and plopped him on my belly. He wasn't like a baby. He was like a little squirmy greasy piglet. I loved him.

Six days later Bruce and I got to bring Sam home from the hospital. We went into our warm room and took off all our clothes. We lay on our bed together and enjoyed what it felt like to be a family.

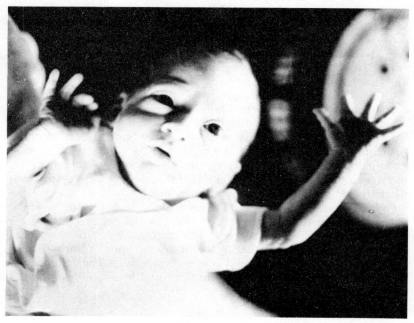

Erinna—A Surprise Breech

Mona: Our birthing began on a Tuesday night when my water bag broke. My husband stayed home with me all Wednesday and by Wednesday night I was feeling some uptight wondering how come I hadn't had the baby yet. I had already had a daughter seven years before. It had been in the hospital and although I felt all right when I went into labor, the hospital scene hadn't been very good; they wouldn't let me sit up, get up, walk, or do anything but lay there until finally I got put to sleep.

By Wednesday night, Eugene and I were quarreling and he went to call a midwife to come over. Two ladies from the midwife crew (Mary and Catherine) came over and started to sort out my and Eugene's relationship pretty intensely. The outcome was that we practically felt like we had to start over again. They said that I didn't give Eugene much real energy, that I needed to really give him some, for instance, by rubbing him out good and strong. They also said that I came on low key and whiney to him which made him come on macho and cold. On top of all that, I had been afraid of the birthing during my whole pregnancy, not just because of my previous birthing in the hospital, but also because my mother hadn't talked about birthings much and the little she did had left me with negative and afraid feelings. These feelings were also increased much by movies I had seen and things I had read which portrayed painful natural births. When Mary and Catherine left, I wasn't sure whether I wanted to do it on the Farm or in a hospital. Mary called Pamela and told her I was chicken. They decided to check back with us in the morning and then left.

Eugene went to sleep and I spent the rest of the night sorting out things in my head that had been bothering me. I was scared and felt stiff as a board. I was so nervous I couldn't sleep. Towards Thursday morning, I felt more relaxed and slept a little. As soon as Eugene woke up, we started talking and I told him I realized there were a lot of ways I hadn't been nice. Eugene liked that and we felt real happy together.

About nine o'clock, Pamela came over to see how we were doing. I was still scared, but told Pamela I wanted to do it here. Pamela said that birthing was like water skiing, that the energy pulled you along, and you had to learn how to get on top of it. She was very compassionate, and said she could help me do that.

Pamela left and Eugene and I were alone together for a while. Eugene went up to get lunch about 12:30, and I began crocheting a baby blanket. While he was gone, I began having very mild contractions which I figured were hardly worth my attention. When Eugene came back, I wasn't hungry, and kept on crocheting. The contractions felt stronger, but were still short and three and four minutes apart. I told Eugene once in a while when I'd have one, but I didn't want him to call anyone, because I thought I had about twelve hours to go.

Around 3:30, I was still crocheting, but the time had gone by fast. Every time I had a contraction, I'd pay real good attention to not drop a stitch, but it was getting stronger, and I felt tired. I told Eugene I was going to try to sleep and he laid down with me. I had read a lot of the birthing tales written by other Farm folks and had picked up what I thought to be a lot of good suggestions. One lady I'd heard about had gone to sleep about half way along and woke up fully dilated. So that was my idea too. As soon as we lay down, we started making out, and the rushes starting coming on really strong, but still short. I had been feeling psychedelic for a while and now with every rush I got high. Eugene would squeeze me really hard whenever I felt pressure. Every time he would squeeze me, it would feel so good that I would just concentrate on how good it felt and forget about everything else. With every rush, I thought that that one wasn't bad, and that I still had a while to go, so I felt like I could still handle it, because it was going to get heavier. Mostly I just felt really grateful for every rush and was glad that they were getting stronger.

All of a sudden it was 4:15 and Pamela was there. She had just stopped by to see how we were doing. We said we were glad she'd come by because we thought I might be in labor. Pamela didn't have any instruments with her, and called around for her things and some help. Then she started setting up.

Pamela: I decided to go over to see how Mona and Eugene were getting along because I knew she was going to have her baby soon and I wanted them to feel good with each other. When I got there, Mona was having pretty heavy rushes. I sent for my kit and for a couple of other midwives to help.

Pamela came up to my loft to check me and she said I was about five centimeters dilated. That was about where I felt I was at too. Marilyn and Kathryn arrived to help. Eugene and I were still making out and taking turns squeezing each other.

Pamela asked how I was doing. I told her fine, but that I thought I was kind of changing techniques a lot; sitting up, lying down, squeezing. She told me that when she was having her last baby, Stephen had told her to just sit through on a few rushes, so I laid there and just let a couple come on. That was fine too, and I felt more relaxed. For a while now, I'd felt like I wanted to get up and go to the pot. I told Pamela and she said to go ahead. I went and squatted on the bucket. I really felt

Pamela: Mona was sitting up for her rushes and said that she felt like she had to take a crap. She sat on the pot and I knew as soon as I saw how she was pushing that that was the baby she was working on.

like I had to go, and as soon as I squatted down, I felt myself go 8-9-10. I knew I was as wide open as I could go, but I still felt like staying there and pushing. Pamela asked me if I was crapping or pushing a baby out. I said I didn't know, but I thought I was just crapping and told

115

her I really liked being there. She told me to come lay down or I'd have the baby in the bucket. Eugene held a flashlight for Pamela. She looked and said, "There's the head." Eugene looked and was amazed. Then the head moved slightly and a brown dot appeared and started crapping. "It's a butt," Pamela said. Then she said, "It's a girl." I was really happy. She and Kathryn, who was hanging on the ladder to the loft, looked at each other. They discussed whether or not they should get the ambulance and get me up the hill and to the hospital. Kathryn said she didn't think there would be time and I agreed. I was feeling like pushing, and not traveling. Pamela told me that there had never been a breech delivery on the Farm before, which I knew, but that she had just finished reading about it and would give it a try. I felt like Pamela could really do it, and told her okay.

Pamela began cutting me, saying she didn't have time for Xylocaine. I told her I'd hold a few pushes back, if she could give me some as it hurt a bit, and she had more to cut. She said okay, and I held a few for the shots, then pushed while she cut. In a few pushes, the butt, legs, and arms were out.

Pamela: I gave Mona a large episiotomy because I wanted to make sure I could get the head out fast after the baby's body was delivered. I had just read about delivering breech babies about a week before in Benson's *Handbook of Obstetrics and Gynecology*, which I was really grateful for. I did just what the book said and the baby came out just like it said. It started crying right away. A very pretty pink little girl, five pounds, one ounce.

Then Pamela reached up inside and put her fingers in the baby's mouth and made an air passage. Then she pulled out the head. Pamela had only been there forty-five minutes. It was five o'clock.

Just then Margaret and Thomas came running in. Kathryn came down and Margaret came up to help Pamela stitch me up. The baby weighed only five pounds, one ounce, but felt strong. Shortly after that, everyone left Eugene and me with our new daughter. Eugene was astonished and we were both very happy and grateful to have had such a wonderful and spiritual trip together. I was glad I'd done it on the Farm and said if I would do anything over, it would be to not be afraid for nine months. I felt like, if God had made birth to be such a Holy passage, He meant for all our major passages including death, to be Holy, and that there wasn't anything to fear. I was grateful too, for my mother's sake, so that she would have that karma worked out for her and especially for my girls, who wouldn't have to carry a lot of sub-conscious around and be afraid of birthings like I had been. I felt like I'd made love with God and was grateful and humble from the experience. And I especially felt like Eugene did at least half of the actual labor. He was patient and tantric with every change I'd gone through and every rush I'd had, and the whole experience felt equally his.

116

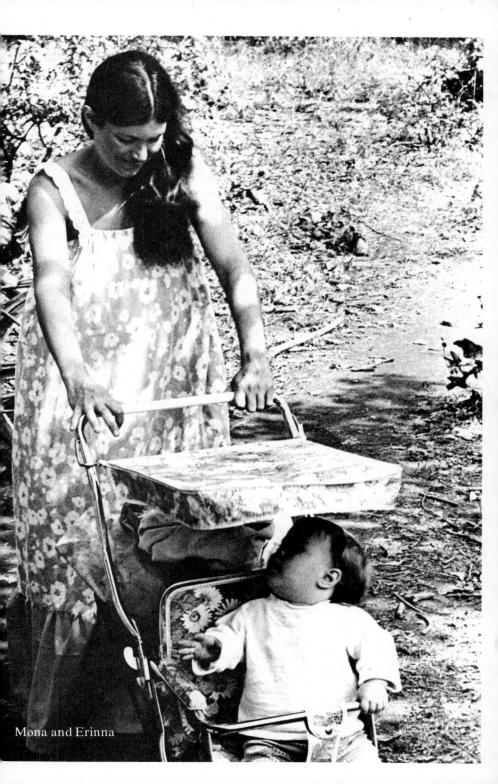
Mona and Erinna

Even though Roslyn had done fine without general anesthesia, Dr. Williams still believed it was the only way to deliver a breech.

A Hospital Breech

amela: We knew Nancy was going to have a breech birth well before her delivery.   We had Dr. Williams check her and we made an agreement with him to deliver the baby at our local hospital. The doctor who had been helping us with our breech babies had quit practicing obstetrics by this time, so we made our agreement with our family doctor.

Nancy started her labor and when she was about four centimeters dilated, we took her into the hospital. Dr. Williams checked her and said he would be back when she was about eight centimeters dilated. It's the kind of hospital where the lady in labor can come out to the waiting room and be with her husband until her labor is pretty heavy, so Nancy was able to be with her husband a lot. Every few hours Kay Marie and I would go back to the labor room with Nancy and check her dilation. When she got close to fully dilated, Dr. Williams came and said it wouldn't be long. He also said he would have to put her to sleep. I didn't like this idea at all but when I asked him about it he said that with first breech babies that's how they had to do it, because they were usually hard to get out.

At that point there didn't seem to be much I could argue with. I still thought Nancy could push the baby out and I didn't like the idea of putting her to sleep, but it was on Dr. Williams' ground at his hospital.

I talked with Nancy and told her I would be able to stay with her the whole time and tell her all that happened.

It was amazing what happened. When Nancy was fully dilated, we took her into the delivery room. She was having excellent pushing contractions and was very cooperative. With every push you could see a little more of the baby's butt. Nancy was having a good time, smiling and looking real pretty. Then Dr. Williams said it was time to give her some gas. The anesthesiologist did this. At that point everything changed. Nancy stopped smiling and her color wasn't so good. The colors in the delivery room, which were previously very pretty and bright, turned kind of a metallic grey. With every rush Nancy would lift up her butt and do the opposite of push. It was like she was asleep and her rushes still happened but she didn't do anything about them. Dr. Williams worked very efficiently and in about three minutes he had given her a large episiotomy and had pulled the baby out. Another ten minutes and he had sewed Nancy back up.

Kay Marie and I stayed with Nancy and helped wheel her bed back into a room where she started to come to. As she did, the auras around her began to get some color in them again. When she asked how her baby was, we knew she was back with us, and we told her she had a lovely baby. She was happy but very tired.

It was interesting to see that putting a lady to sleep does not help the lady at all and is hard on the baby too. This baby was basically healthy; however, for an hour after it was born it was having retractions. That's when a baby kind of grunts when it breathes and has a hard time breathing. It is common for this to happen if the mother has been doped up for her delivery. The baby gets some of that dope too, through the placenta.

I'm sure Dr. Williams saw all this. After this birthing we talked with him and he told us that he would rather come out to the Farm and help us with our breech deliveries with a local anesthetic instead of gas.

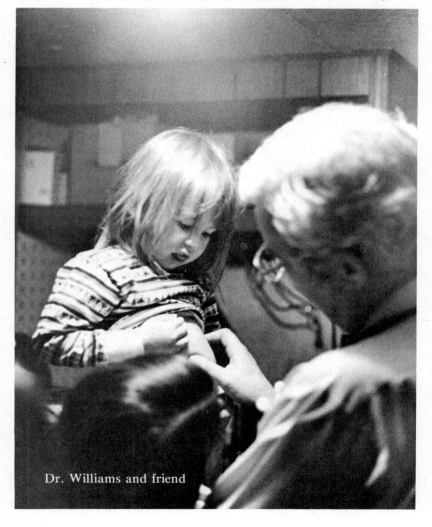

Dr. Williams and friend

Rear Entry

inda: Michael and I decided to come to the Farm to have the baby because we liked the way the midwives delivered the babies at home. We had been planning to go to the hospital, but when some friends sent us a card at Christmas time and told us to come to Tennessee to do it, we came right down. My due date was April 6, and we got to the Farm in the last week in February. I was just about seven and a half months pregnant.

The first time I went to pregnant ladies' clinic, the midwives could tell the baby wasn't in the usual position, and the second time, Ina May confirmed it. She could feel the head way up high between my ribs. I got a little teary-eyed when she told me. The first thing I thought of was that Michael couldn't be with me in the delivery room because the local hospital didn't let men in.

It was very important for us to be unattached to being at home and to realize that all birthings are fun and that the baby was the neatest part. We were really grateful to be here, too, because a midwife would get to go into the hospital with me and help me out.

Michael and I were also trying to decide whether to live here or not after the baby was born, and that made me uptight right around then. I got emotional and teary again, and later Ina May and Margaret came over and said they wanted to know where I was at, because both times Ina May had seen me I had been upset and crying. Ina May said that the Farm ladies had a really good reputation with the local hospital because of how they had their babies, and if I started blubbering at everything, how was I going to have a baby without anesthesia? I realized right then that I had to stop being self-indulgent and straighten up. I promised them right there that I was going to do it right and they trusted me. I really believe that any lady has the option to chicken out or not. I felt like I had made a vow to have a good time at my birthing, and I knew a month ahead of time I was going to have fun. That left the rest of my pregnancy to look forward to it. We were even getting a little excited about the adventure of going to the hospital and I was embroidering a birthing shirt for Michael to wear.

At the beginning of April I saw Ina May again and she said she was going to try to arrange to have a doctor come to the Farm to deliver the baby.

A few days later I met Dr. Williams and he checked me out. He didn't believe a lady could deliver a breech baby without being knocked out. A lot of the midwives were there in the clinic and everyone told him we wanted to do it here, and he said, "Well, Ina May and I have different ideas where you should have this baby and right now she's winning." Dr. Williams didn't think a lady could relax enough without anesthesia to let a breech baby out as quickly as would be necessary. [*I thought a lady with a good attitude would be able to relax better if she was not on anesthesia. Roslyn had been able to.—Ina May*] I just stayed quiet and tried to be unattached but actually I wanted to get him to come here because as I got nearer to my due date I felt strongly that I'd need Michael with me when I had the baby. Now there was a possibility he could be there.

Michael and I waited to see what would happen. Ina May made sure that I understood that I had to impress Dr. Williams when I had my baby because if we convinced him that we could deliver breech babies naturally on the Farm, other ladies could do it later on. Finally he agreed to do it here, but insisted on having the ambulance parked right outside. If there were any complications, he would whisk me off to the hospital. That sounded very safe and sane. It felt like he was going to take good care of us. The baby waited until we got adjusted to this new plan.

On April 24th, two and a half weeks after my original due date, I woke out of a strange half-sleep, having to pee. "Michael, the mucus plug!" I yelled, and he jumped out of bed. It was 5:30 in the morning and we knew it was happening. I went to the outhouse and when I got back I was having steady rushes four minutes apart. We called the phone lady, and Carol—one of the midwives' helpers—came over, and at 6:00 I was five centimeters dilated.

As I got into labor I was awed at what was happening. My body was going through incredible changes and I watched and felt and got very high. At first I moved around a lot. I walked around, but very gently. I felt like walking on my tiptoes and whispering. My memories are all sensual. There was a skylight and the windows were wide open. It was warm and sunny. I remember the swirly lights and shadows and colors of the room. It was very psychedelic.

I kept dilating more and more and I grew to trust the midwives completely. They kept checking me and decided to call the doctor. When he arrived, it really amazed me that although he had never been to a Farm birthing before he was very telepathic with us. He sat in a chair and smoked his pipe and watched us do it. He respected the midwives and they respected him, too.

At one point I got to a place where I was getting on my hands and knees and shifting position to sitting cross-legged or lying down and then standing up, and I told Carol that I couldn't seem to get comfortable anymore. She said that I probably wouldn't be able to get very comfortable from then on until the baby was born. I began to get anxious to meet the baby.

I was lying on my back on the bed by this time, and Michael was sitting by my head holding my hands. It seemed like hours that we looked into each other's eyes, and we felt like one thing as we rode through the rushes. He gave me so much and was steady and sure the whole time. He was an infinite well of energy to me.

121

Carol was down by my feet, and at just the right time she told me to blow out my belly very full on my in-breaths. That really relaxes and opens you up more and also gives you something to put your attention into. It took about three rushes to get the knack of it. You don't need to practice ahead of time, because you can learn it on the spot.

My time sense was gone that day, so I have no idea how long that went on, but then Dr. Williams stepped up to the bed. He was crisp and clean-looking and smelled real nice. He checked me out and said I could start pushing on the next rush. I was amazed we were so close. Slow starting—tried to understand where these pushes came from. Then hands clasped under knees, and heavy pushing began—pushing and grunting loud.

Then the doctor started his fancy dance. He cut me as I pushed, all the while encouraging me and flattering me on my pushes. I kept on doing it, really chugging along, and pretty soon it seemed like he was up to his elbows in me getting the baby born. He was really working hard, and I was really impressed. He knew exactly what he was doing. Everyone watched and seemed to hold their breaths. The baby's balls presented first, and then the legs and body were born, and I heard a gurgle. He was breathing before his head was out. Dr. Williams stuck his hand in and cleared an airway and delivered the head. There was sort of a pop as his head came out, and he was upside down and blue and yelling.

Michael and I laughed and cried and hugged, and I was shaking all over. It was 2:45 p.m., a nine-hour labor.

Michael and I looked at the baby. We all hung out and took a nap and loved each other a bunch. It was the most beautiful, perfect day of our lives. Cody was with us, and we were so grateful to be all together on the Farm.

A few days later, Mary Louise came over, and I told her how incredibly happy I was, and she said that's because having a baby is your ultimate fulfillment, and that's absolutely true.

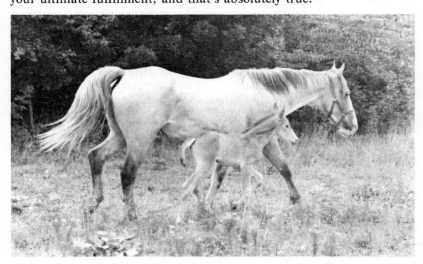

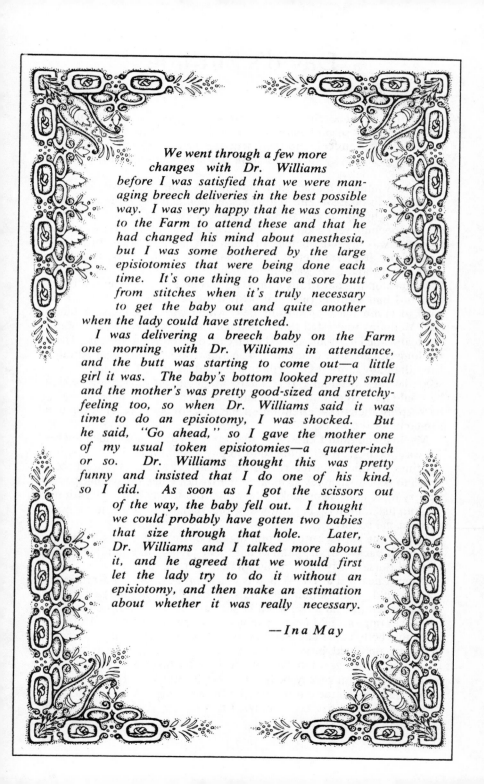

We went through a few more changes with Dr. Williams before I was satisfied that we were managing breech deliveries in the best possible way. I was very happy that he was coming to the Farm to attend these and that he had changed his mind about anesthesia, but I was some bothered by the large episiotomies that were being done each time. It's one thing to have a sore butt from stitches when it's truly necessary to get the baby out and quite another when the lady could have stretched.

I was delivering a breech baby on the Farm one morning with Dr. Williams in attendance, and the butt was starting to come out—a little girl it was. The baby's bottom looked pretty small and the mother's was pretty good-sized and stretchy-feeling too, so when Dr. Williams said it was time to do an episiotomy, I was shocked. But he said, "Go ahead," so I gave the mother one of my usual token episiotomies—a quarter-inch or so. Dr. Williams thought this was pretty funny and insisted that I do one of his kind, so I did. As soon as I got the scissors out of the way, the baby fell out. I thought we could probably have gotten two babies that size through that hole. Later, Dr. Williams and I talked more about it, and he agreed that we would first let the lady try to do it without an episiotomy, and then make an estimation about whether it was really necessary.

—Ina May

David's Birthing

Deborah: I had known for about a month that my second baby was breech. Dr. Williams was going to come to the Farm and deliver. I felt grateful and lucky to get to have a Farm birthing with a breech baby.

I did my laundry that morning having very light rushes. As soon as I decided I was doing it, and William came home, it started moving right along. We hung out and smooched. I had long juicy rushes when we were smooching real good. I loved having good strong rushes because I knew it was my baby being born that was making me feel that way.

At about five centimeters (about half-way dilated), my rushes got pretty strong and there was almost no time at all between them. When I sat down on the pot I fully dilated and when I stood up my water bag broke. I had a strong rush that pushed the baby down a little. It was hard to climb back up on our bed, which was raised up on blocks (Dr. Williams requested that it be high for the delivery.)

Meanwhile Dr. Williams had been called and was on his way. It was the longest half hour of my life. The midwives said they wanted me to keep the baby in until Dr. Williams arrived. I had to remember every second what I was doing. If I let loose at all and let the rushes come on he would have come out. All the ladies in the room were helping me out by keeping their total attention on me. I kept eye contact going with someone all the time.

My husband didn't know how to keep it together in so much energy. He was nervous. It felt more solid to pay attention to the midwives at the time. William started rubbing my belly. I asked him a couple of times to cool it since it was making the rushes come on stronger and I was trying to hold them back. Mary told him to pay better attention to me and listen better. The midwives told William to sit behind me and support me solidly.

By now the baby's butt was bulging out during the rushes. Cara was holding it back with the palm of her hand. It was like holding back a team of horses. My baby really wanted to be born.

When I heard that Dr. Williams was approaching the Farm's gate I was so glad. The ambulance outside had him on the radio. Dr. Williams felt like an angel when he walked in. He took one look, put his gloves on, and told me to go ahead and give it all I had. I did and his whole body came out on one push. His feet were still inside. Dr. Williams unfolded him. It reminded me of a bird just hatched, unfolding its wings. On the next rush, I pushed his head out. Dr. Williams put him on my belly. He was beautiful. My cup runneth over. He checked me out to see if I had torn. He was amazed to see a breech with no tear or episiotomy. I had stretched while his butt was bulging out. Ina May asked Dr. Williams previously to see if I could stretch enough before he went ahead and cut me.

I loved Dr. Williams for helping me out.

David's birthing was a turning point in my life. It showed me how strong you can be when it gets that heavy.

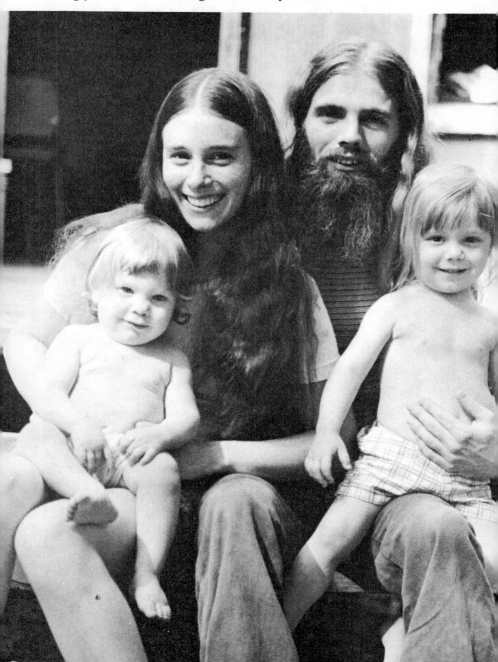

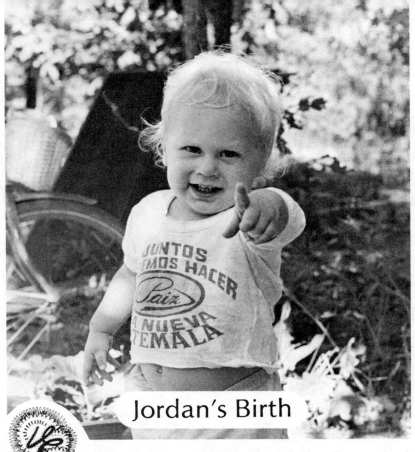

Jordan's Birth

llen: I was pretty dilated and feeling like maybe I needed to push, so Denise called Mary Louise and Pamela. As soon as Mary Louise got there, the whole room got psychedelic and I realized I could've called her sooner—she only lived across the road. She got someone to crank up the stove and I got nice and warm and took off my nightgown. It felt really good to do that. Naked seemed like the right way to have a baby. The room looked really pretty and all the ladies looked beautiful and glowy. I think someone lit some incense. Mary Louise was real pregnant and she looked like a lovely fat Buddha sitting between my legs. As I pushed, the ladies cheered me on—it was really fun. Mary Louise rubbed oil on my puss and stretched it and pulled at it and pretty soon the baby's head came out. I wanted to see if it was a boy or a girl so bad I didn't even wait for a rush—I just pushed and out came his body. His eyes were open and he was looking at me and I just loved him a whole lot. I heard organ music playing and the light that came in through the window was all pink.

Willa May

oberta: On Thursday I went to the clinic and Carol told me I was two or three centimeters dilated. I had been rushing a lot the past week and was feeling really good and open so I wasn't surprised. My mother had come three weeks earlier to help me with the baby. She and I waited together. By this time I was already two weeks overdue.

On Friday I stayed home all day; I felt like I was getting ready. Early that evening I went to Joel's office, spent some time with him and my mom there and brought him home. I decided to go upstairs after dinner and told Joel to do the same. We hung out for a long time, feeling really in love. Around 11:00 I told Joel to go to sleep. He seemed tired. I was rushing—not strong or regular rushes. I didn't tell Joel. I didn't want him to get excited too soon. I got out *Spiritual Midwifery* and read my last birthing tale. It seemed to have all the instructions I needed for this next birthing. It stuck in my mind the part where Cara said if I smooched Joel it would open me up. Also to keep my sense of humor.

I lay in bed for several hours just feeling the rushes come on. I had to use the toilet a lot that night, so I went up and down a flight of stairs at least five or six times. I looked at the clock around 3:00 and flashed I would have the baby around sunrise—but I couldn't possibly see how. I went upstairs, and soon after that a thunderstorm began coming up. Joel rolled over and said that maybe this was the energy I needed to get going. I knew I was well on my way. We hugged tightly through the storm and I could feel the baby real strong. The rushes were still coming. They weren't regular or very strong yet. Around 4:00 I went downstairs. This time I lost my mucus plug. I knew I was beginning labor. I went upstairs and woke Joel up. At first I said wait before getting Ruth, a midwife trainee who lives with us, but in another minute I told him to get her. Suddenly the rushes came on strong and fast. Ruth and Marilyn came in, all excited. We'd all been waiting for a while; the last weeks seemed the longest. Ruth checked me. I was three centimeters. I was a little disappointed. It seemed like the rushes were getting strong fast. Ruth and Marilyn went to get things together and call Carol, who lived down the road.

Joel: Marilyn then came in and she and Ruth began getting things ready. From their conversation and from our experience with Louey, I was getting ready for a two or three hour happening. Roberta and I smooched and hugged and Roberta started squeezing my back during her rushes. It was great—Roberta could squeeze my back as hard as she could to help her through her rushes, and it was loosening up my back. Roberta seemed pretty experienced about what to do, this being our second birthing and her assisting at other birthings.

127

Roberta: Me and Joel had a good time. I got into a position where I could squeeze Joel's back really hard and at the same time keep my bottom relaxed. It seemed like a long time that Ruth and Marilyn were gone. Suddenly I panicked. I wondered if I could continue. It just took a second and I almost fell apart completely. Ruth and Marilyn walked in. I told them about where my head was at. They chuckled, and told me I was way past the point where I was freaking out the last time. It blew my mind so much I quit panicking and continued squeezing Joel's back. I kept remembering Cara's advice to give Joel a lot and to keep my sense of humor. Ruth said I could have an enema when I was four centimeters. Marilyn said I could get up and run around the block a few times. I laughed. I knew the rushes were strong but I decided to get up and walk around. I joked with Joel about how he was calmly sitting on the bed and I was pacing the floor. The rushes were really strong and I was sweating. But I felt on top of them, even in control. I felt like I had learned how to "surf" on them and really bring it on. I knew I was opening up with each rush. During one rush I had a vision of a girl.

I asked Ruth if I couldn't have that enema soon. It was only about five minutes when I squatted down and told her that actually I felt like I had to push. She told me to get on the bed and checked me. Fully dilated. It blew our minds. It had only been thirty or forty minutes since I first called Ruth. Marilyn ran to call Carol. Ruth joked with me, held her hand up and asked me to please wait for Carol. I thought about my mom. Should I call her now? It was all happening so fast. I decided to wait.

I had a good rush when Carol came. While she was washing up I asked her if I could push. She said go ahead, watching me the whole time. A rush or two and the water bag broke, splashing everyone. Another few rushes and there was the head. The cord was tightly around the baby's neck, so Carol clamped it and quickly cut it.

Joel: Carol's hands were fast and sure. As she brought the scissors to the cord it looked like the baby's ear was right next to the cord and would be cut too. But in the next instant Carol had her finger between the cord and the ear and made the cut. Carol reached in and grabbed the baby's shoulders and pulled heartily a few times until the baby was out. More meconium spritzing everywhere. As the body came out it was bluish-purple and deflated. Carol and Ruth started working on her immediately. Carol had brought her out and covered her up and started working so fast I couldn't tell if it was a boy or a girl. Ruth was syringing the baby's mouth and throat so she could breathe. The baby was blue-purplish-green around the face and extremities but I could see that the baby was pink around the chest area. I could also see a strong white glow around the chest area and I knew that we still had to bring this baby through but it was strong and would make it. Carol was reassuring as she worked away. The baby whimpered slightly but couldn't get out a strong cry. I felt as if I was one huge sigh caught in my throat as I watched Carol and Ruth work. There was nothing I could do physically to help them so I zapped the baby and them with my love and attention. Roberta was doing the same. Instant by instant I could see the baby was getting stronger. The action slowed down some and one of the ladies asked if it was a boy or a girl. Carol said she noticed it was a girl as she came out. Ruth checked again and reaffirmed it. Wonderful. Our hearts delighted.

Roberta: Suddenly my mother came running in, jumped on the bed, leaned over Joel and gave me a big hug and kiss. She was glowing. In the meantime Carol asked for some oxygen: the baby was breathing but her cries were still scratchy and she was some laid back. When we gave Willa the oxygen she got pinker and her cries were stronger. When I first saw her I knew she was Willa May. It seemed to be written all over her face. She looked like Uncle Bill, who had died this past year. Carol put Willa on me. She was beautiful. Then Carol gave her to Ruth, who kept syringing her nose and mouth, then cleaned her and dressed her. Carol delivered the placenta and stitched me up. We were all so happy. I'm so grateful to Carol and Ruth and Marilyn and all the midwives for helping my children have a safe and stoned entry into the world.

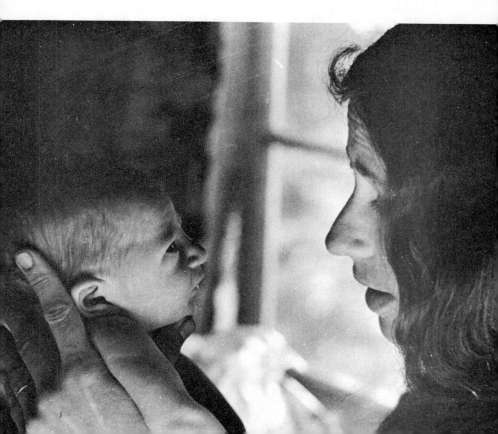

Birth of Michael

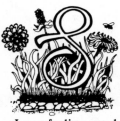

hirley Ray: When Ina May arrived at my bus, I was all clenched up knowing I was going to hurt any minute. [*First baby.—I.M*] My water bag had broken a couple of hours earlier. She came over and showed me how to breathe differently and soon I was feeling good. She said I was supposed to be having a good time. I found it easy to do what she said. It was like making love to Ina May.

I had to get along better with John. I didn't want to. I found myself being mad at him (he was tender and kind to me) because I knew he couldn't help me now! We got friendlier. He was the nicest man I knew and I was ashamed at being angry at him. John reminded me that this was what I had always wanted and Ina May seconded that. I was twenty-eight years old and this was my first baby. I was glad the midwives were so nice to John. They seemed to make up for all that I lacked so it was perfect all the time.

The midwives lay down to get some rest. John and I smooched and cuddled through my rushes, and we had a good time. Ina May told me to say when I felt like I needed to push. When I spoke up, all the ladies woke up, and I was amazed at how busy and efficient they all were. I knew we were in business. They turned me around on the bed and sat me up more. Now I was to push the baby's head out. Ina May massaged my puss—which seemed stretched to its fullest capacity—with baby oil. She said she could see his hair and I was so happy.

I made a noise—thought I'd explode into a thousand billion pieces—and his head was out. The most wonderful moment. Then he slipped out, wet and warm. A beautiful big baby. [*He was big. He weighed ten pounds, a moose like his father.—I.M.*] Just what I had always wanted. He was blue but I knew everything was all right. John wept, he was overcome. Extraordinary peace pervaded my whole existence.

I watched Ina May pat his feet to start him off. Then they handled him and got him all pink and John got to hold him while they cut the cord. Margaret cleaned him up and Ina May showed me how to get him to nurse. I was tired and very thankful.

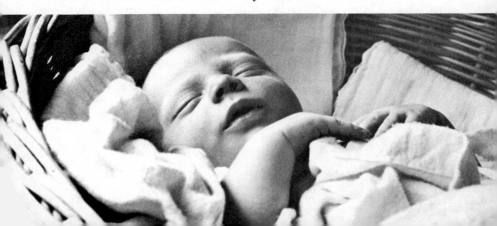

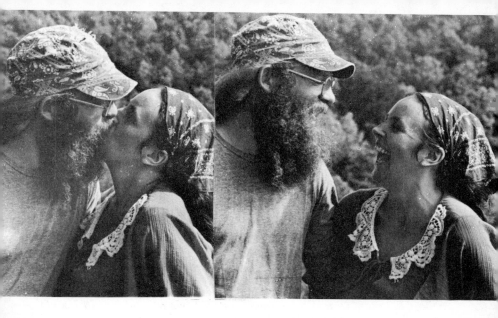

Our Two Ten-Pounders
Followed by Fifteen Pounds
Worth of Twins!

ohn: Michael's birth was happening and we were uptight. Ina May, Louise and Margaret came onto our bus and I was relieved. They went to sleep on the floor while Shirley Ray and I smooched and got to know each other.

Michael was born the next morning. As we came up on his birth, my body went through a lot of changes. I sweat a lot and my sinuses drained. I felt like an athlete just before the birth. I didn't see Michael being born, because Shirley Ray needed my attention. When he came out I felt him reel from the sensory input. My emotions rose up in me and I began to cry. There was a human being who wasn't there before, coming to life, breathing, turning pink. Then my vision began to flash, like someone was flashing a flash-bulb complete with popping noise. I struggled to stay on top of it. My vision was changing with the baby's heartbeat. I felt like I was going to pass out. I didn't want to pass out because I would fall forward into the birthing fluids. I asked the closest person to hold my hand. I didn't pass out.

When David was born, I was determined to be more together. It never seemed like Shirley Ray and I were together enough to have a baby when her labor began. We had to hustle and get it together every

131

time. I like to smooch then. It feels good to enjoy the time together. My lady looks so pretty then. After we worked at it all night, David was born. We thought he was a girl, but he's a mellow, calm boy. He was born in the Adobe, our hospital at the time. We weren't totally, one hundred per cent, look-'em-in-the-eye, hold-no-grudges straight with everybody in the house. We didn't share our thing with everyone. Our birthing was strong, but it didn't spread out very far, like it could have.

Then I found out we were going to have twins.

I was delighted. What a blessing to have two babies! I really liked our boys and I knew it would be even more fun with two the same age. We had one week's advance notice. I was nervous when Shirley Ray went into labor. I wanted to share our experience this time not frivolously but lovingly. There was a crowd at our birthing. All the midwives, our doctor-to-be (Paul) and Dr. Williams, plus some more clinic ladies. We had such a good time. It seemed like everybody knew we'd love to have twins and they loved it with us. Ellie-Megan was born first. She was a small fat girl. We had known each other for a while. About a week before the birthing I had a dream. *A very pretty young lady came into a bare room and sat down at a table. All I could really see were her eyes which were full of life and love. Then she turned into a baby.* I woke up. Ellie-Megan was that baby. Everyone cheered. There was one more baby. Dr. Williams felt up into the womb and said he was butt first. He had felt the baby and knew what sex it was. He tried to get Paul, our student doctor, to bet him what sex it was. He looked at his watch and said he had been in long enough. He reached up and pulled down two legs. Then he pulled George out. It was stronger than a contraction from Shirley Ray's face. George's nose was flat like a pig. I loved him anyway. Later on his nose stretched out like everybody else's. A boy and a girl. I loved him as much as her. She looked from one person to the next and then she screamed. She comes on strong like Michael and Shirley Ray. George was also bruised about the chest from his rapid journey through the birth canal. He was quite nice about it. He's good-natured and likes to laugh.

We are so happy with our twins. They have their own thing and lots of times they have it together when the adults don't have it so together. Twins are especially beautiful—they'll smile together, move as one thing and be really in tune with each other. They are an incredible amount of work. They'll teach you to be fast and efficient. About three days after they were born, I laid both George and Ellie on my stomach while I lay on my back. I was really glad they were here and I got to be with them. They felt the joy I felt. I began to feel blissful like everything was heavenly and I reached out with my head and I could feel a long way. I felt strong, like I could move mountains. Then I felt more joy. I floated in this ecstatic state for a long time.

ns

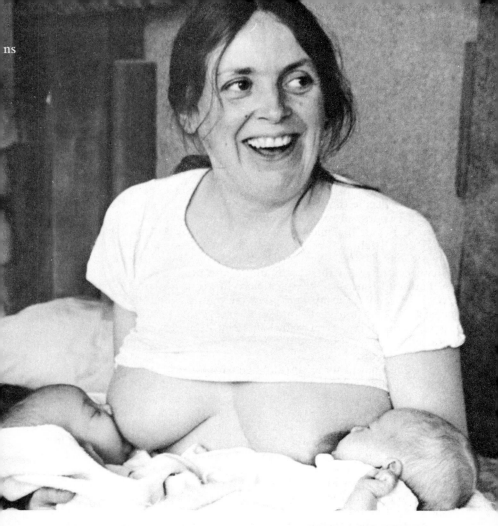

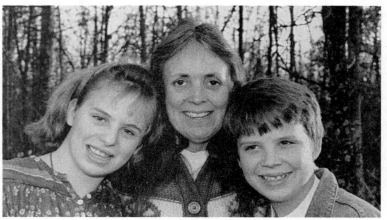

Ellie-Megan and George at 14.

Leonna

Debra: Having my baby was the most wonderful thing that ever happened to me. It was the best psychedelic experience yet. I could really feel God's presence and I was really aware of how cause-and-effect works. A couple times when it got heavy I started to get a little frantic and it was obvious immediately. I knew I had to calm down.

If you decide that you want to keep yourself together and get high on the energy of your kid being born and have that agreement with your man and the midwives, it can easily be the most Holy day of your life. I felt so much love and support from the ladies and Paul, my husband, that it was hard to complain. I saw that a lot of what I concern myself with is really dumb and piddly.

Paul and I arm-wrestled a bunch during my labor. When I got a rush, I would reach up and press my palms against his as hard as I could. It helped a lot to put some energy out as all that energy was going through me. Paul really helped me keep my sense of humor. If it started to get hard he would "moo" at me or do something that would make me laugh. I was really glad I was at home with my husband and friends and not in some hospital bed with nurses I'd never met before.

Mary Louise and I fell in love. She felt real soft, but strong and sure at the same time. She really felt the baby's presence a lot. She was very compassionate with me; I could feel her feeling what I was feeling. One time I asked her, "How much longer do you think it's going to be?" She laughed and said she couldn't answer that because she didn't know. She said I had to welcome every rush and not think about how many there would be. I realized I generally get impatient about a lot of things, and I knew I had to let go. One time I felt like maybe I couldn't really do it. I told Mary Louise that and she just calmly told me that she knew I could and I knew she was right and felt a bunch better.

One time when she was checking out my dilation she had Lee on the phone telling Barbara that I was almost fully dilated and to start to get ready to come over. All of a sudden I got this big rush of energy. My whole thing started to open up; it almost felt like I was coming on to an orgasm. I said, "Oh, Mary Louise, that feels outrageous." She said, "Wait a minute. Tell her she *is* fully dilated and to come right over." Her touch felt so heavy that my whole self just opened up. It blew my mind. I could really feel the baby a lot then. She was right there, her consciousness was strong. Thinking of her helped me a lot. I knew she was ready to get born and I wanted to help her do it.

Pushing was a lot more work than I thought it would be. I had heard ladies say it took them three pushes and their kid was out. I had to learn how to push and then got into it for a while. I felt like a cow and started to make these really loud, low bellowing noises. I had no idea I was going to do that. It just felt completely natural and it just came out. At first it seemed a little embarrassing and I asked Mary Louise if it was okay. She said yes, it was helping move the baby down and just keep my voice low. I could feel Leonna moving down and coming out. All the ladies would push with me and breathe deep and it really helped me out a lot. I could just look into their eyes and breathe deep and almost forget about myself. It was in the afternoon and really hot. Janine kept putting ice on my body and in my mouth. I was sweating and they said I was red as a beet. While I was pushing I was really connected to Mary Louise. Paul was at my side and she was at my feet. It was intense feeling Leonna's body move down a little on each push and her head bulging out. I could hardly believe that I had to put out so much energy. I had to push for about an hour and a half.

Finally I could feel her head really close and I knew she was almost out. One more push and her head popped out. What a rush! She had her cord around her neck and Mary Louise said pant. All the ladies started to pant together at the same instant. *It was a timeless moment.* Mary Louise was hustling, clamped and cut the cord, turned her and pulled out one shoulder, then another, and pulled out her body. I was completely amazed when I saw her. She was so pure and perfect. They cleaned her up and suctioned her out and gave her back to me. She was beautiful. I felt totally elated and high. I just couldn't believe my eyes. Wow, we really did it, we had a kid! It was a miracle.

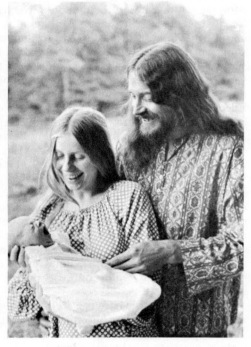

Mary Louise: Paul really helped Debra out in a very monkey, non-conceptual way. Any time she'd get into high-pitched, tight sounds, he'd just laugh and do some nice deep grunts and get her to talk back to him and they'd sound like two monkeys talking and having a good time. When Debra was pushing, she started mooing like an old cow—sounded great. At first she thought it wasn't okay but we all loved it and she and Paul and their noises really moved that baby out.

Debra, Paul and Leonna

135

Eileen

artin: Somehow I couldn't get behind shoveling shit. The manure crew's wit was sparkling, the soda flowed freely, but something was keeping me distracted. People kept telling me I ought to work harder, and I'd say, "Yeah," but I kept feeling out of place. When we rolled through the gate, I found out why. "Go home, Martin, your wife's havin' a baby!" Bonnie was about a month early. I went and washed the horse shit off. Bonnie's rushes were quite light, and we slept lightly. The birthing was easy and Eileen was born the next morning. We made out a lot, and I kept Bonnie rubbed out. The baby was small and came out without a lot of pushing.

A little girl, just what we were hoping for. She slept and cried and sucked, and we watched her closely, because she was under six pounds. When she was just over a day old, she lost her voice. It was kind of haunting, hearing such a pure voice go out. Laa, laa, laa, she would cry, each *laa* a little scratchier and fainter than the one before. She didn't seem to want to suck so much. That was Sunday, and so Monday we took her to the doctor's. No sign of any infection, he said. She just seemed really quiet. We had a little soft toy elephant that you could wind up and it played, "Frere Jacques, Frere Jacques, dormez-vous, dormez-vous," and she lay there on her belly and looked at the sound with no-mind baby eyes, and we lay there watching her, wishing she'd nurse, wondering what she was doing. Lying there quieter and quieter, sleeping more, scarcely breathing, *is* she breathing? "Martin, Eileen's stopped breathing!" I've got to hop on the phone and call the ambulance, *quick* into the ambulance, slapping a little, Kathryn and Matthew saying, "C'mon, *breathe!*" Forced air in her lungs, Eileen occasionally cries a little, hope is alive, Eileen is alive. Hospital room, watching a doctor working *hard,* like I never saw a doctor work before. We are noticed, asked to leave. Sitting in the waiting room, with all the normal emergency room traffic. Fat sullen lookalike family, the youngest boy put his hand through a window. Two workers from the carbon electrode factory, very dirty, one fell and broke his shoulder, the other is helping him out. We talk with them about the Farm, and start feeling optimistic. Possibilities and phrases drift out of the operating room; blood transfusion, steady pulse, transfer to Nashville. Finally the doctor walks out the door: "I'm sorry, but we lost your baby."

What can I say? There is a feeling you get when somebody who was near you is gone, gone beyond, gone to the other shore, completely gone, departed. If you know, you know it; if you don't, you will. We walked out onto the hospital lawn in the warm May moonshine. We cried a lot. "Life," Suzuki says, "is like going on a boat which is going to go out to sea and sink." The factory worker comes out, says, "I'm really sorry...I know it's hard to accept, but these things happen for reasons...sometimes you can't see right off why, but God has reasons for everything." Yes, we tell him, yes, we know. Yes, we know.

The drive home. A friend's drive-in, just closed for the night, provides Coke and french fries. Bonnie's tits ache with useless milk.

A carpenter built a little plywood coffin. No need to see her. We bury her in the Farm's churchyard. Ina May tells us, "You were lucky to have someone so very pure come and stay with you, even for such a short while." Her own baby is barely a week old.

Yes, we were. Lucky to see how fragile and precious and pure life is, lucky to get beyond tears and remorse and come closer together with each other, our other children and everyone around us, all so lucky to be alive and well. I would have been glad for Eileen to have lived; and yet I know it wasn't bad that she died. I know everyone did everything they could. I know how lucky we all are to be here.

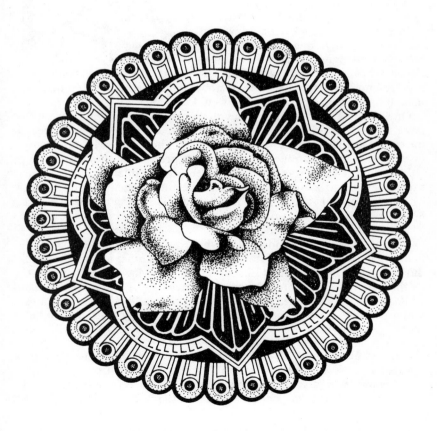

Abner

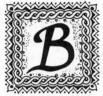onnie: We got pregnant again about six months after Eileen's death. We'd decided we really wanted another baby again soon. During that six months, we got to know each other in a whole new way; it was the first time in our relationship that we hadn't been pregnant or had a little baby.

All during the pregnancy, our bodies felt a lot alike. If one of us rubbed the other, we both felt better. About four or five weeks before Abner was born, I started getting rushes steadier and heavier than the Braxton-Hicks* contractions I'd had earlier. I quit my job and slowed down a bunch because I didn't want to have this baby early.

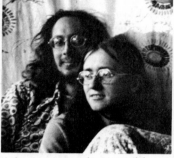

In a couple of weeks Ina May said our baby was big enough to do okay if born, so I was ready to have it any time. Whenever another lady would go into labor, my rushes would get regular and heavier and I'd debate about calling a midwife. Then I'd usually fall asleep and the rushes would slow down.

One morning after having rushes all night—I knew two ladies were in labor at the time—I did call Mary Louise and asked her if she'd check me out. The rushes I was having were heavy enough that I didn't want to babysit if they continued, though I was pretty sure they'd stop.

Mary Louise said I was nearly three centimeters dilated, so we called Martin home and set up for a baby. I was still skeptical. At one point we were all upstairs in our bedroom. I said I was going downstairs and Mary Louise said, "Oh, no. You're the guest of honor. You're going to sit down on this bed and have a baby."

We talked with the midwives a while, as the rushes kept getting heavier. Then Martin and I started rubbing each other and making out during rushes, like we had at Eileen's birth. Ina May came around two in the afternoon and brought an obstetrical nurse whom she'd met while on tour at Albuquerque. She'd worked in a hospital at birthings and was mind-blown to see us do it our way. I really liked having her there, because she enjoyed it so much and learned a lot. Finally, it felt like I was nearly fully dilated.

Earlier, at the end of each rush, I'd get a rush of energy from opening up. Now, I felt energy like that almost all the time. Ina May said I could try a push, and sure enough, I could feel the baby's head wedging in between my bones. After that, my only interest was in

*These are irregular, painless contractions that occur throughout pregnancy, increasing in intensity during the last month.

getting the baby out. I pushed harder than I'd ever pushed with my other kids, who were smaller.

At one point, the calves of my legs cramped suddenly, and no amount of rubbing would relax them. Ina May said, "Why don't you just push the baby out?" So I did. At 3:45 p.m., Abner was born—all eight pounds, two ounces of him. It felt good to have such a fat, healthy baby.

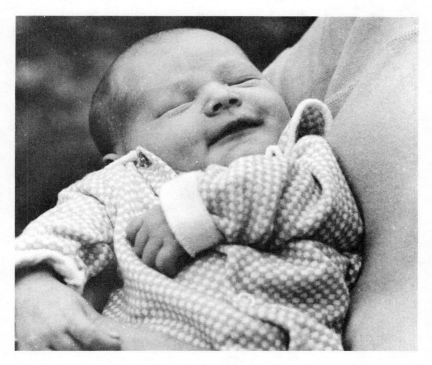

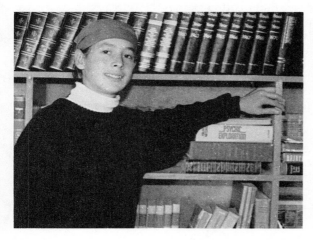

Abner at 14.

Short Notice

na May: The shortest notice that I ever had that I was going to deliver a baby came one day with a phone call from Leslie, the head of our gate crew, that a panel truck from Florida had just arrived at the gate with a lady inside having contractions two minutes apart. Living on a farm that gets anywhere from fifteen to twenty thousand visitors a year, we often get phone calls at our house from the gate crew, reporting that we have this or that interesting guest, but this was the first time we had a lady already in the process of having her baby land on us. Stephen was away from the Farm so I knew that this one was completely in my hands. Leslie told me that the lady's name was Janice, and I remembered that she had called me two weeks before from Florida, telling me that this was her first baby and that she had been told by a couple of doctors that she would have to have a cesarean because she was too small to have her baby naturally. She was very much against having a cesarean if there was any way to get around it and wondered what did I think. At the time she was four weeks away from her due date, so I told her that if she and her husband could come up to Tennessee right away, I'd check her pelvic measurements and her baby and see what I thought. I didn't really think about her again, and now here she was at the gate about to have a baby on me.

Leslie and I chuckled a little together after he had given me all the information he had. He was fully aware what he was handing over to me. I hung up the phone, grabbed my midwife bag, got in my truck and headed for the gate.

I pulled up to the gate and Leslie was there smiling and pointing to a dilapidated little Chevy panel truck. I got out of my truck, went over to the panel truck, and looked in the window. It was an authentic hippie truck—made-in-India cotton paisley bedspreads draped over the ceiling, brilliant color pictures of Hindu deities pasted here and there on the walls, handmade macrame thingies hanging in the corners, food storage racks on the walls with little bags of granola and edible seeds, and a couple of potted plants in holders bolted on next to the windshield so that they would get enough sunlight. In the driver's seat was David, who introduced himself as Janice's husband. He was big and blond and in his late twenties. The entire back of the truck was a platform with a mattress on it, and Janice was lying on it with a worried-looking friend crouched beside her, nervously massaging her belly. The friend explained that he had come along to assist in the delivery of the baby, but that now Janice just wanted to go to a hospital. I understood how she felt. I thought that if I was in labor with my first baby and had someone that nervous rubbing on me, I'd probably prefer a hospital too.

My first impulse was to get in back with Janice and examine her to see how much time we had to work with. I asked the friend to come forward while I examined her. He didn't like me asking him to move, but he did get out of the truck.* *Sometimes people will get attached to getting to observe a birthing.* I rather laboriously climbed into the back (I was seven months pregnant myself). Janice was thrashing around on the mattress and crying. She was like a frightened animal; her eyes were rolling around showing white on all sides. My heart was pounding along with hers and I knew what she was feeling. I sat beside her and began to rub her legs and belly while we talked. She said that the pain was unbearable and that she didn't think she could go through with the birth without anesthesia. Her body was rigid—her legs were stiff and shaking and her belly was hard as a rock even between contractions. I told her that the reason that she was hurting was because her body was uptight and that she would feel better as soon as she was able to relax some. All this time I was squeezing the rigidity out of her belly and her legs and feeling great rushes of relaxation come over us both.

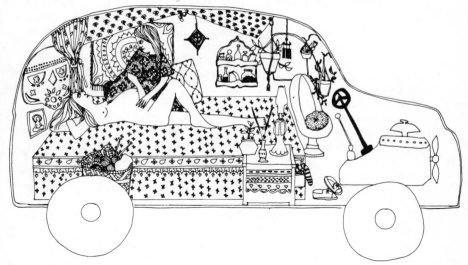

When I had got Janice to where she could hold still, I examined her and found that she was about half-way dilated. I could tell by examining her that she had ample room to let a regular-sized kid out, which this one was. While all this was going on, David was telling me the harrowing story of their trip, how they had left Florida about sixteen hours earlier and that Janice had started having rushes after a couple of hours on the road. By the time they had got to Birmingham her rushes were pretty heavy and quite close together and they were wondering if they were going to be able to make it up to the Farm in their bumpy truck without having the baby first, so they stopped at a

*The friend was attached to being there at first, but later he understood why I had made the decision I had. — I.M.

hospital to get a doctor's opinion. The hospital folks told them that Janice's cervix was about half dilated, but they didn't want to deliver the baby after hearing that David didn't have enough money with him to pay the bill, and sent them on their way with a small delivery kit in case the baby decided to be born before they got to the Farm. They had driven the last two hundred and fifty miles of the journey as fast as they could with Janice doing her best to keep the baby inside till they got to us.

The more I squeezed Janice's belly and legs, the more relaxed she became, and she began to think again about whether she really wanted to go to a hospital. David was very much into having us deliver the baby and I felt in good communication with him, but I told him that it had to be her decision since she was the one actually having the baby. I wanted to help them, but didn't want to try and deliver Janice unless I was sure that I would have a good level of cooperation from her. I explained that if she did go to our local hospital that she wouldn't be able to have David with her, as they had a regulation against having husbands in the labor and delivery rooms. She thought about it for a while and then said that she would rather stay on the Farm and have me deliver the baby. She wasn't frightened any more and she had felt so responsive to any help that I gave her that I felt like she would be able to have a nice time having her baby.

The next thing to do was to find a suitable place for the birth to happen, so Leslie and I got David and Janice the use of someone's place for a few days and we got them settled. I arranged for a place for their friend to stay while he was on the Farm.

Once Janice was in the bed where her baby would be born, she felt much better and began to enjoy herself. I showed her how to breathe deeply during her rushes in order to get the most she could out of them. She became soft and melty to my touch, the way a lady ought to feel when she's about to deliver. She and David cuddled with each other now that he wasn't having to be her chauffeur, and that helped her relax even more.

Seven hours after their arrival at our gate, a seven pound boy was born to David and Janice. She had a beautiful delivery and looked radiant when she first saw her son. They named him Michael.

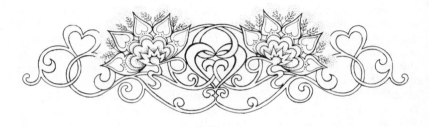

Miguel Ari

anet: The head was out. We all panted while Cara checked to see if the cord was around the baby's neck. He was breathing but mucusy. Cara told me to glide his body out on the next rush. It was a boy, slightly blue-tinged under his skin. He started crying right away. Kathryn suctioned out his mucus. Cara clamped and cut the cord. I held him and he looked at me, and looked around, coming into this world.

All of a sudden, for a few moments I was in a pure chamber of sound, where there was no head or background static. Each sound was magnified as it happened. This was the baby's hearing.

I stayed up with the baby for most of the night. It was too stoned to sleep. His head radiated white energy.

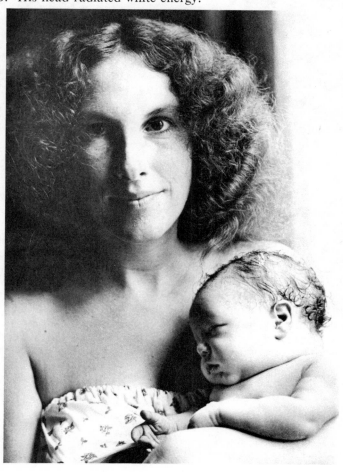

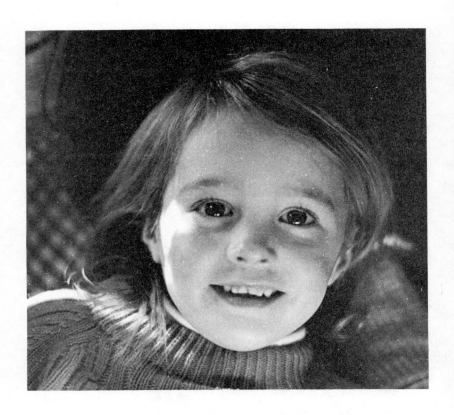

Timothy's Birth

Anita: Clifford would touch precisely where I needed it, when I needed it, how long and at what pressure I needed it. It was like he was feeling everything I was feeling and we were one thing, too. It felt like we all knew the same thing and I felt one with everyone there.

When the baby came out, there was just a flash of an instant that was neither death nor life, just sort of a pre-conscious, before-life-awakening state, the point just before he started breathing. *It was like everything in all space-time suspended for an instant in this transition state.* It blew my mind.

Anna's Birthing

Ellen: Anna was my third baby so I figured that by now I should know how to do it real good—big mama and all. When I had Sarah Jean, my second child, it was fun and went real fast (four hours or so). So it seemed logical to assume that this one would be easier and faster. However, it took me at least twice as long and I had a harder time.

With Sarah Jean, I just lay down on the bed and got it on and had her. With Anna I tried that and not much happened, so I got up, walked around, took three cold showers, and did various other things, but still not much was happening. I started feeling uptight that it was taking so long. Somewhere, I thought that (being my third kid and all) if I didn't have it in less time or at least the same amount of time as my other one, that I just wasn't making it as a baby-haver.

Once it started happening, I forgot all about that other stuff and *experienced a whole other level of consciousness that seemed eternal and timeless.* I especially remember a unique feeling I had *in-between* the contractions; the sense of relief and relaxation made it seem like I was melting. I remember my mouth hanging open, drooling, and feeling very warm and psychedelic and light-headed. (One of the reasons for that, Pamela said, was because a lot of blood and energy was centered at my bottom and left my head light.) Laying there, I felt One with everyone in the Universe.

Two pushes and she squirted out. Baby girl! I was glad to see her and she was the fattest girl I ever had.

Anyway, I just wanted to share with y'all what I learned and tell you not to have any preconceptions about how your birthing is going to be, or try and make it go a certain way because it blows your mind *every* time and it's new and exciting *every* time and it's the most ultimate here-and-now experience you can ever have.

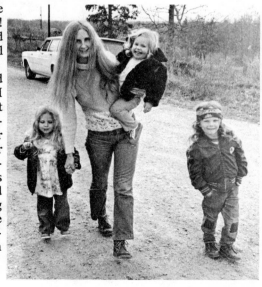

145

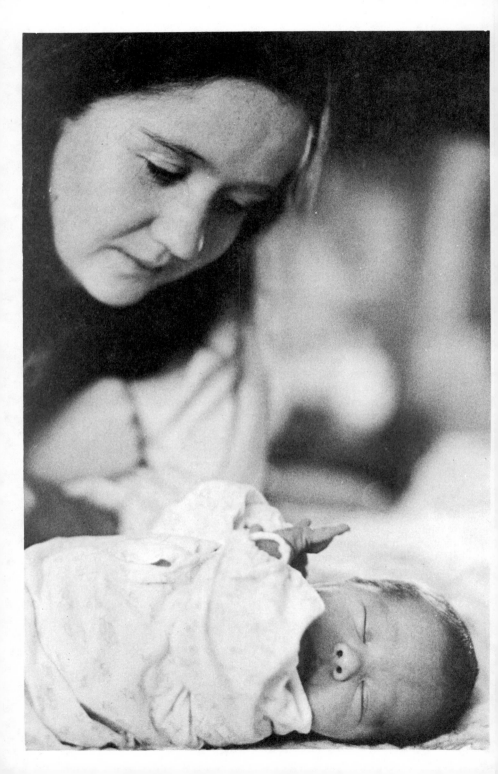

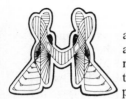arilyn: At seven months pregnant I started bleeding and having some rushes en route to the Farm to have my third baby. At first I was scared. I wondered was the baby coming out now or what. I'd had two normal pregnancies and this one had felt the same way. I tried not to put any attention into the rushes so they would go away. They did, and the bleeding stopped after a day of rest and we continued to the Farm non-stop (after the bleeding had been stopped for 24 hours). As soon as we came onto the Farm's bumpy dirt roads, it started happening again. After two days in bed, a midwife went with me to the doctor. He thought maybe the placenta had partially separated but was not covering the cervix. He couldn't examine me internally at this point to tell for sure. I was to take it easy and try to keep the baby in for at least a month longer.

Ten days later I was bleeding again and this time stayed in bed until the birth. I bled quite often during the next 3½ weeks, sometimes profusely and passing clots which we first thought might be pieces of placenta. I was told that the placenta might be covering the cervix and how much would determine whether or not I would have to have a cesarean. That would have to be decided at the hospital when I was in labor. The important thing was to make sure the mother and baby were okay in the meantime.

Whenever I'd bleed, we'd call a midwife who'd come check out the baby's heartbeat. A lab person, usually my sister, would come to get some blood to check my hematocrit. We felt like we got to have a continuous birthing. Sometimes a midwife helper would sleep at our house and wake up every two or four hours to check the heartbeat. Douglas learned to use the fetoscope and we were given one to use whenever we felt like it. Mary Louise came over and called a lot. Her constant love and compassion were an immense source of strength. I felt so well taken care of that I never once thought the baby wouldn't make it. Whenever there was a question, I'd get a strong kick from the baby and know everything was all right. It didn't occur to me until later that this was a serious complication of pregnancy and that most ladies would have had to spend this time in a hospital. I'm so grateful I got to be with family.

Five weeks after the first bleeding, I started bleeding more than I ever had. Mary Louise and the ambulance came and we were off to the hospital. The rushes were strong and from 5-10 minutes apart. With each one, I would bleed quite a bit. They took me from the emergency room to the labor room where I couldn't be with Douglas. He had been a big part of our other birthings. Thank goodness for Mary Louise. We were calm and strong in our faith that everything was just fine. The nurse in the labor room was nervous about how much I was bleeding. I passed one big clot that reminded me of having a baby. Finally the doctor came and examined me and told me it'd have to be a cesarean.

From there it all went very fast. When the doctor asked me if I wanted my tubes tied, as long as he was going to be in there, I started to cry. I'd known that a cesarean was a possibility but I still had hoped that I might get to go home. I'd loved having my other babies and was afraid I wouldn't be able to have them again naturally. The thoughts that everything was okay and whatever it took to get this baby out gave me strength. I felt telepathic with the baby who was about to be born (one way or another didn't matter that much), and with my mother, who had an emergency cesarean having me.

Mary Louise got dressed in surgical clothes but at the last minute they wouldn't let her come into the operating room. I was just wondering who would be receiving the baby as it came into the world when Dr. Williams came in and connected with me, smiling. They were ready to give me anesthesia and now I was ready too, knowing the baby would be in his good hands.

The next thing I remember was feeling very groggy, very thirsty and someone saying you have a healthy baby boy. It barely registered I was so out of it. I didn't get to see the baby for 12 hours. I was told he would be in an incubator for 24 hours. When I finally got to see him we fell in love right away. He was a sweet, strong boy. I only got to see him every 4 hours for 30-45 minutes, and Douglas could only see him through the nursery window. What a change after two home birthings. It felt so different; I could hardly wait to go home. I got up and was walking around the next day. The hurt in my belly was no more than the episiotomies I'd had before, it was just in a different place.

Mary Louise, his Guardian Angel, came to Owen's homecoming. He really knew he was home. He stretched and opened up and relaxed as I'd never seen him do in the hospital. He looked like a flower opening up. It felt like the real birthing as we all shared and appreciated his new-born consciousness. It was truly a blessing.

A year later, Owen got critically ill and spent 5 weeks in intensive care and 2 months altogether in the hospital. We had a strong telepathic connection and I really believe we are bonded together even though we didn't spend those first hours of his life together. I remembered those kicks of reassurance I had gotten while lying in bed to keep him in, and every day he was sick, at least once, he would look in my eyes and say the one word he knew and we'd both know it was cool. Owen is a healthy fatso now, but there's not a day that goes by that I don't remember and be grateful he's here with us.

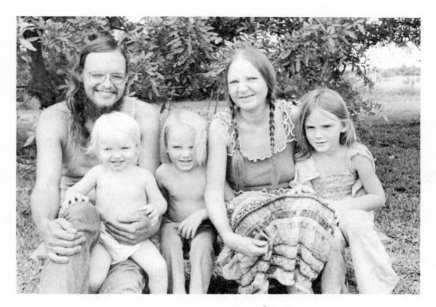

Tana's Tale

Tana: Having Paul, my second baby, was the heaviest thing that ever happened to me. I'd had my first kid, Eve, in a hospital. I was completely knocked out because that was how I wanted it. My doctor said doctors who practiced natural childbirth were crazy, and I believed it, not having been informed otherwise.

So I went into my second birthing full of faith and some fear. I found it hard to integrate the rushes. I'd look at my man, and say, "Oh, Timothy," and he'd say, "Oh, Tana," like it wasn't heavy, which sort of helped and sort of didn't. I had a good time but I wasn't very connected with the midwives or Timothy. I was somewhere on the astral plane, feeling all the forces of the Universe, it felt like, pounding my body. I flashed on wild stallions, thunder and lightning, and the ocean. I felt like my brain and upper body were separate from the rest of me, and were looking down on the action. Also I felt like Marilyn Monroe or some sex symbol writhing around.

It was like my body was its own thing, and I was pushing really hard and putting everything into it. I made outrageous elephant-like grunts. I just put my attention out the window on the trees, like I was looking away from something happening to me. I realized later I should have kept my attention on the folks and the here and now, and I would have been much more grounded.

149

I felt like I was in a car wreck or some heavy karmic situation as I was instinctively doing all I could to push the baby out. I felt strongly that when I got through having the baby, I would never complain about anything again.

I gave another big push and prayed this would do it. I said, "Can you see the head?" Then pretty soon, with my puss feeling like it was coming apart, out came this big blue boy. I was really hoping for a boy, and it felt like I already knew. Pamela started rubbing and massaging him and he came to life. He was beautiful. Timothy looked at me and said, "Paul?" and I said yes, because we had hoped to have a boy and name it after Timothy's father. It felt good to christen him only minutes after his birth.

The midwives said he was big and took him to be fixed up. Then they handed him to Timothy, and he held him, sitting across from me as Pamela stitched me up. Paul lay in Timothy's lap and looked around with big blue eyes. Weighing in at eight pounds, twelve ounces, he was born at 6:47 a.m. just as it was getting light. My labor had started six hours earlier.

I was in paradise with my new baby; I was mindblown by his beauty and my love for him. I felt I was so privileged to spend so much time with him. The trees and the early morning light just flashed and reverbed like a strobe-light, and for several days I would have a flashback at every dawn and sunset. I was ecstatic for two weeks.

Even so, I did spend all day integrating the experience. I felt like I wasn't sure I'd want to do it again but that I was supposed to feel different. I knew I wanted more kids, so I thought I had better change my attitude. By talking myself into it all day, I did come up with a change of attitude through will. But I was still afraid of childbirth and I carried that fear through my third pregnancy.

I was, however, in much better shape physically after the natural birthing than when I was in the hospital. After I had Eve, I was so doped up, I felt like I was climbing out of a pit. When I got to my room and settled in my bed, I realized I had to pee really bad so I made the incredible walk across the room and did it all by myself and managed to get in bed. I was very proud of myself and a nurse said later I shouldn't have done it.

I had planned to nurse my baby around the clock and now I found I was so exhausted I wasn't that interested.

As a contrast, when I had Paul, I felt fine, my head was clear and my body felt great. I wasn't too sleepy to enjoy my baby and I got to see my newborn baby go through many beautiful changes the first day. His skin turned from bluish to white and then gradually to pink. He also changed in other ways, and I realized what I had missed with Eve. Also, I couldn't believe the strong bond I felt for my new baby and the overwhelming maternal instinct. I knew I didn't take him for granted as I had my other baby because I knew what an intense experience it was to get him.

Also, I was more telepathic with him, such as when he would scream about getting his diaper changed, I couldn't take him too seriously because I knew we both had some relativity on what was serious.

I loved Eve a bunch, but I never hovered over her much or thought too much about her conking out. With Paul, while I was very happy, I also would feel a little uptight or nervous that something might happen to my newborn. I knew I wasn't supposed to be uptight so I started to identify these feelings as hormones, a perfectly natural and miraculous method of protecting the baby, and I felt better. In fact, I was the happiest I'd been in my life.

❀ ❁ ❃ ❀ ✿ ❀ ❁ ❀ ❀

I was a little uneasy as I went into my third pregnancy. Timothy said I didn't give him much attention during the last birthing and I was also told that I complained. So I decided not to complain and to give Timothy some and keep my attention in the here and now.

I was born with a rare genetic defect of my skin called *Epidermolysis Bullosa* which causes it to tear easily and blister badly with any trauma. [*Before Tana got pregnant the third time, we sent her and Timothy to a genetic counselor who said that there was no chance of her children inheriting her skin disorder.—Ina May*] I went to see a dermatologist in the last months of pregnancy. When he heard I was going to have a natural delivery on the Farm, he was quite alarmed and advised against it. He said I might have emergency complications. I told him that we didn't expect any problems and that I hadn't had any trouble before. He did put a little doubt in my mind which had already been conditioned to be scared of childbirth.

This doctor felt uptight about sex in general. I think it's male chauvinism to make a lady feel she's too neurotic and not strong enough to do what almost all other ladies have done before her, and are simultaneously doing around the world.

The day I had baby number three, I kept thinking I might do it anytime, because the baby felt so low. I sat in a big armchair all day, relaxing. Around dusk I felt a little bit of energy and went and took a hot bath. Then I really got relaxed. I forgot all about my body and felt really comfortable. As I came out of the bathroom, Timothy was lighting the lamps and the light was very golden and beautiful. I thought it was amazing that the vision changed before I had any rushes.

Just as I thought this I sat down and started having some light ones. I timed them fifteen minutes apart for an hour as I folded laundry. They weren't at all heavy. Timothy asked me if I wanted to have some friends come over, and I said yeah, because I wanted to see them and I thought it would be nice to have company during the early part of labor. I thought it was going to be several hours.

When Steven and Kristan walked in they both kept saying it felt like Christmas. It was November 16. I told them I was having the baby. Kristan and I had had our last boys one week to the day apart, across the street from each other. She had just had another boy about a month ago.

I asked Timothy to call the midwife. I had to go to the pot and felt good and laughed and felt a little nervous on the energy, but determined to stay centered. Then it started seeming like it wasn't going to be so long and we made arrangements to get our two kids to a neighbor's house.

When the midwife came in, there were Steven and Kristan and the man who was going to keep our kids and a man with a car who was going to carry everybody and the stuff. It looked like a party. Susan came in and said, "You're doing it, huh?" We sat around for a while and she asked me what I thought it was and I said I sort of hoped for a boy, but would be grateful for either. She said she flashed on a boy, too.

Then she said she'd like to check me. We went upstairs and she checked my dilation and said it was almost five centimeters. She said she was amazed that I was integrating the rushes so easily and that I was that far along. I told her I was having fun and I was happy and glad she could come.

I had a couple of strong rushes standing up and standing up helped to integrate them. It was getting heavier and I wasn't sure I could take it, but each one wasn't too bad. It was a lot like real heavy menstrual cramps I had had in high school. I felt like I needed to push and get everything out. I was grateful for those cramps for they felt like a practice run.

Then came a big rush and I wanted to stand up for it and I got off the bed and stood up and had a big whoosh—splat! My waterbag broke with water all over the place. It felt like a lot of pressure was released and I got back on the bed.

It was coming fast. Two other midwives had arrived and Timothy was with me. Then I started to feel afraid and worried. Ina May walked in. I said, "Help me, Ina May." Then I said, "You can't, can you?" feeling I had to come up with it myself. I put my hand down to my puss and felt it coming out. I thought, "I've got to get it together now." Ina May said to pant and that I was going too fast. I panted on the next rush and his head came out and I looked at it and was so moved because I had not wanted to miss that part as I had last time. It looked like his head was covered with little ringlets. I don't even remember another rush and out he came, looking beautiful, pink and breathing.

I had made it with hardly any pain and not much fear. I think maybe if Timothy and I had smooched more during the birthing, I would have gotten over my fear sooner, but my fears of childbirth are over. I know having a baby naturally is one of the greatest joys of existence and also our natural birthright.

We were so grateful. It was a miracle. We just rejoiced it had gone so well and so easy. It was like a dream. I thanked God for taking care of us and giving me such a beautiful boy. His name is Vernon. He weighed seven pounds and five ounces and was born two and a half hours from the first rush.

He was a wonderful baby. "Rosebud" we called him from his healthy flush and beautiful little mouth. The midwives were entranced with him and so was I. You just nursed him and changed him and put him to bed. He hardly cried.

I wish I could have lots more babies for the fun of it, but we need to stop where we are for a while. I can't understand the ladies who think fulfillment lies only in a career or a position of wealth or power. Maybe a career can round out your total life, but I feel that a career alone can in no way measure up to the real fulfillment I experienced in being privileged to feel that birthing energy, which I never felt anything like before, and to see that beautiful creation, so perfect, which we have a small part in, but which is mostly done without us. I just feel so wonderful when I'm nursing my baby or taking care of him that I know that this is heavier than being a corporation president.

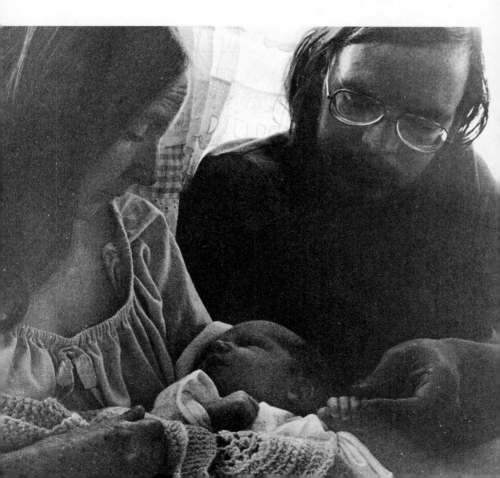

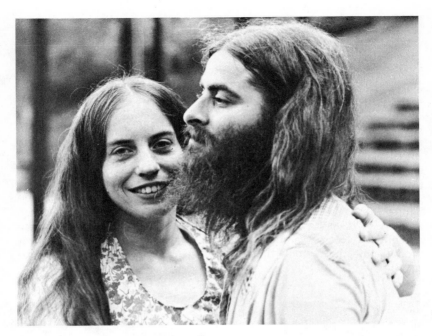

Katherine

ean: Katherine's birth was so easy and psychedelic, so quick and exciting that I highly recommend second babies even if you had a difficult time with your first. With the birth of Patrick, my first baby, I had gained the reputation for being one of the worst baby-havers on the Farm.

One morning I had some irregular lower stomach twinges, but Leigh talked me into letting him go to an appointment he had in a town twenty miles away. I figured maybe they would go away so I went to work sweeping and cleaning. But they kept coming around. I laid down in the afternoon and noticed they were getting stronger. So I went to call the midwives but our phone was dead and I had to go to a neighbor's to call. On the way home I hugged the big old oak trees along the path with each psychedelic rush. Kathryn arrived soon and determined that I was fully dilated already, so we had to hustle to get ready. Then she quietly held my hand and calmed all my fears about whether I was going to do it right. She said I was doing fine and it was okay to push if I felt like it. I did.

From my first birthing I had learned what kind of thoughts made it work and I felt so good that all I could think was what a miracle it is to be alive, and how much I loved my baby and everybody, and that I wanted to make it quick and easy for the baby to come out.

I thought of Leigh too. One of my greatest fears seemed to be happening, that he'd be gone when I had the baby. But it didn't feel good to be attached (tight throat). So I just loved all these lovely ladies who were helping me out—Kathryn and Mary—instead.

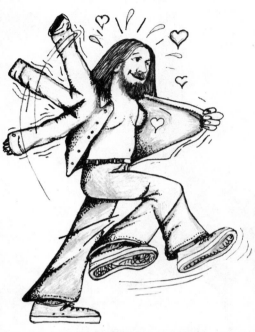

We had just given up hope that Leigh would arrive before the baby when he threw open the door, took off his coat and shirt, and jumped on the bed. (My hero!) We kissed and I was rushing and pushing the baby. I could feel the head moving down the birth canal and it felt so good to push in tune with these strong tantric rushes. They were the strongest I'd ever felt. It took only about two pushes to get the head out. It wasn't hard at all. It was fun.

She was fat and rosy and we all got very high. (And we loved the midwives so much we named her Katherine Mary.)

Next time I plan to call the midwives whether I think it's heavy or not.

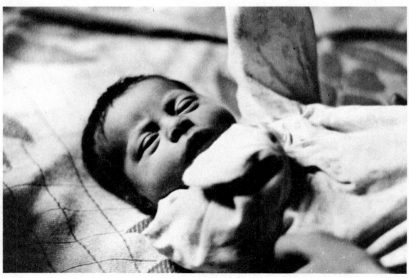

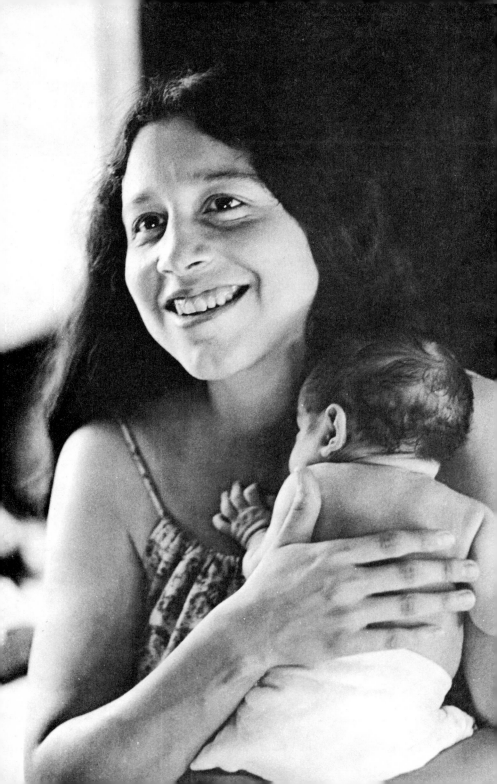

Sasha

ee: Sunday morning I woke up feeling good. My head was clear, my body felt psychedelic and Holy.

During Services I kept having slight menstrual cramp-like feelings. I'd felt them every so often in the past few weeks, so I thought of them as "Previews to the coming attraction." I supposedly wasn't due for another month.

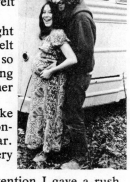

After I got home, I kept having those cramp-like feelings until I had to admit they were really contractions and they were getting strong and regular. I lay down and timed the rushes . . . they were every five minutes.

As I was timing them, I realized the more attention I gave a rush, the stronger it was. I also felt that the initial response I would have to a rush was to tighten up in the backs of my legs and my bottom. I knew from the birth of my first kid that getting tight slowed everything down and made it no fun. So I immediately made an inner vow to stay as loose as possible, especially from my waist down. As soon as I thought that vow, I felt my body relax and I had a good strong rush. It made me very happy to remember that I was in control of my body, not my body in control of me. I giggled thinking of that old saying, "Mind over matter."

I went into the living room to let Alan know my rushes were regular. We laughed and were having a good time when Mary Louise, a friend and midwife, drove down the road. As she was coming back up the road, I asked Alan to tell her I was having regular rushes. Alan and I were still being nonchalant about it all—there was a part of me that just wasn't believing it was happening.

I was glad to see Mary Louise and curious to know what she'd find out after checking me. As she felt my dilation, I felt open and very strong. She pronounced with a smile that I was three and a half centimeters dilated—well started. Knowing I was that much dilated made me start rushing even more. I had no desire to lay down at this point, even though during a rush I'd have to hold on to something. I was involved in packing up clothes and a few other things for Melissa, our daughter, who was going to spend a week with another family.

It felt good to be doing something while starting my rushes. During my first birthing I'd really made it harder and longer by thinking it had to be a certain way—thinking I had to lay down and have my man and the midwives rub me. It was not until I started massaging Alan

Lee and Sasha

that I realized . . . that was the key—I had to open up and put out the energy.

After Mary Louise had checked my dilation, she called two other ladies to come help. They arrived pretty quickly with sterile packs and a baby scale. They set up the instruments and baby preparations and soon had me on a chamber-pot after an enema. It felt like the enema allowed more room inside for the baby to move down. It sure brought on stronger rushes.

The midwives had arranged a bunch of pillows for me to be propped up on. Alan was on one side of me and Cynthia on the other. As the energy mounted, I'd hold their hands and pull. This channeled a lot of energy out my arms and chest and allowed my bottom to stay loose.

In between rushes, Alan and I made out and felt a whole lot of love for each other. We were glad to be having a good time. The vision was very clear and psychedelic. *Time became suspended—eternal. There was an ageless feeling about everything that was happening.* I felt connected with every woman who had ever had a child, connected with all of mankind.

The contractions increased in intensity until my cervix was near to fully dilated. Mary Louise suggested I try bearing down on the next rush, while she was feeling the dilation. I pushed, but didn't open any further, so Mary Louise said I should wait through the next couple of rushes.

My face tingled, my nose was numb, and my eyes felt like they were crossing. *It was feeling very ethereal . . . felt like I was going to float away.* All the energy was down moving the baby out.

Mary Louise said to expand my belly* during my next rushes. Doing so, I could feel my puss opening up more with each rush. Blowing out my belly seemed to open up my whole pelvic area.

Then it got to the point where I felt that all I could do was push. I told Mary Louise and she said I could try pushing again. Next rush I took a deep breath and pushed with all my might. I could feel the head coming through the birth canal. It felt absolutely fantastic to be exerting all I could to push the baby out.

The baby's head was crowning when Mary Louise told me to stop and start panting. To put the brakes on at this point was like doing a couple of back-flips in the middle of running. I gathered all my strength to stop from pushing. Kay Marie got my attention and helped ground me by having me slow down my breathing . . . what I experienced was like a reversal of the flow of energy—it felt like a fountain erupted from the top of my head and shot out from there and my face.

Mary Louise, meanwhile, had slowed the baby's head from coming out with one hand. Then she told me I could push, and out came the baby's head. She had me pant while she checked around the neck for the cord. Next rush out came Sasha hollering until she was bright red!

---

*This is a standard yogic breathing exercise in which the mother breathes inward as deeply as she can, expanding her abdomen and relaxing her muscles.

This was Cynthia's first birthing. She wrote down some of her comments:

My butt felt loose the moment I walked into the room. Cara dropped by to check things out and she felt good to me—very heavy and strong and motherly. Several times I flashed on my mother when I looked over at Mary Louise, too. After Kay Marie gave Lee an enema, she sat on the pot and rushed and looked like she was really having a good time. You could tell it felt really good. She and Alan kept it feeling very nice. Alan would say something funny and we'd all laugh.

Only a few hours after we arrived, Lee was ready to push. We were all amazed at how fast and easy everything had been so far. Lee was looking forward to having this kid and I think her kid was just as eager to come out. Sometimes it looked as if her kid was pushing on her ribs when she rushed. Mary Louise had Lee push once and her baby's head popped out. It changed color from white to purple and turned around and opened its eyes and looked at me. She was totally right there all the time. One more push and out came a strong, healthy baby girl. After Kay Marie cleaned her up, I held her for a while while Mary Louise gave Lee a couple of stitches. I was really grateful to have been able to be at this birthing.

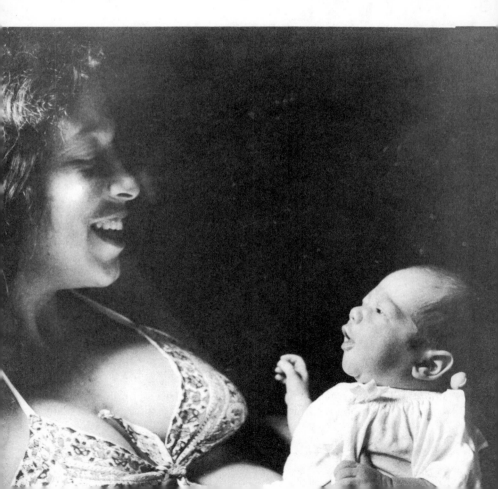

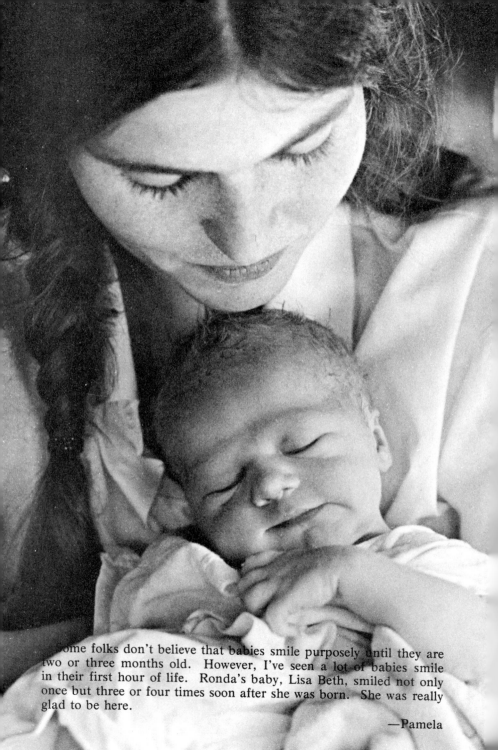

Some folks don't believe that babies smile purposely until they are two or three months old. However, I've seen a lot of babies smile in their first hour of life. Ronda's baby, Lisa Beth, smiled not only once but three or four times soon after she was born. She was really glad to be here.

—Pamela

Melina Marie

Janet: Edward and I took a walk down to Joseph and Mary Louise's the night before we had Melina Marie. It was three weeks past my due date, and I was very big. It kept feeling more psychedelic as the baby grew and that night I felt very calm and high, but I kept feeling a cramp and after a while Mary Louise said she'd check me before we left.

We all settled down in the living room and we were feeling incredible energy—lots of love. Later she found I was one centimeter dilated and she said I might be starting.

We walked home and went to bed knowing that it would be good to sleep. Through the night my belly would cramp and Edward would grab it and it would feel better. I had decided that I wouldn't complain at my birthing because I knew where it was at about that, but by morning I started feeling like someone hadn't told me it would feel like this.

At six in the morning I was having rushes every five minutes. Then my water bag broke. It was a warm loosening, watery feeling. When we called Mary Louise she said that was great, and keep doing whatever brought the rushes on. I felt like, "Are you kidding?" I was still trying to get comfortable with the feeling.

Mary Louise came. She was getting stuff together and I was rushing and started noticing that when I looked in her eyes through a rush I got some strength to feel it as a force that was intelligent and courageous. I noticed that when I looked at Edward through one I felt it as a pain. When I asked her about that, she said that it was because she wasn't believing that it was painful and that I needed to keep my sense of humor and be nice to Edward. That clicked and with the next rush I laughed, and started laughing as they came.

That got the energy up higher and of course the rushes came on stronger. It was far out to keep on integrating each new level of it. This is a part of the birthing that I'm really looking forward to experiencing again just to see what it will be like when I do it again knowing about it already.

Edward: We'd found a spot in the middle of Janet's back by her waist, which, when I'd grab it, would whoosh a bunch of energy up her back. So we continued making out and playing around and got the knack of it to where we were riding the rushes like a surfer rides the waves. The energy would swell up and Janet's eyes would grow deeper until it seemed like I could look through them like peepholes, and see the vastness of the cosmos out beyond her pupils; *endless space.* I told her that, and she rushed, and smiled, and looked really beautiful.

Janet: Stephen and Ina May came in and I felt something about the

161

rites of passage as natives initiate their young to adulthood—that had a whole new meaning to me, this being the passage of my first kid. Another rush came and, as I looked at Edward, Stephen said, "Don't look so tragic, Janet," and I realized that I had slipped back into complaint. He pulled on my toes and told me that it would get a lot heavier. Wow! What an amazing trip it is having a kid! It totally blew away all my conceptions.

Edward: As the time approached for Janet to start pushing, we went back into the bedroom. By that time Carol had joined us, as well as my sister Lee, and there was an intense warm feeling of family. Janet and I just kept on with our end on top, while the midwives took care of keeping her bottom stretched and oiled. As Janet opened up further, it got to where we had to hold up just a little because the rushes were coming so fast. Then Mary Louise asked Janet to start pushing, and soon she was saying, "Harder," and Janet would push harder and Mary Louise would say, "A little harder," and Janet would push harder yet, with a mounting intensity, until I was astonished at the sheer effort. I'd never seen anybody work as hard before—her face would contort and turn red then sometimes purple, and her eyeballs would bulge until finally she looked like a psychedelic frog or something. She was beautiful. I understood more clearly what Stephen had meant by the phrase, "Great pure effort."

Janet: We kept passing the energy between us, and Mary Louise knelt near my legs and Carol and Edward were on either side of me. I'd rush and the energy would move up their spines and they'd arch their backs and straighten as they'd rush. When Mary Louise checked me again, she said I could start pushing. That was great. I really wanted to get this baby out now—no matter how strong the rushes got or how long it took.

Edward: I'd occasionally take a look down to see how our baby was doing until I noticed what appeared to be a little head with a slippery tuft of black hair on it. Finally on one push, out came Melina's head, and I was face to face with a good-sized head, not little as I'd thought, for the little part I'd seen was actually just a scooched up part that had kind of bulged out like a bouffant yarmulke, like a two-storey head so it could fit through the bones.

Janet: Her head popped out and I panted while Mary Louise unwound the cord on her head and when I pushed again she popped out. There was a warm, rubbery, alive, slippery little being on the other end of this cord still inside of me.

Edward: On the next rush, whoosh, she was out and into Mary Louise's hands—all wet and covered with meconium, and scrunched up with folds of flesh, blue-colored, like in those Hindu posters of Krishna. She didn't start up right away, so we all took to coaxing her along with shouts of encouragement. "C'mon, baby, let's hear you now," and for a little bit all she'd respond with was opening her eyes, looking around at the new world around her. Mary Louise worked on her for a while; we continued calling to her, "C'mon, let's hear you." Finally Melina let loose with a strong full cry, and we all laughed, almost cried, and quietly in my heart I felt a deep wordless gratitude. I said, "Welcome aboard, baby, welcome aboard." As she cried, she breathed; and as she breathed, a pink flush of life started spreading from her heart out to the rest of her. I sat watching, astonished and amazed, and must have had my jaw drooping because Mary Louise looked at me and chuckled, "You look absolutely mind-blown, Edward." I laughed, closed my mouth and looked at Janet full of love and gratitude for the blessing that the whole thing was, and for the grace with which Melina had come to us.

Janet: It was a bright, early spring afternoon. All the dogwoods were in vibrant white blossoms. We had a girl. She looked like an old Aztec. She was beautiful. We were stoned and grateful she was here.

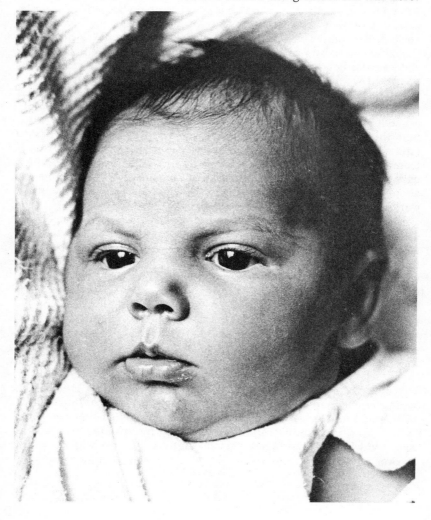

Sarah's Birthing

Cara: Betsy's rushes didn't get strong until she was about eight centimeters dilated. Betsy is a big, warm lady who was really sweet to everyone. A few times I've delivered ladies who are real nice to the midwives but snappy to their husband, or who are all smiles on the surface but who are subtly complaining. But Betsy was truly nice. We could tell she really loved her baby.

We dozed on and off—Betsy was making slow but sure progress. When her rushes got strong, we all woke up to help her out. I checked her and she was almost fully dilated. She stayed like that a long time. After a while, I helped her cervix back over the baby's head with sterile gloves, and she was ready to push the baby out. Each time she pushed, we could see a little more thick, dark hair. We had been checking the baby's heartbeat all along—a good, steady ticker. We checked the heartbeat again when she was pushing, and the baby's heartbeat sounded definitely slower, around 94 beats per minute.

I decided to call Ina May. She called our doctor who said that if we had any doubts about how the baby was to get Betsy in to the hospital, a good half-hour's drive away. Ina May and Stephen felt like the best thing to do was to get the baby out. They arrived minutes later. It was really a psychedelic experience to watch them work as a team to deliver the baby. Stephen got right up beside Betsy and just gave her a bunch of energy and really appreciated her. We could see about a silver dollar's worth of baby head down in Betsy's puss, working its way out.

At that point, stretching the lady's puss usually helps her open up and make more room for the baby to come out. But Ina May put her whole hand over Betsy's puss and her touch was so tantric and relaxing that Betsy could just open up behind that. The baby's heartbeat was still some slow but was real steady and the color of the baby's head was good.

At one point, Stephen helped Betsy's husband John to realize that he really loved Betsy and cared about her and wanted to help her out, but that he could be more relaxed and not so formal. That had been subtle but was so true that when Stephen said it and John understood it, we could all feel our bottoms open up and the baby moved down more.

We were all enjoying being with Betsy. Her family is Dutch and sometimes her expressions seemed almost old-fashioned but just right. "Oh, I do want to see you, beautiful little baby." One time she said, "Oh, this is just grand!" Stephen and all of us just loved how sweet she was, and what nice noises she was making. I fell in love with everyone all over again.

The baby's head eased out, and the cord was wrapped around her neck, but was loose enough that Ina May let it be, and the baby slid out, showing us a nice seven pound, fourteen ounce girl.

It was really good to see her and she started real nice. She worked real good—all systems go. Betsy didn't tear at all, which I know was because of such good feeling vibrations. Ina May cleaned Betsy up and she and Stephen said goodbye and left. I felt so grateful to be able to see them deliver a baby together; it felt good and helped Betsy out so much.

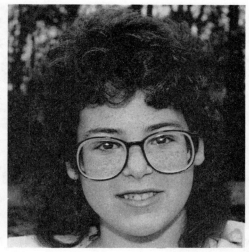

Sarah at 14.

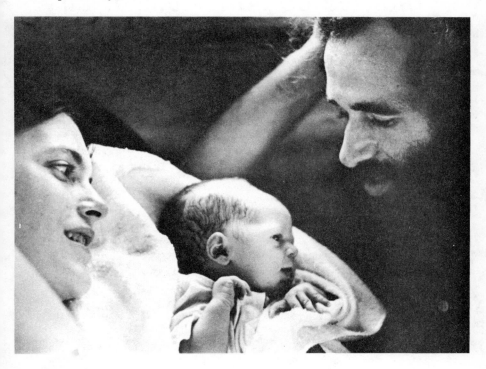

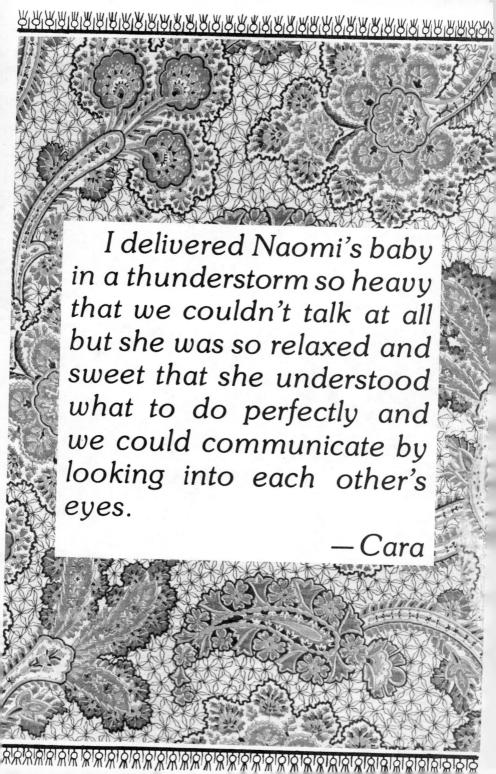

I delivered Naomi's baby in a thunderstorm so heavy that we couldn't talk at all but she was so relaxed and sweet that she understood what to do perfectly and we could communicate by looking into each other's eyes.

— Cara

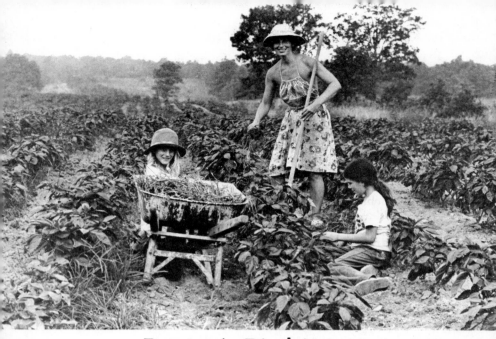

Benno's Birthing

Marion: Benno borning on a summer morning. I remember bits here and there. Waking up early, walking up the path to the outhouse—lying back down next to sleeping Alexander—suddenly a very intense sensation—tightening—took me away somewhere dark with a pinpoint of light—when coming out of it, thought came with, "I've got to get myself together if this ain't even the real thing. Wow!" So somewhere around then Alexander and the boys woke up. They started getting ready for workday. Made oatmeal. I did nothing, just sat in bed. Occasionally another rush—not so intense—I kept looking at the trees' leaves. I touched my fingers to my puss and they had blood on them. Could it be? I told Alexander. He hesitated to believe. It's something to believe! He and the boys continued to get ready to go, eating oatmeal. I felt a flash of angry complaint—I just realized that the two are the same and the next thought was, "Don't keep doing *that* one," and didn't. I put my attention out to the leaves and everything was fine. After a couple more rushes, uneven in interlude, thighs shaking—I convinced Alexander to stay home, he got all excited and he went off to call for a midwife. He came back saying someone was coming and then he got the kids ready to go. I felt a reluctance to send them away—it felt too automatic—but I did anyway. I felt how much I loved them.

Alexander was sitting beside me rubbing my back and holding my hand. I felt glad he was with me. A couple more unevenly spaced rushes, thighs shaking—Cara comes walking down the path with her baby under her arm. I moved to a different position and she told me to keep my hips down flat and to not wriggle around, which I kept trying to do. She examined me with a sterile rubber glove and couldn't find my cervix. Mary Louise came just around then—she had ridden her bike—and checking it together they figured that my cervix was fully dilated. Wow! Kathryn came. Alexander was sent off next door to call Ina May and let her know. He came back and said she was coming. Sometime in there, after trying not to push, I said I had to, so they said okay, go ahead, and I started having deep sounds coming out and they said okay. The upper part of my tube felt open. I started losing control of my legs—when I was told to hold them I needed help getting my legs up to my arms. I think I once said "help" and got it right away. I felt really grateful—Kathryn and Alexander each on a side. (Borderline note—I have thought since then that when I was aware of doing it, I was in transition stage already.) Once I felt like wanting everything to stop for a moment. Saw the absurdity of that and dropped it. Ina May came and standing there gave me instructions for the last couple of rushes.

Out he came and then shoulders and then I saw him—between my thighs—all blue and pink and white coating and purple with a deep scowl between his eyebrows and quivering deep red lips—lower lip stuck out and down. He felt and looked immense. My vision had gone through a change and he took up the whole. I had no feelings or thoughts that I can recall other than everything was intense and happening and amusing and amazing and oh oh—he was taken to be taken care of and checked and the placenta came out and they saw I had torn some when his shoulders had come out. Ina May instructed and helped Cara stitch me together. I lay there feeling wonderful and kissed Alexander with everything all. Benno came out in Mary Louise's arms. She and I connected very strong right in there. Benno was so into sucking that he'd sucked the rubber syringe while Mary Louise was suctioning out his mouth. We put him on tit and he sucked. And continued to do so for two and a half hours. Ina May showed me some exercises to get my stomach back in shape. Everything felt very relaxed and it was sunny and breezy and warm. After the ladies left we just stayed there looking. He slept for an hour and then sucked for another three hours. Then he slept for a long time—almost through the next day. I was grateful for such a beginning with him.

Marion and Benno

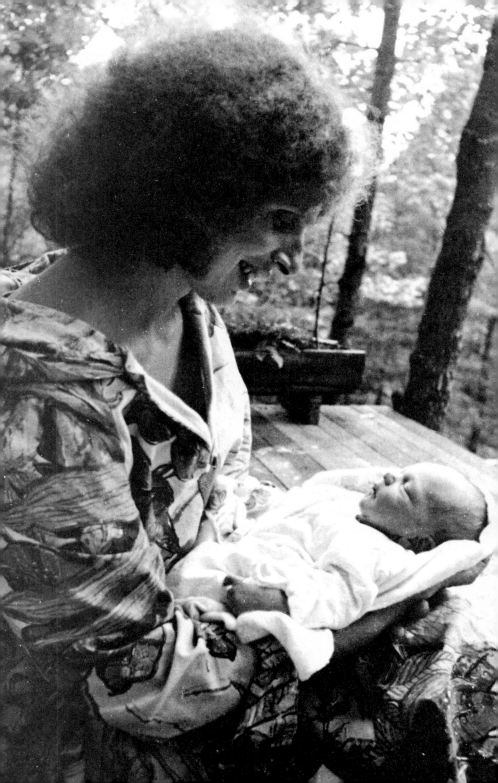

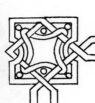

Every once in a while there is a baby who is hard to start. Teresa's second baby, Jessica, was like that. When she finally took her first breath and her cheeks began to get a pretty rose color in them, it was one of the nicest things I'd ever seen. The room got all glowy and I really felt God's presence and that He was helping out.

— Pamela

Jessica's birth was the third Farm birth I'd been at. The baby came out and was very pale, sort of grey-blue. The thing that looked different from the other babies I'd seen was that the baby was very floppy. She didn't seem to inhabit her body at all. I hadn't seen enough birthings yet to know if this was considered normal, but it felt very heavy. Pamela breathed into the baby and gave her heart massage. After about two or three minutes, we felt the first faint response from the baby. After that, with Pamela stroking and handling her, the baby came on and on and on, getting pink and very much alive. Thank God. It was a prayerful moment. I felt so lucky it went the way it did.

— Mary

Avram's Birthing

Cara: The fastest birthing I ever attended took a minute and a half. Amy's labor with her first baby had lasted only half an hour, so we were prepared for some fast action.

Amy called me, saying she was having no labor but felt in a condition of heightened awareness similar to what she'd experienced when she had her first baby. Not waiting for any more information, Kathryn and I jumped into the truck and tore down the road toward Amy's place. At the same time Michael, my husband, rushed Amy's husband down from the tractor barn. As soon as we arrived, Amy's water bag broke and the baby started coming out. I had Amy lie down, washed my hands and delivered her nine pound son. The whole thing took about a minute and a half. The baby's face was a bit bruised from such a fast passage, but he was fine.

It's birthings like Amy's that really keep the midwives on their toes.

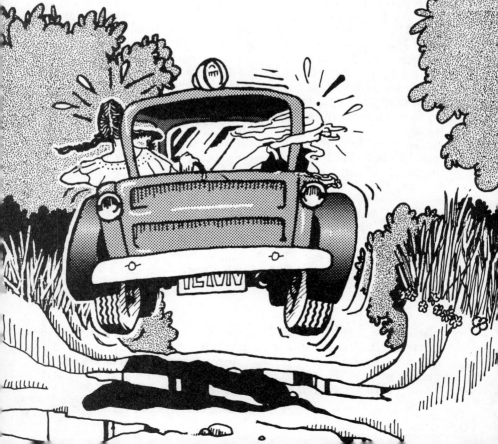

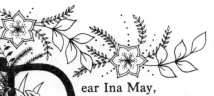

ear Ina May,

I wanted to tell folks about our baby that didn't make it because I learned that you can keep it together even when you think you can't, and Paul and I learned to love each other more.

I was seven and a half months pregnant and one day the baby stopped moving and I could feel the life go out. I had to go to the hospital to have her delivered because there is danger of infection and hemorrhage in a case like this. The hospital folks wouldn't let Paul be with me, but they did let Mary, who is a midwife and who lived next door to us. I am really grateful they let Mary be with me because she just tripped with me the whole time and kept me together. When I would have a rush, she would look straight at me or hold my hand and her whole face would go pure and she would just give me her very best one, and all her energy to help me through. It would get really high and I would see white light around her face.

Sometimes I would say something about the cold bedpan or how long the rushes were and she would say, "That sounds a little complainy to me," and I could see it and stop doing it. It was not time for complaining. The only thing to do was keep it as high as we could. Other times I would think something during a rush and Mary would say, "How was that?" and I'd say, "Well...it hurt!" and she would say, "Oh, I know, when I was having Ernest..." and tell me how to handle the rushes better. Sometimes when the rushes were real long and intense and I would be hanging on to Mary's hands and looking at her so hard, it would feel really dramatic and we would both crack up laughing.

Once I was fully dilated, the baby was really easy to push out. She came out fast. She had flipped over so many times inside me that her umbilicai cord had got twisted up into three kinks, and the doctor figured that this had cut off the circulation between me and her. She was really beautiful. I thought that when they die inside you like that, their body and soul don't separate. She looked intact like that and really pure. Paul got to carry her home to the Farm to bury her and he said he could feel her good bones.

We loved her a lot even though she never made it to us. We learned to be nicer to each other and love each other more because to get to be alive at all is such a precious thing.

Love,
Cornelia

Paul: It was quite an experience for us—we were looking forward to and loving this baby a lot. I was sad that it happened, but I was glad it was nothing hereditary. We had to readjust for a while after that, because we were all geared up for a baby. I figured that how she died was a real freak accident and we'd get pregnant right away.

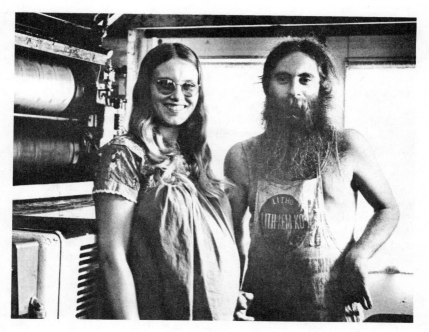

Cornelia and Paul

aul: Two months later, Cornelia was pregnant again. We were both really happy. The first few months we were feeling things like not wanting to get excited because you never would know what was going to happen; and we didn't want to be attached to having a kid. After a while, I noticed that the whole pregnancy felt different. Cornelia felt strong and healthy most of the time, and I just kept feeling better and better. As soon as Cornelia got past eight months, we both got really high and believed that this was really going to happen.

On Saturday, Cornelia started to have rushes and Cara came up to check her out. She was one and a half centimeters dilated. It started to get very psychedelic. After a while, her rushes stopped happening and we went to sleep. Sometimes when Cornelia would rush, I would get really tingly all over. It was really telepathic. Cornelia and I felt connected. After a few days, it seemed like nothing was happening, so I started going back to work, even though my interest was not really there. I kept expecting to hear from her any minute to come home. After a few weeks all the folks on the Farm (which had eight hundred folks then) would say, "Hey, did Cornelia do it yet?" It felt okay because I knew everyone was real anxious and excited about seeing this kid, after losing our last one.

173

I started noticing Cornelia looking a little sallow and asked her if she was worried about losing the baby. She said, "Yes," and started to cry. We talked it out and got feeling better. That thing seemed to trigger me off to being afraid that I'd have to keep Cornelia together, getting her straight for her birthing. Well, we went on like that for a few days. The vibrations started getting strained between us.

One day, Cara came over to me and said she noticed Cornelia looking really psychedelic and having a beautiful white aura around her and that I should give her more energy. Well, this surprised me. She said I should be a strong source for her and not lecture her on how to do it. Just give her a lot of love and encouragement and do whatever she said.

I walked into the printshop pretty amazed. I picked up the telephone and called Stephen. I told him what was happening and what Cara said. I said I wanted to do the right thing, and asked him if he could help me out. He said he'd noticed Cornelia looking really good and me looking a little paranoid and laid back. He said Cornelia was very high and thought she could have her baby any time. He suggested I take off from work for a few days and just smooch and be nice and we would have our kid.

I went home and told Cornelia and the rest of our household what had happened and started doing whatever I could to help out.

Cornelia: That afternoon I went to the clinic to see Dr. Williams supposedly about swollen ankles but when I got there Cara said, "Will you check out her baby?" I told him I was overdue and he listened to the heartbeat and tried to check the baby's position but he said he couldn't tell because my uterus was hard. I told him that was because it gave me rushes to have my stomach rubbed. He said, "Oh ho! Want to have this baby tonight?" And he started rubbing my stomach and did an internal exam and loosened my cervix with his fingers. He kept asking, "Does this hurt?" and I answered that it felt great because it opened me up and started so much energy flowing. He said, "You'll have a seven-and-a-half-pound boy the day after tomorrow."

That night I started having rushes. It was really exciting but I didn't wake Paul. I slept for a little while and woke up at sunrise and it was still happening. I was really happy. Finally, I woke Paul and told him and we stayed in bed and tried to laugh quietly so as not to wake up the other folks in the house. I went and took a bath and felt my stomach and thought about the name Zachary. I asked Paul how he liked it and he said, "Zachary Jacob."

Paul: A few hours later we called Cara. She came over and checked Cornelia. She was still one and a half centimeters dilated, was having strong rushes and it was for sure going to happen. We spent a while enjoying the rushes. After a while, Linda Lou came over—Cara had sent her over to help out. We all felt glad to see her. At one point, she said, "Why don't you hang out and smooch for a while," and left the room. We lay down and made out. The rushes started coming on stronger and Cornelia thought maybe Linda should come in. She had opened up to about four centimeters. We all thought that was great.

Cara came over. She felt real heavy. By this time, Cornelia was really into it. Cara told her when it would get intense to breathe deeply and relax.

Cornelia: I tried to clean up the kitchen but the rushes were too strong and I ended up just sitting on the couch cross-legged. My belly felt beautiful and round and I felt like one of those Buddhas. I kept laughing because the room was just rushing on the energy. I would watch my belly during a rush. It would strain down in a psychedelic ball, all streaked with blue and white and red with a brown stripe up the middle. Then Linda left us alone and we cuddled and Paul rubbed my stomach. The rushes were quite strong so Linda called Cara.

Cara felt really solid when she came in, like she could carry the responsibility for getting this new life out. She checked me and I got a strong rush and looked in her eyes and she looked back with that same look that Mary had had.

It felt good to hang onto Paul and have Linda rub my back. Paul suddenly looked strong as an ox to me. I would pull on his arms and look in his eyes, and when the rushes would peak, he could feel it and he'd smile or laugh. Once I got a rush that was much stronger than before and I said, "Cara, I don't think I can integrate this," and she was right there saying, "Breathe deep, slowly," and got me back in control. I got up on my knees one time for a rush and I roared like a lion, it felt so much like that Lion yoga position. We all laughed.

Sometimes the rushes were really intense and I'd get a little untogether. I just put my head in Paul's lap and shut my eyes. Cara was really nice, and she kept telling me it was okay and that I wasn't supposed to have any brains in my head, they were all in my bottom at this point. So I just kept talking to her during a rush and told her how it felt and she just told me exactly what to do. I kept looking around at her and Paul and Linda, and thinking, what an amazing experience.

Mary came in, and I barfed. Stephen and Ina May came and checked me out but I was still only about five centimeters, so she said to call her when it was time and she and Stephen left. Mary Louise came in and I barfed. Throwing up felt great.

It got to feel like pulling on Paul tightened me up instead of loosening me. After a while, Ina May called and said to don't pull on Paul, that we should just smooch and get it on, because the lovemaking energy was what would open me up. So the midwives left, which scared me a little. We ended up scrunched in a dark corner of the bed with me hanging on to Paul for dear life and mashing his mouth with my teeth. It was definitely not high. After two rushes of that, we called Cara and asked her what to do. She said that usually they have the lady come on strong to her old man but in our case maybe I should just lie back and have Paul lay it on me. He was kissing my neck and hugging me and doing everything he could to help me out and give me some energy. It was great. It seemed like only a few rushes and Cara said I was enough dilated for her to burst my water bag. We all cheered. She popped it and I barfed and after the next rush I felt like I'd have to push. Cara said, "Wait just a few more rushes," and she called Ina May. She could feel the baby's head now and when she touched it she said, "Hey, baby," and we all felt telepathic with her and the baby.

Ina May came in with Stephen and Margaret. Stephen bent over me and looked into my face and there was a long heavy rush, real quiet and bright with his face all blue and white light and dazzly. He said, "Really stoned, huh?" Then he grabbed my belly and squeezed and pushed down. It scared me because even a light touch on my belly gave me such strong rushes, and then it opened me right up. I told him I couldn't let anyone else but him do that to me. I was still talking about it during the rushes and suddenly I realized that I was shouting and asked if that was okay to do if I kept my vibrations together, and Stephen said yes, if I didn't get too fast. Then he said, "Ina May, I'm going to let you do your thing now," and left.

I started to push hard on the baby to get him out. I made a lot of noise. I remember telling them that the louder I talked, the better I felt. Ina May was sitting right in front of me between my legs, and her face looked really clean. She talked to me in a real calm, even voice and showed me what to do with all that energy. One time she told me not to run all the energy out my mouth. Another time she said, "If you be really graceful, the baby will come out gracefully." That was a helpful one.

I could tell he was big, and it stung, but it was so good to feel him coming. I could push really hard and I could feel him move. My body felt really strong and I could push as hard as I wanted. Margaret had her arms around my shoulders and was whispering in my ear and Paul was saying excitedly that he could see the hair on his head. Ina May told me to go real slow to get his head out, and then it was out.

Paul: The head started squeezing through now and when it came through, I could hardly believe it. I thought I had seen this person before. Then I felt like it was me. Then he looked like my father. *It all felt timeless.* I knew it was a boy.

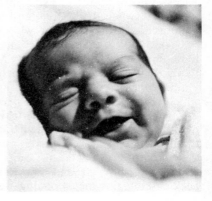

It took another two pushes, I think, to get the rest of him out. He just kind of popped out. I noticed I was quickly checking out if he had all the parts of his body. He started up real quick. I was so happy that he was alive and all there. The midwives took him out and weighed him and cleaned him up.

When they came back, he was wrapped in a blanket. He looked like an angel. He also looked just like my father. He weighed nine pounds, ten ounces. I held him while the midwives fixed up Cornelia. Everybody was real glad to see him.

Cornelia: Later me and Paul realized that now we weren't just married. We were related, we had a common relative: Zachary.

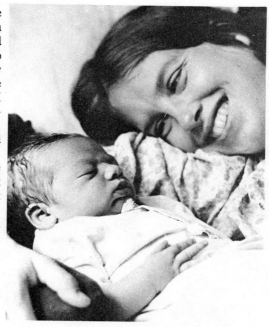

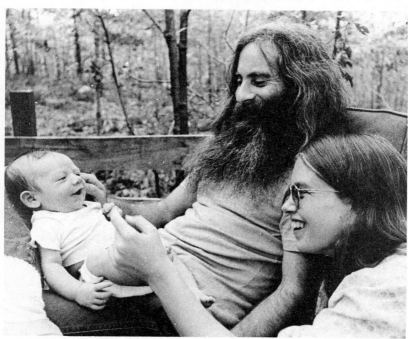

Zachary, Paul and Cornelia

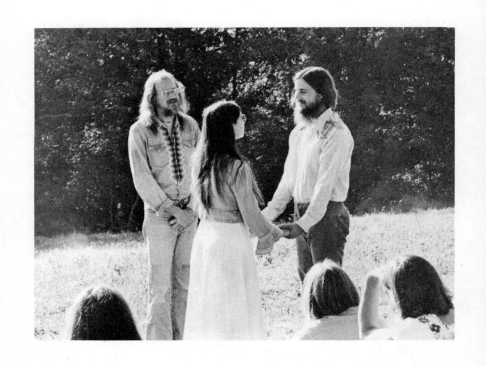

A lot of what being married is about is that your mate is your touch partner, your laboratory, and that's when you can really discover where touch is at, and go through the changes and discover where you're at.

—Stephen

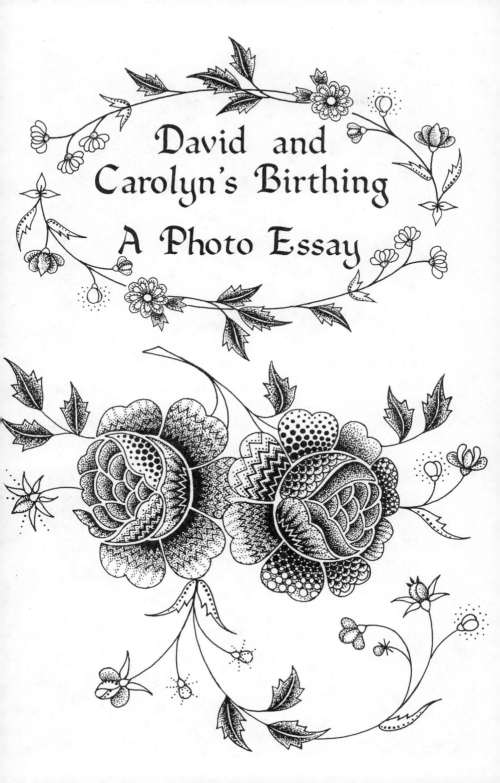

David and Carolyn's Birthing

A Photo Essay

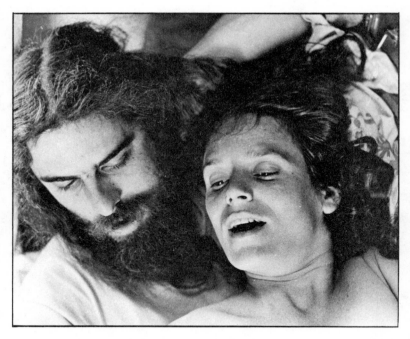

It was my first baby, after several years of trying to get pregnant. We had finally gotten unattached to having our own genetic kid, and applied to adopt an orphan. I conceived within the next seven to ten days.

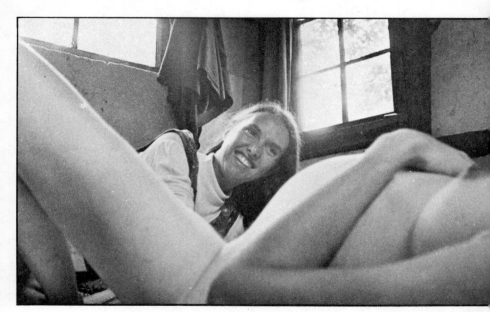

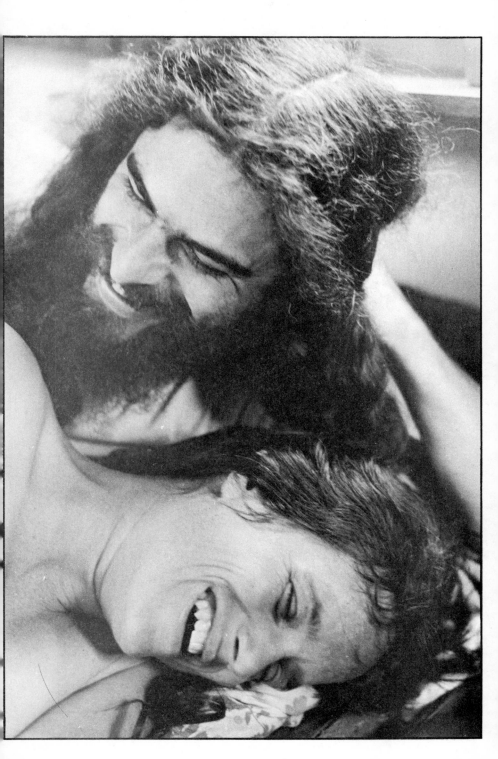

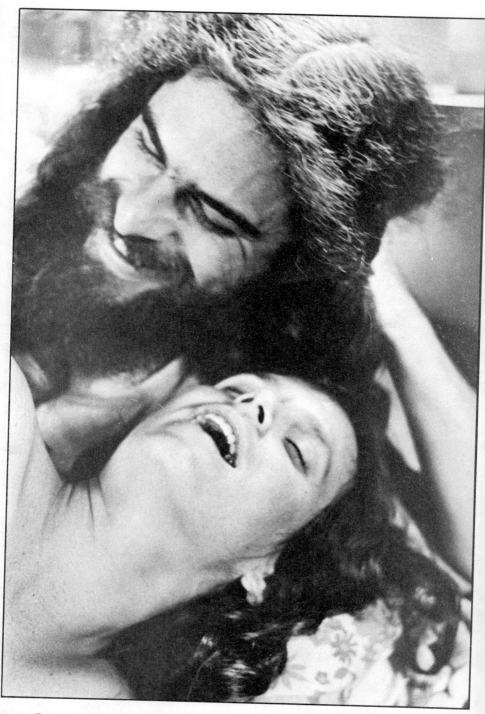

It was such a new feeling. It was as if we were newly-weds again or something.

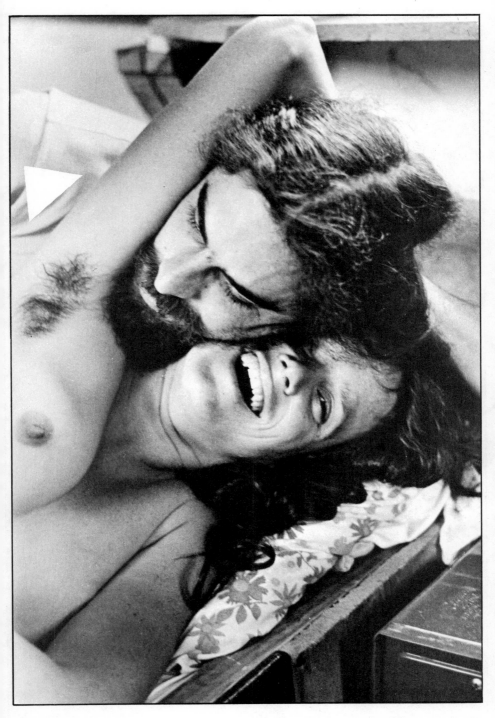

Everything was bright and sparkly; everybody's eyes were wide and intense.

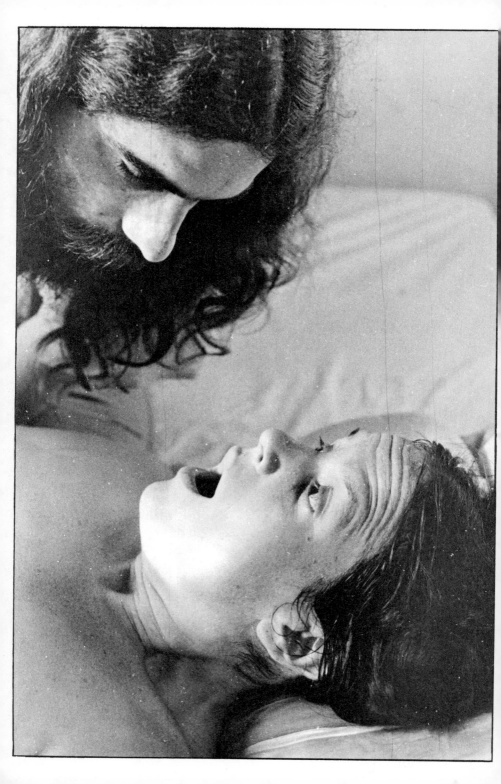

It does a man good to see his lady being brave while she has their baby . . . it inspires him.
— Ina May

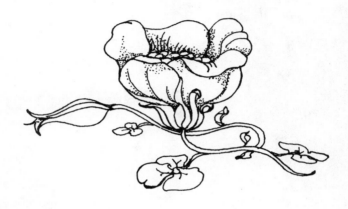

At each push it felt like I was pushing as far as I could, only to find out those weren't real limits and I could set my goals further ahead.

I really discovered I had to believe I could keep setting ahead my previous threshold of what I felt I could do and what I could handle. And the miracle was, that in believing in the leap of faith, it became real—I could push still harder and open further, and stretch more. I just had to concentrate everything on that total effort, and grunt and push. And sometimes I had to override brief temptations to interpret that powerful earthy push as pain instead of as life force, something greater than just me that I was only a part of. I guess you could say it was really down to the nitty-gritty.

Now it was the head moving out against the bones and tissue around the final opening, the baby's gateway to the outside world.

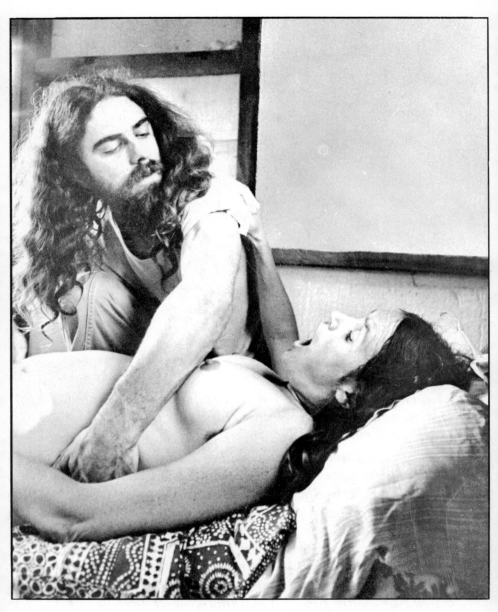

David was helping me integrate the muscular cramping sensations by rubbing me, especially at the small of the back. Cara showed me how to breathe with the rushes, pushing my belly out as I inhaled. I would look at David as a rush started to come on and then he would press under my back as I pushed my belly out. It was a far-out sort of see-saw effect, a tantric exercise, pushing and then relaxing, gliding on the rushes together.

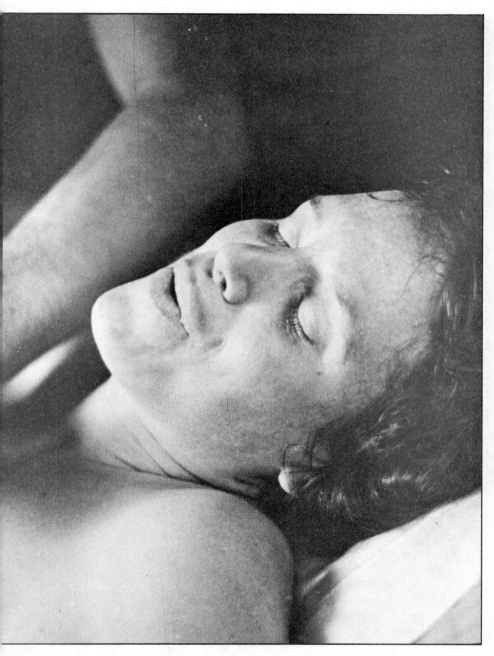

I flashed on all the mothers around the world who must be having babies at the same time, and felt telepathic with them. Then I felt it all go back in time to include all mothers. It just felt like giving birth is such a pure, eternal thing, always happening somewhere, always Holy.

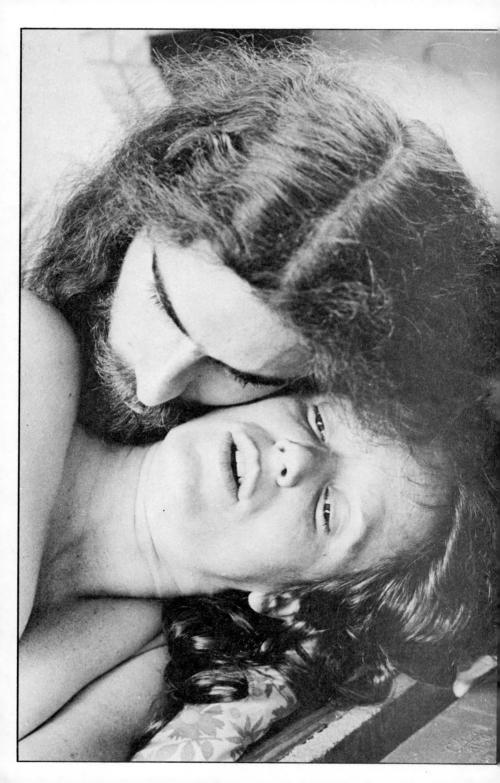

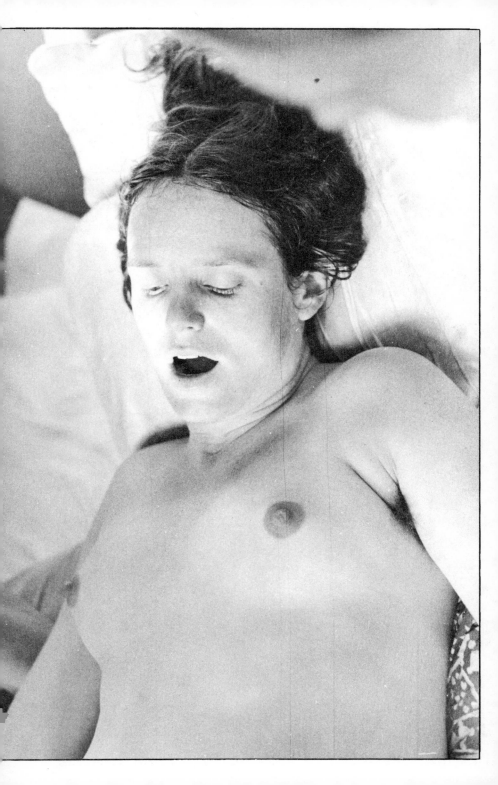

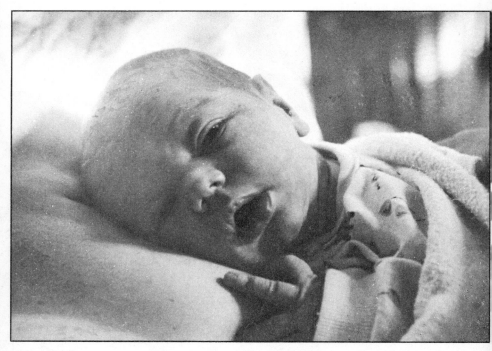

I got to look at him and hold him for a while. What a stoner, so fresh and new.

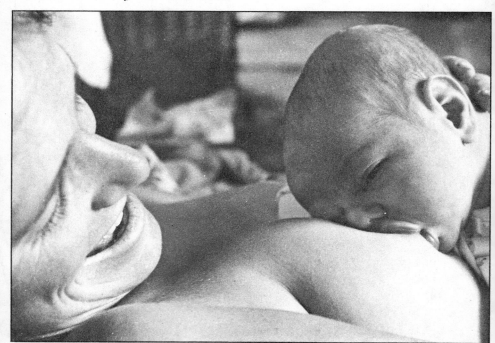

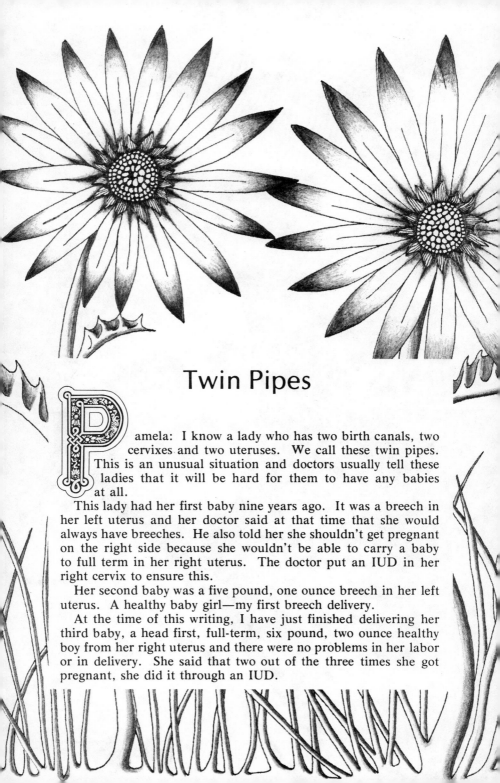

Twin Pipes

Pamela: I know a lady who has two birth canals, two cervixes and two uteruses. We call these twin pipes. This is an unusual situation and doctors usually tell these ladies that it will be hard for them to have any babies at all.

This lady had her first baby nine years ago. It was a breech in her left uterus and her doctor said at that time that she would always have breeches. He also told her she shouldn't get pregnant on the right side because she wouldn't be able to carry a baby to full term in her right uterus. The doctor put an IUD in her right cervix to ensure this.

Her second baby was a five pound, one ounce breech in her left uterus. A healthy baby girl—my first breech delivery.

At the time of this writing, I have just finished delivering her third baby, a head first, full-term, six pound, two ounce healthy boy from her right uterus and there were no problems in her labor or in delivery. She said that two out of the three times she got pregnant, she did it through an IUD.

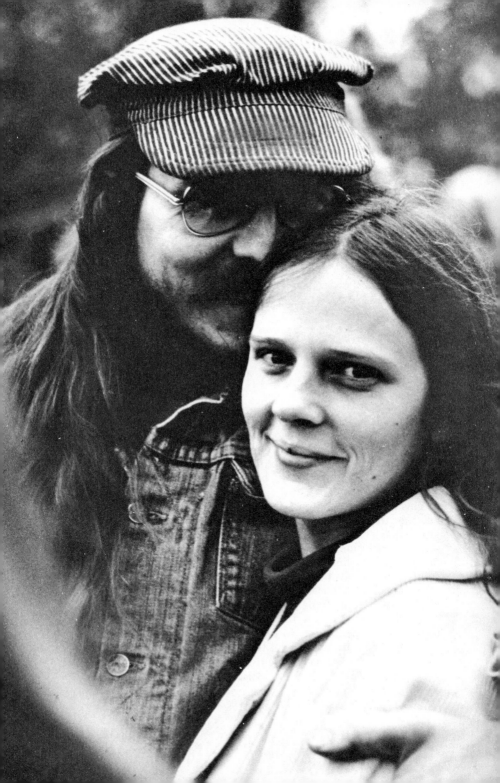

James Tells It Like It Was

ames: Abigail arrived about two weeks before we expected her. Judith and I were getting the Scenicruiser ready for a trip to Washington, D.C. [*James is a mechanic and maintains the bus that the band travels in.—Ina May*]

I had a lot to do to get ready and hadn't been thinking of the possibility of having a daughter at the time. I had just finished replacing a side window when Judith went to see Ina May about gas pains. She'd been having light pains like that most of the day. Earlier we'd gone swimming in the creek to relax and Judith got relaxed and sort of glowed. It was all very crisp and pretty around her.

So we went on home which was about the farthest out in the woods that anyone was living at the time. I did what I could to get things together—got water, cleaned up some, made sure the phone worked, stuff like that.

Well then things started happening, although Judith didn't think it was very much at first. She was rushing pretty regularly by now so I asked her what intervals and she said, "Oh, about four or five minutes," and I said, "I'm gonna call somebody," and she said, "No, not yet, don't bother anyone." I said, "What!" See, I'd seen the cowboy movies with birthings in them, so it was time to get a midwife. So I tried the phone which wouldn't work at all.* Then I hollered over to Wilbur's and no one was home, so I hollered to Leigh's and no one was home. By now I was getting OUT THE LOUDEST, NICEST HOLLERS I EVER MADE IN MY LIFE, so I tried yelling across the hollow to Philip and Ellen's or Kay Marie's place and no one answered, so I hollered back over to Wilbur's and Pamela answered. She was coming out to check on Judith. Well, we were happy we'd gotten some help with all this and very glad to see her. She checked Judith out and she said she was pretty far into it. So we let it roll along for a while and Stephen and Ina May came out. They weren't leaving for Washington for a few more hours. Stephen and Judith hugged and kissed. Then he left and Ina May stayed.

Well, we'd gotten so comfortable by now that Judith was starting to lose her steam. Ina May checked her out and said that somehow she'd gotten her cervix to contract and was actually regressing. Well, I got behind Judith and leaned her head on my chest and kind of cradled her and rubbed and kissed her and did stuff to turn her on again. We got her going again. And shortly she was rushing all kinds of pretty rushes and color changes. She changed colors in waves usually starting in heavy pink at her head and moving on down in about an eight-inch wide wave followed by a gold and a white, the pink one being very physically visible and the other being more like shining light around her.

*This happened in 1973, before we had reliable phones or C.B. radios.

She got into pushing and I even helped some but she said she'd rather I didn't help so I rubbed her and grabbed onto her tits very strongly and rubbed and squeezed pretty hard, until Abigail's head popped out. It wasn't long after that that she was all out and yowling mildly. Well I was blown out by now and felt very elated so Ina May told me to get myself back together so I did. It was all very much fun.

Ina May: I learned something new and interesting about what a lady can do with her body when I delivered James and Judith's baby, Abigail Rose. Judith looked very psychedelic when I arrived at her place after getting the word that her labor had started. Pamela was already there and had been coaching Judith about how to handle the early part of her labor. Her rushes were pretty close together and after she would have one, she'd look at me and raise her eyebrows, communicating, "Wow!" It was amazing to see her looking so mindblown because she usually looked like she had everything so covered. I checked her and found that her cervix was dilated about four centimeters. She wanted to know about how long it would take to get fully dilated, and I told her that this varied a lot—sometimes a lady would open up steadily, a little bit at a time, and take several hours, and another might dilate all the way in just a few rushes. It looked like Judith was glad to know it was that variable.

I noticed that whenever Judith would laugh at something, she'd have a very good rush right afterward, which would dilate her cervix a bunch more. So we all sat around and had a good time talking with each other, and after a few more rushes I checked Judith again and found that she was fully dilated and ready to push the baby out. I was very excited about her dilating so quickly and easily, partly because the energy was so high from her opening up like that and also because it looked like I was going to get to catch the baby (I was scheduled to leave for Washington, D.C. in about three hours, and I hadn't really expected to see the baby before leaving).

Judith, though, on hearing that she was fully dilated, became very sober, very serious. If someone said something funny, she was the only one who didn't laugh. She didn't seem upset at all, just serious. She coughed once, a shallow, polite little cough that obviously didn't get anything done. By this time I was getting curious as to what was going on, as we had just been so stoned and now there didn't seem to be much happening. So I put on another sterile glove and once again checked Judith's dilation. She was only four centimeters dilated! I was amazed. I had never known before that a lady could go backwards and undilate herself. When Judith heard what she had done, she admitted that she had been worried that the labor had been coming on so fast that it was getting out of control. I told her that it was supposed to feel like that and that she shouldn't hold back—that if I needed her to slow down I would tell her how to put on the brakes. She relaxed and in one or two more rushes she was fully dilated again and after a few good pushes, Abigail was born, a bald, pink, tender, young thing. We were all amazed and happy to see her.

Judith: It was as loose and open, Holy and pure, as it had been intense a minute before. I felt telepathic with all mothers before me and knew that we were one thing, all come to that same consciousness. I felt like I learned what trying is and what it is to put out all the energy you've got. It felt like such a new thing to push against something with all my strength. It made me feel strong and healthy and like I had a new place to work from.

James and Abigail and me felt like one thing, and I understood what Stephen said about bringing the sacrament of birth back to the family. I felt blessed to be home and with folks I loved and trusted.

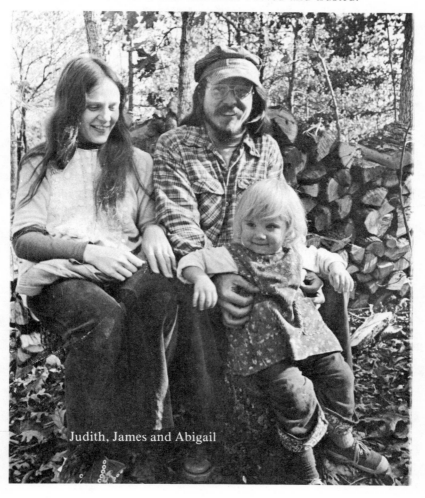

Judith, James and Abigail

Angus Luigi

Mildred: I started having rushes down low after coming home from Services. They were stronger than usual and five minutes apart, but I could still sleep, so Michael and I lay down for a nap.

My friend Mary Jane called and said she was coming over to visit. Michael and I thought that we'd stay in bed, but when she got here she walked in saying how she'd made a baby blanket for me, and I got right up. I thought I'd like to check with a midwife and found out that Mary Louise was at the laundry. Michael and I went up there, she checked me, and I was three and a half centimeters and doing it. It was very exciting.

Mary Louise came around six o'clock. As the rushes got stronger, I found lying on my side most comfortable. Michael was at my left side the whole time. I would tell Mary Louise how it felt and she would tell me what to do. Carol would rub my back and it felt like waves going down my back. At one point I had a rush that felt like a lightning bolt. (I thought he felt like a boy then.)

When I had to push, it felt like he moved down two times. He was face up and it took about an hour to get him through the bones. I had real fast rushes. Every time Mary would take the heartbeat, it would come on. [*The heartbeat was somewhat harder to hear because the baby was face-up.—Mary*] It felt best with Mary Louise's hand just right there pulling and rubbing my puss. Mary Louise would tell me when to breathe and she would wiggle her mouth if mine was tight. Every time I pushed she would tell me what happened. I had to push with all my strength. Once he was past the bones and Mary Louise told me he wasn't going to slip back, I was relieved. A little bit longer and his head was out, pointed on top. Then his whole body was out and he was going, "Wahhh," and he was a boy and all together. Mary would just say, "Oh, how pretty," and gushed and cooed the whole time we could see anything. It was really nice energy. She felt like an angel just putting out nice motherly vibrations.

I really kept thinking the whole time that I was glad to be doing it at home with everyone there. If I would have been in the hospital, I wouldn't have had the slightest idea what to do or what was happening. Having folks rub me really helped it go as fast as it did. I liked having Angus next to me so we could check him out. I also like having Michael sleeping next to me.

Angus Luigi was born fast and easy. It was after he came out that was hard for us. Ina May will tell you about it.

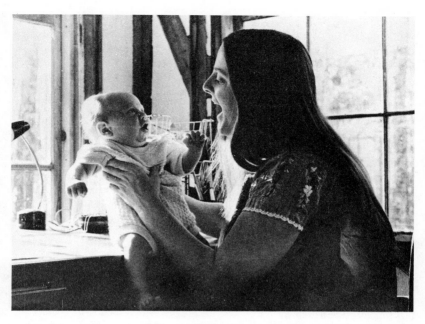

Ina May: Angus' mother, Mildred, was the financial director for the Farm at the time, one of the more high-pressure, demanding jobs one can have. She continued her job right up until the time she went into labor, took just two days off after the birth and then went back to work.

Angus began life plump and creamy. I went over to see Mildred and him when he was less than a day old. He was very juicy and beautiful and I understood why Mildred looked so pleased. I didn't see them again for a week, but the next time I did, Angus looked all different— more like an old man, and leaner. I saw him several different times during his first month, and each time he looked thinner—not unhealthy, but definitely smaller. Mildred looked more concerned each time, although she was trying not to worry. I tried to set her mind at ease about Angus. We sent Mildred to the doctor with Angus three times, and had lab tests done to figure out what was wrong. The doctor found nothing wrong but recommended that Mildred put the baby on formula. Margaret and I didn't feel that she needed to give up breast-feeding, but we did tell her she could supplement somewhat with formula if he would take it. Angus seemed basically healthy, but was almost four weeks old and still hadn't gained back his birth weight, which usually happens by ten days. Mildred's first baby, Angela, had started out plump and had stayed that way. Mildred had never had any problem getting her to eat. There was nothing wrong with Mildred's milk supply either; she was dripping milk every time I saw her. It was just that Angus preferred sleeping to eating.

197

Not only was Angus being puny—Mildred had other things on her mind as well. It rained several days in a row, keeping the Farm's carpenters from working, which meant Mildred wasn't getting a large percentage of the money that she was counting on.

When Angus was a little over a month old, Margaret and I conferenced to see if we could come up with any ideas about how to get Mildred and Angus to where they were doing it good. We both felt that Angus' failure to thrive had something to do with his being a boy. We talked with Stephen, who agreed, and said he thought that Mildred was inhibited about nursing Angus, where she hadn't been with her daughter.

The next day I happened to be with Mildred and Angus for a stretch of several hours. By now Angus looked like an invalid old man. His eyes were sunken and he had his lower lip drawn up so that you couldn't see it at all. His skin was mottled and sallow. It was shocking to see how much he had changed from the juicy kid he had been.

Margaret and I talked with Mildred for a couple of hours. I told her that we thought she was hung up about giving Angus any because he was a boy—that she didn't seem to think it was cool to let it feel good while she nursed him. She listened and thought it over. Meanwhile, Stephen had come by where we were sitting, heard what we were talking about and said,

"Look, Mildred, a little incest is cool up to about age twelve. Somebody's got to give him some."

Mildred cracked up laughing. It was just what she wanted to hear.

I told Mildred that instead of holding Angus out in front of her and looking at him with a concerned expression while trying to figure out how to get him to eat (which worried him), that she ought to smooch him and cuddle him—let him know that she found him attractive just as he was. She picked him up out of the car bed he was lying in. He looked like a sour old ascetic—resigned to a life of none. Then she planted a kiss on his cheek and looked back at him. Angus looked startled but interested. He looked out of his eyeholes. Mildred kissed him a couple more times, once on each cheek. Angus loved it. The vision got psychedelic and Angus turned from yellow to pink. Over a few seconds' time, he went from looking like an old man to looking his age. It was amazing.

Then I showed Mildred how to exercise him. Sometimes a mother will handle her new baby so delicately that she doesn't attract his attention to his body, with the result that his consciousness exists only in his head. Angus was like this, and when Mildred grabbed his ankles and "ran his legs" for a while, he looked amazed. Margaret and I left Mildred that day telling her she shouldn't weigh Angus for a week.

We didn't see Mildred and Angus for a couple of days after this. Then Margaret saw them and reported that Angus already looked fatter. He had round cheeks. When Mildred weighed him after a week had passed, Angus had gained three quarters of a pound—two ounces

198

a day. Everyone who knew Mildred, Michael and Angus relaxed along with Mildred.

Everyone said this was coincidental, but when Angus started gaining weight, it stopped raining, the carpenters were able to go back to work, and the money started coming in again.

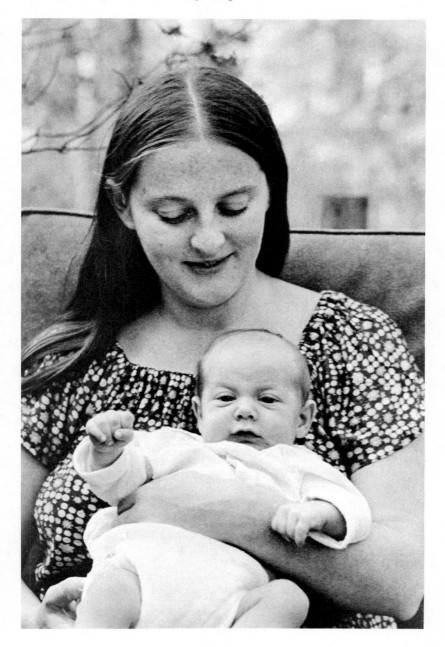

Alice's Birthing

Kathy: The first rushes felt like menstrual cramps. After about half an hour of these, I felt or heard my water bag break, and I stood up out of bed, so it would run on the floor. I laughed and felt relieved, because now that it was starting to happen, it was really different from all my weird anticipations of the past weeks. Doing it was much easier than thinking about it. Pamela and Cara came after what seemed like a good while—I had expected them to come running over in a *big* hurry. The first part of the labor was like heavy menstrual cramps, and I began to have thoughts like, "How long is this going to take, anyway?" At that point I couldn't remember that the baby was going to come out and that I really wanted to be there to see it. The rushes got stronger and my consciousness changed so that they were easier to integrate. I became unable to think about them or experience them as pain in a certain part of my body. I became more like an animal, like the cat having kittens that I watched one time. The rushes just grabbed my whole body and rolled me under. I felt like I was treading water, and that the midwives' voices were there—like the sky to look at—to remind me not to go all the way under. They said, "Stay connected," "Don't whimper," "Smile," "You're doing fine." Pretty soon we were through the cervix, and then we could push. I say "we" because Rupert gave me his body to do it with too.

I began to make all kinds of sounds when I was pushing out the baby. Rupert made some too. They were like pre-human sounds that I ordinarily couldn't make. The midwives were cheering us on, saying, "Push, push, push," "Good one," "So much of the head is showing," (showing me with their hands), "Some hair is sticking out," "This kid will be out in a few minutes." On the last push, I felt the baby come out; first a sting, because my skin tore (I didn't care, though), then bumpy, squish, run, slither—that was the baby's body. At this point Rupert started laughing and almost crying; the midwives were saying, "Big kid," "A girl," "Look at that hair," and then I heard Kathryn say, "On your own," when she cut the cord.

A few minutes later, they handed me the baby. Her eyes were wide open; she looked me in the eyes, held my finger in her fist, and opened and closed her mouth—an unmistakable "Hello" that made me forget what pain I had felt, laugh, and be grateful for getting to be there.

What I felt like I wanted to tell folks was that you don't have to be an unusually brave person to give birth without drugs. I'm something of a paddy-ass myself, but childbirth is a drug in itself. It changes your consciousness just like it stretches your skin. It all takes care of itself and just happens. And that "sacrament of birth" is a life and death tunnel that you go through with your husband that makes you both remember that you're one thing, in case you've forgotten. That seems like a good thing to be reminded of before you're entrusted with another life.

Rupert: Seeing Alice slide out, coughing and crying, was just a rush beyond words—a new, pure consciousness—I started laughing, it was so beautiful and funny and outrageous at the same time. I can't really imagine what it would be like waiting in a separate room to hear how your lady and kid were. Being there to help out is where it's at.

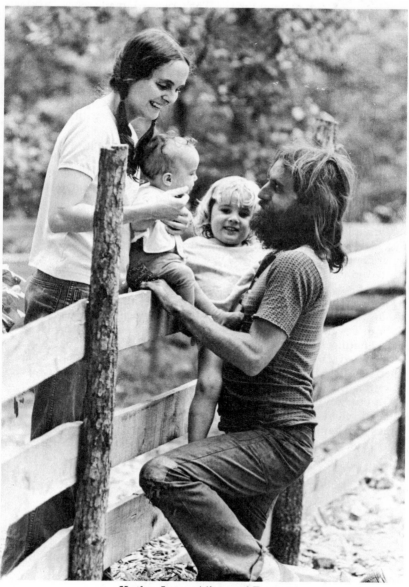

Kathy, Lucy, Alice and Rupert

A Telepathic Experience

inda Lou: I got called one night to go to Nina's birthing. Nina and I had known each other for about four and a half years. Her relationship with her husband, Richard, was about the best I'd seen it in a long time. They seemed really close to each other. Nina was very relaxed and beautiful when I got there. Denise and I got there early, so we were able to be with them for quite a while.

Nina and Richard were having a good time and it felt real good in their tent. Cara came when Nina was about half dilated. I've known Cara for a long time. She used to live in a bus near mine when we both had our baby girls a couple of weeks apart, three years before. We had both changed a lot since then, and it felt good to be with Cara again at such a Holy occasion.

We were all sitting on Nina's bed. Nina was looking outrageous—pink cheeks, dilated eyes—obviously bursting with energy. She would look one of us in the eyes and the room would get really bright and still, and you could see the energy in little waves like heat waves that come off the roof of a car on a hot day. [*Ina May: What Linda is describing here is called a "contact high."*]

Cara and I were sitting back-to-back on the end of Nina's bed. At first, I felt like I was leaning against her, like we were holding each other up. Then it started to feel like we had one back between us and I started to get heavy rushes going up my back which was Cara's back too. I thought, "Wow, I wonder if Cara is feeling this too." I felt really telepathic with Cara, but it wasn't the kind of thing you talk about while it's happening. So I just let it happen and figured I'd ask Cara afterwards if that had happened to her too or if I'd just been hallucinating.

Nina had a beautiful dark-haired boy, which really made her happy since she already had two girls. It was a smooth birthing because of how stoned it felt the whole time she was in labor.

On our way out to the truck, I asked Cara if it had gotten really stoned in there when our backs were touching. She said that the same things had happened to her and that she was going to ask me about it too. I really love Cara and Nina and I'll never forget that birthing.

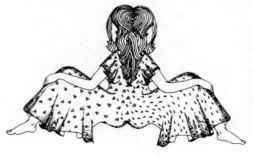

Paul Benjamin's Birthing

*I*na May: I have babies too—in fact, I had a baby in the midst of putting the first edition of this book together.

I started having some convincing-feeling rushes one night about three weeks before my due date. I knew my baby was big enough and done enough, so I was quite ready to go on ahead with it. My last baby had weighed nine pounds, fourteen and a half ounces and had been ten days early. After having a few consecutive rushes a few minutes apart, I told Stephen that I was going to have the baby pretty soon. He said, "I thought you were looking pretty psychedelic back there." We already had two kids together, but he hadn't been able to be at either of these birthings. It was about ten o'clock at night and we had all had a long day, so Stephen and I agreed that it would be nice to get a few hours' sleep before I started getting really serious about having my kid. That felt nice to me because then I really knew it was okay for me to take my time—which of course I would do anyway. Stephen had been telling me that I was prowling around the house like a mother cat looking for a place to have my litter. He kept telling me that I could do it any time, that I could have my kittens in his dresser drawer if I wanted to; which I thought was a funny thing for him to say to me. But I was glad he was so accommodating.

So we went to bed. I was pretty excited, knowing that I was really on that train and was actually going to see our kid soon. I was pretty sure though that I could sleep, at least for a little while. We both slept all night. Whenever we would roll over, I would be aware that I was still having light rushes quite regularly.

In the morning we woke up early to have a baby. We talked about whether it was a boy or a girl—Stephen had dreamed that the baby was born and that it was a girl, but he didn't seem to believe the dream. He had already said a few months back that this baby felt like another boy, and I kind of felt that way too.

After a few minutes of being awake I had a couple of rushes that began to remind me of what it felt like to have a baby—that it's heavy every time, no matter how many times you've done it. I was pretty sure after these two rushes that my cervix was open a little. We called Mary Louise to tell her that my labor had started. Stephen was going to deliver the baby, but we both wanted to have Mary Louise there too. My good buddies Margaret and Louise were already with me, helping me get nested and getting my three other kids settled.

Mary Louise arrived about fifteen minutes later with a big grin on her face, her birthing bag in one hand and a sterile pack in the other. She checked my dilation. "Yup, you're going to have a kid. You're four centimeters dilated," she said. My rushes were pretty mild but very psychedelic and I could tell that it would be a few hours before the baby happened. I have always taken at least twelve hours to give birth.

I told Stephen that it would be all right with me if he went out on the Farm for a while to do some business while I was still in the early part of my trip. Us ladies were having a nice time with each other, and I thought it would be nice if he could get out on the Farm and see what was going on.

I spent the next several hours having rushes, writing letters and talking with Margaret, Louise and Mary Louise about the kind of stuff we thought ought to be in this book. Mary Louise read some of the stories that other ladies had written about their birthings and sat down and wrote about hers. Every now and then we would all get curious about how much I was dilated and Mary Louise would check me. I took a few pictures of her while she was doing this, thinking it would be nice to have some shots of a midwife from this point of view.

Stephen called home a few times to check on how I was doing. All this time there didn't seem to be much hurry—my rushes didn't take all of my attention, so I decided to just do whatever I felt like doing, as long as it didn't slow down my labor any.

When lunchtime came, I considered whether or not I ought to eat anything. Someone had brought us some good-looking sandwiches that had me pretty interested. Most folks don't seem to feel like eating at five centimeters' dilation, but there I was—hungry. So I ate. I figured that eating would either make me strong or make me sick. I could use the strength if that's what I got, and if I got sick, it would cause me to open up faster and that would be nice too.

At about three o'clock in the afternoon I was between five and six centimeters dilated and starting to feel like it would be nice to have Stephen around. He called right then and said he was on his way home. My labor picked up as soon as he arrived. It felt like I could handle the energy best if I looked at him while I was having the rush. Each one was heavier than the last, and by this time I didn't have any attention left from dealing with my rushes to write letters or eat or anything. Louise and Mary Louise sat on either side of me and rubbed my legs and my back. Stephen wanted to know if it was okay with me that he was sitting in a chair at the foot of the bed, not actually touching me. I knew that he would move if I wanted him to, but I felt best with him being where he was—I felt very high and one with him just looking at him. I felt very grateful that Stephen and my friends were there helping me do this; I loved them all a lot for being with me while I was tripping so heavy.

In between a couple of my rushes, the baby began punching me with its fist at regular intervals, not very hard, but very steady, and I was sure it was a boy. I suggested that we think of boy names. We all liked the names Paul and Benjamin, but didn't come to any final decision. Mary Louise checked me again and said that I was seven centimeters dilated now. By this time I was beginning to long for the time when I

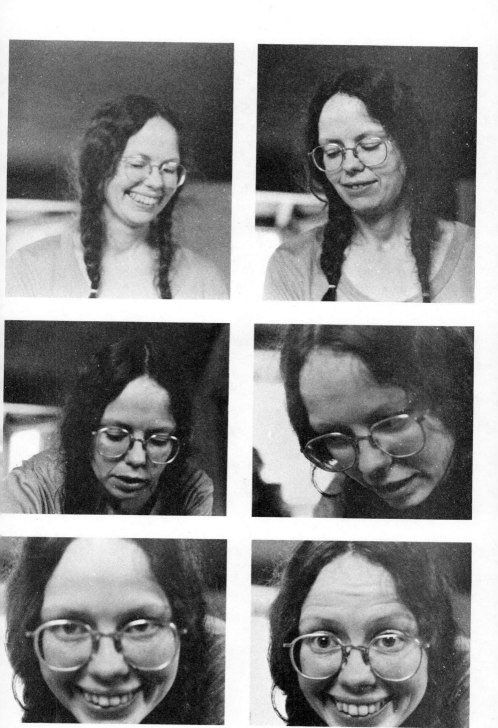

would be fully dilated and could push the baby out. I felt like I would like to get clean and cool before having the baby, so I asked Stephen if he'd pour a bucket of water over me while I stood on the porch. He did, and it felt great. The baby moved down lower while I was standing up, and I knew it wasn't going to be long now. I hoped that I would have the baby before dark so that we'd be able to get some pictures after he was born.

Mary Louise checked me again as soon as I laid down and said I was almost completely dilated. I was glad to hear that because it certainly felt like it and I did want to push. On my next rush I tried a gentle push during the strongest part of it to try to move the baby's head on through my cervix. I could feel the baby's head come through my cervix and move into the birth canal. That's always an amazing feeling. Stephen cut his fingernails and got all washed up, ready to catch our kid. It took just a few short pushes to move the baby's head down so that he was crowning. Stephen, Margaret and Mary Louise kept telling me that I had plenty of room to stretch around the baby's head, so I kept trying to move it farther. I looked down and could see the baby's head when it was halfway out and decided to push it the rest of the way out. Stephen checked and said there was no cord around the baby's neck and began to pull gently on the baby's head to stimulate another rush, which was exactly what I wanted him to do.

It felt really beautiful to push his body out—just a beautiful feeling of fullness and then relief. Someone picked up the baby's legs and I saw that we had another boy. He started moving and sputtering and crying all at once and turned from a pale purplish color to a beautiful rosy pink. I reached down and touched his hand, and it felt really nice. I felt so good and so grateful to have another live healthy baby. I just overflowed with that for a while. Everybody there looked really beautiful and alive. We named our boy Paul Benjamin.

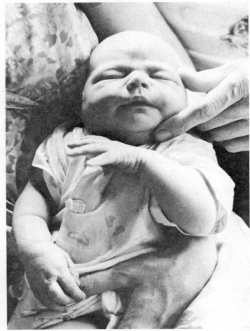

Paul Benjamin

206

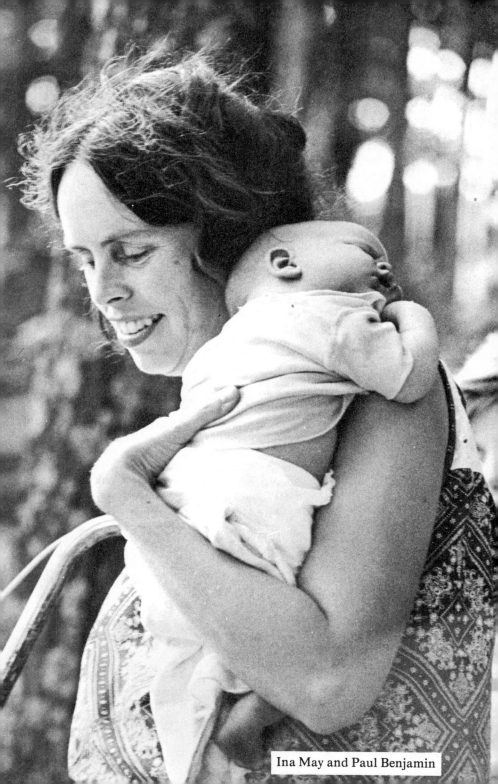

Ina May and Paul Benjamin

Jeffrey and Sarah's Kids

Sarah and Jeffrey had three babies in between the time when he left, with Stephen's blessings, to do his medical training and when he returned seven years later to be our doctor. Coincidentally, we found out later that the doctor who had backed up Jeffrey when he delivered his first child as a medical student was the same doctor I had met on the Caravan who gave me my first instructions in midwifery.

—Ina May

Sarah: I want to say a word about how we learned that a strong loving agreement and trust relationship is mostly what gets a baby out without it "hurting."

When Jeffrey and I had Samuel, our first boy, we didn't know too much about spiritual midwifery and just used breathing techniques to stay relaxed. It was a nice birthing but in retrospect I was scared at times, wondering how I'd ever get through this.

With Nell, we had read *Spiritual Midwifery* and only partly believed hugging and smooching and staying connected with each other would get me through.

Then we had Harry and we knew Ina May and Stephen and all the midwives were right. Jeffrey and I really fell deeply in love at Harry's birthing. One thing I always kept running in my mind during my rushes was, "They are an interesting sensation that gets your baby out."

Jeffrey: Birthings are so obviously spiritual because such strong love and great heart and good faith have come from them. At the birth of each of our children Sarah and I experienced teachings that have made our lives happier.

When Sarah went into labor with Harry, our third child, we just knew that it was going to be fun. We were in South Carolina at the time, living in our bus. A bunch of folks had been visiting that evening to listen to a tape of Stephen's Sunday Service. I could tell that Sarah was having rushes by her glow as she was working around the kitchen. After a while the folks had to go and it felt good to put the kids to bed and know that by morning we would probably have a baby. For a while then, we just spent time together rubbing out each other and feeling the rushes. Around 9:00 p.m. we decided to go visit our neighbors Sam and Margery. We had asked Margery earlier to help us out at the birthing and Sam was an intern with me at the time, who I needed to talk to since he was going to take care of my patients for the time I'd be home.

We boogied together to some rock and roll music for a couple of hours and laughed a lot to a song that goes, "Can't keep it in—gotta let it out." When the rushes got strong enough we went back home and finished cleaning the bus and sorting some beans.

Margery came down to the bus and I got the bed ready and set up a table for the instruments and stuff. When Sarah felt like lying down we smooched and hugged right up until Harry was born. It surprised me to feel how hard Sarah could squeeze me. I squeezed her back the same way. It was a way we could share the rushes and it was painless and timeless. It was so fun and so incredible that it kind of surprised us both when Harry was suddenly crowning. I had to hustle to get it together to wash up and glove in time to control his head. He came out so nice and easy. It was a joyful blessing for us all and we knew that our love and good faith made it happen that way.

Margery watched over us sleeping until the sun came up and our kids, Sam and Nell, woke up to see their new brother.

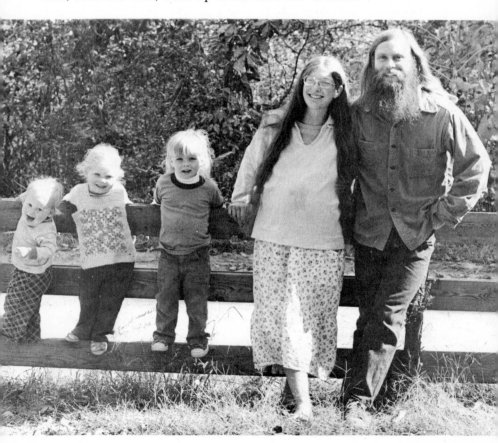

209

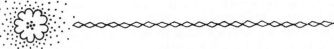

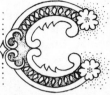ynthia: I'm seventeen and making it good with a nine month old boy. I came to the Farm when I was five months pregnant. My parents had felt very strongly about me not having him at first. They put a lot of pressure on me—they even put me in a mental institution and told me that any time I would consent to having an abortion they would let me go.

I realized that this was a time when I was going to have to be strong and stay with my moral beliefs, because even though they had taken that physical part of my freedom, it was still actually my decision, and I had to stay smart about it and keep my wits about me.

They had folks come in, psychiatrists and (hereditaryists-geneologists???) and they told me all kinds of things to sway me—even to the point of telling me that my kid was going to have a two-thirds chance of being deformed, or that I wasn't going to be a good mother (you can always work that out).

One day after I'd been through this for two months, I sat my parents down and said, "Look, I know about this safe place where I can go and have my baby, where they'll take good care of me and deliver my baby and teach me how to take care of it and I can stay and live there." I just basically told them that I would be safe and healthy, and that my baby would be treated real good and it wouldn't matter to those folks if I was young, unmarried, and pregnant. My parents, too, finally saw that it was my decision and let me come on down.

They really love my baby now and we're all friends.

Amber

avid: At about 7:00 p.m., I first noticed that there were red and blue soft-focus outlines around Valerie's head, and it felt very glowy and warm. I asked her about it, but she was playing it cool and saying it really wasn't anything heavy. She said after a while that she was feeling something pretty regularly. I got excited because I thought the baby was coming, and went in the other room to get a watch from Susan, who was training to be a midwife. I said I thought it was starting to happen and everybody noticed it felt like *something* was happening. She was having light rushes about every two and a half minutes. Susan checked

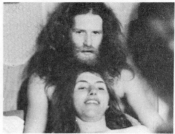

her and her cervix was four centimeters dilated. We were both pretty excited; it was our first kid. Time didn't seem much like standard—it just progressed —and Leslie, who would be delivering the baby, came. I leaned up on some pillows behind Valerie and she leaned back on me and got really comfortable and relaxed. I rubbed her back and tits, and we smooched in between the rushes sometimes to keep it loose. Soon there were seven ladies in our 5' by 11' bedroom: a couple of midwives, some midwife trainees and a couple who lived in the same house as us. I had never seen Valerie put out so much effort as she did pushing the baby out. It was getting us both very high.

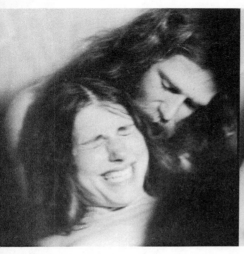
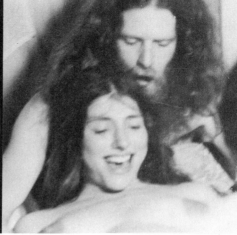

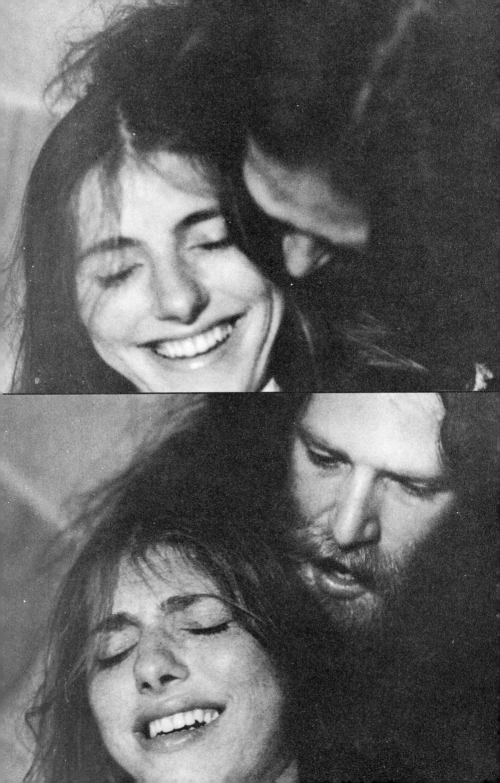

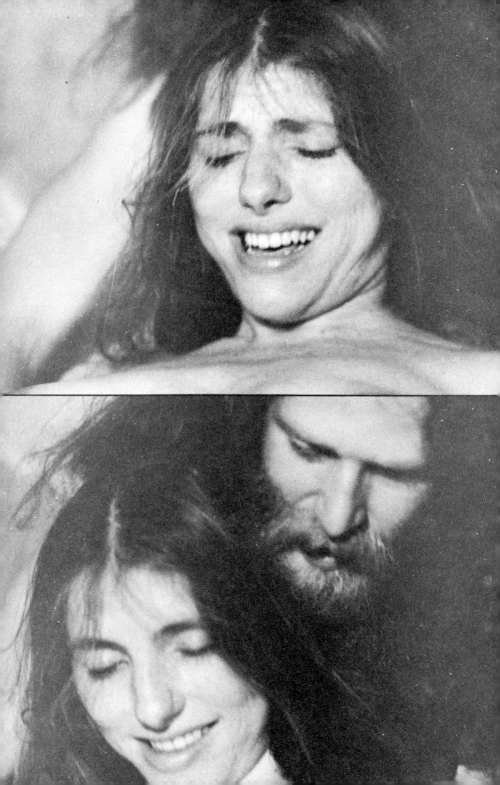

Pamela checked her and said she was nice and loose and doing real good and getting wider all the time. She was letting out these amazing lion roars while she pushed, and kind of giggling and relaxing on me in between. I had to go outside for a minute, and when I came back in she was bright

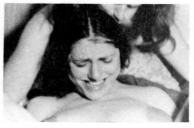

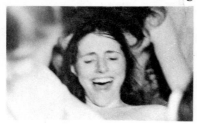

pink and grinning ear to ear. After a while (the whole birthing took about seven hours), Pamela showed us the baby's wet hairy head with a mirror. It was just starting to squeeze out. It wasn't too many more pushes until at about 3 a.m. the baby slid on out, radiating purple and white, then pink as she started up. She was healthy and pretty loud for her size, and just lit up the whole room. I saw her look like my grandfather, then my father (a lot of people say she looks like me).

Valerie was wide-eyed and shining and giggling quietly about how small and perfect she was. We had already decided to name a girl Amber, and her hair matched. In fact, everybody in the room looked golden to me. Valerie and Amber and I hung out and kind of melted into each other and fell in love.

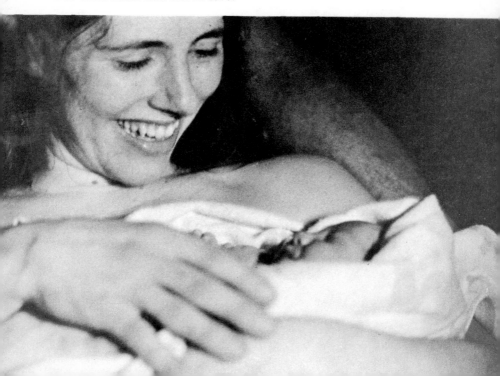

Lyle

arilyn: When I started pushing, it was with my whole thing. With the first push, the water bag broke and got Kathryn in the face. We laughed. "See, you didn't need us to do it," the midwives said. Douglas held up a mirror for me to see my puss and I was amazed. It looked very psychedelic, like the big pink petals of a flower opening up. It was really beautiful. It surprised me and I felt like I had a new respect for my body. I remembered and told everyone how the story of Buddha says he was born from a lotus blossom. Everybody, every Buddha, is born that way. Just a few pushes later he came out, all purple and yelling. He was beautiful, real strong and healthy-looking. I was really grateful to see him. I wanted to hold him right away but I still had to get the placenta out and both of us had to get fixed up. I kept looking at him. He was right there. I was awake all night, too energized to sleep, and whenever I'd think, "How is he? Is he okay?" he'd open his eyes and look at me.

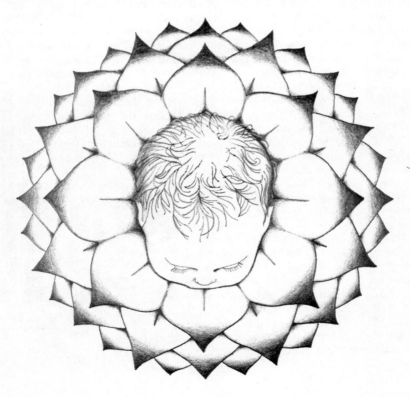

The Story of Theodore

Catherine: I had started labor the week before. I dilated to four centimeters and stopped. Five days later I lifted a heavy pot and my water bag started leaking. It leaked for two days. On the second day I was resting and felt a bigger gush of water and a mild rush. I got the clock to see if any more rushes would come and how often. Twenty minutes later at 3:30 a heavy rush came. It was very strong and I thought it would never end. I hoped it would stop so I could call James and the midwives. It stopped and I got up and called James. I told him not to hurry since it had only been twenty minutes from that first mild rush. As soon as I hung up, another strong rush came. I hoped James would hurry. I then called my dear old friend Kathleen to come over and check me. By this time I could barely talk on the phone. She and James both arrived in ten minutes. Later, at 3:50, we went into our room. Now the rushes were back to back. I was sitting Indian style. I had decided I'd like to try it this way this time. For my last two kids I laid down for the entire thing. Two more heavy rushes and I felt slightly like pushing. Kathleen looked surprised—I wasn't. Another rush and I definitely was pushing. At this time there was no equipment or sterile pack—just Kathleen who had called Pamela five minutes earlier. Then our old friend David walked in with his camera. We had originally planned to videotape the birthing. In fact, the week earlier everything had been all set up, but this time there was no time so we at least wanted pictures. We were all hoping the midwife would just arrive, let alone the video equipment. During the next push I asked if Pamela knew to really hurry. Kathleen hoped so. Me too. The ambulance arrived with supplies. I was never worried because the baby seemed so strong and determined to just come out. He was going to be born whether there was an audience or not.

Then Pamela and Susan popped in and immediately washed their hands. Pamela said to pant so they could get an eye on the situation. I panted for five or ten seconds and started pushing again. The head was crowning. I could feel half of his head come out, then the rest of it. They said his nose and mouth were clear. I asked if I could push his body out. I could do it at will, and I did, and he slid out smoothly. "It's a boy," James said, and that feeling came over me that every woman must feel when she first sees her baby. You feel exhilarated and the love

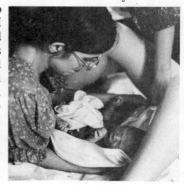

is just gushing out. My baby hollered loud. His mouth was huge. They put him on my stomach. He was wet and sticky and I tried

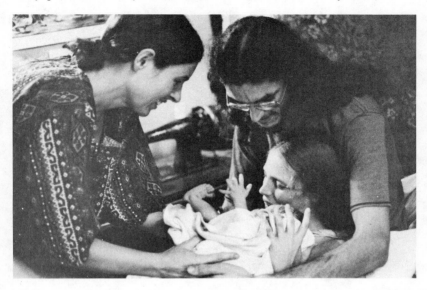

to keep him warm. He was gorgeous and I could hardly believe it was all over. It was only 4:25. It was like the labor consumed me. I had no choice but to groove and go along with the flow and not think. We named him Theodore because it means gift from God.

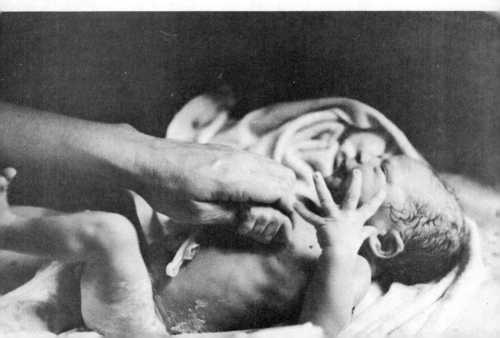

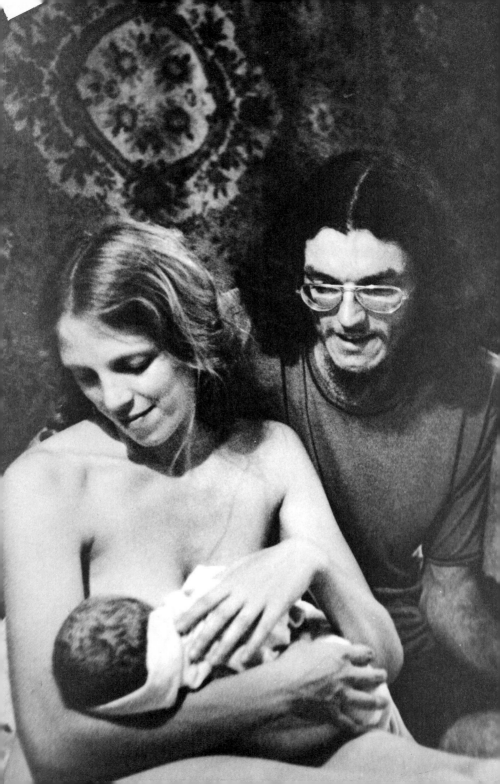

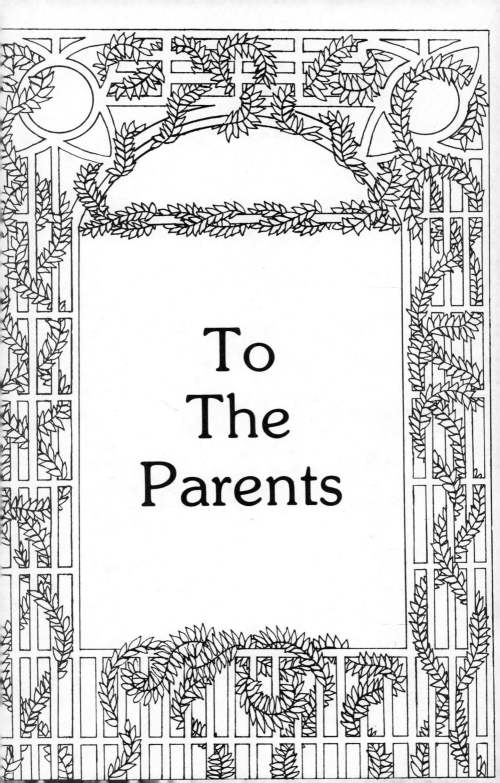

To
The
Parents

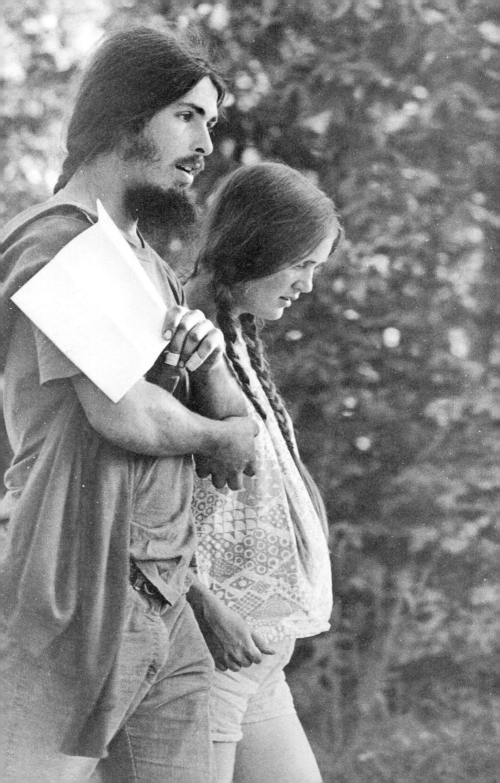

Taking Care of Yourself While You're Pregnant

NUTRITION

Making sure your nutrition is good during pregnancy is the first way you take care of your child. Many people think that babies get all the nutrients they need no matter how poorly their mothers eat, but this is a myth. If you have never before given attention to your diet, now is the time to begin.

Start by checking on your protein intake. Protein is the stuff from which our bones, muscles, skin, hair, nails, organs, blood and hormones are made. We need protein for the proper functioning of enzymes, antibodies, and our blood clotting factors. During pregnancy you will need 60-90 grams of protein a day. There are both animal and vegetable sources of protein. Milk, meat and eggs all contain complete protein, containing all the amino acids necessary to good health. Vegetarians may get protein from nuts, various kinds of dried peas and beans and from soybean products such as tofu and tempeh. If you are a vegetarian, it is important to eat your protein food in combinations with different grains, such as rice, flour, or cornmeal, so that you get all the amino acids you need. Pay special attention to eating enough protein during hot weather, since it is the type of food most likely to feel heavy and unappealing at this time.

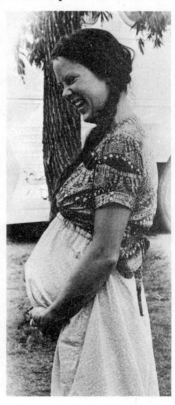

If you eat no animal products, be sure to supplement vitamin B12. You will get all you need if you take a 25 mcg. tablet twice a week; the body stores extra vitamin B12 in the liver but only absorbs a few micrograms at a time. A deficiency of vitamin B12 causes pernicious anemia, a condition that may be masked by eating foods rich in folacin (dark, leafy greens). Vegetables and fruits are important for vitamins and minerals. Raw or lightly cooked vegetables are best. Steaming is better than boiling. Save any vegetable water to use in soups or gravies, so you don't throw away precious vitamins. Alfalfa and other types of sprouts are excellent sources of vitamins and minerals.

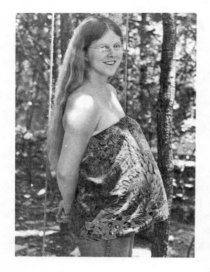

Fats play an important role in helping the body absorb certain vitamins. They also provide you with enough calories to keep your weight up while you grow a baby. Weight gain is better when it is consistent rather than sporadic. A weight gain of 25-35 pounds is desirable for most women. If you start very thin, you may gain even more. Too much weight gain is less risky to a pregnancy than too little. It's important to remember that it's not the baked potato or the home-made bread that is fattening—it's the butter or sour cream you put on it. If you want to eat foods that are rich in protein but comparitively low in fat, you can choose dried beans, peas and non-fat dairy products.

Drink plenty of fluids, especially water and juices. Avoid junk food and drinks, and get in the habit of reading labels. In general, avoid swallowing anything that isn't food. This list includes preservatives, dyes, and artificial flavoring.

I recommend that prenatal supplements be taken, especially by women who eat non-organic foods, drink polluted water and who breathe dirty air. Even if you conscientiously try to eat all your dark leafy greens and grains and nutritional yeast, it is good to be sure. Prenatal vitamins differ from regular multivitamins in that they contain extra amounts of all the vitamins and minerals that you need for both of you, and a generous amount of iron.

Speaking of iron, both the World Health Organization and the National Academy of Sciences (which issues the Recommended Daily Allowance of nutrients) recommend supplementing iron during pregnancy. They feel that the iron requirement of women of childbearing age is already hard enough to meet through diet alone, and that most women wouldn't be able to meet the added requirements of pregnancy. It is good to eat iron-rich foods, such as kale, other dark leafy greens, apricots, molasses, whole grains, beets, parsley and prunes during pregnancy. Even women who try to take in plenty of iron may develop iron-deficiency anemia, since not all women assimilate very much of the iron they take in. Iron supplements may also cause constipation and indigestion. I have had very good results in recent years with giving alfalfa tablets to raise the hematocrit. I have seen (and experienced myself) a dramatic rise in the hematocrit (from 5 to 10 points) in as little as a week. Avoid drinks with caffein, as these may deplete your body of its iron stores.

Calcium supplements and calcium-rich foods are also important during pregnancy. This mineral is most easily obtained from dairy products. Vegetable sources include dark greens, broccoli, bok choy, sunflower seeds, okra and peanuts. Lester Hazell, in *Commonsense Childbirth*, says that calcium should be taken on an empty stomach with the addition of Vitamin C. Lack of calcium may cause leg cramps. If you do take a supplement, take one gram of calcium gluconate or dicalcium phosphate. If you take calcium lactate, you will need about two grains daily, as it is not so easily absorbed. Take two 500 mg. tablets or three 5 grain tablets to make one gram. Your baby is calcifying his bones in the last half of pregnancy, and if there is not any extra calcium around, it will come from your bones. Be sure to continue the calcium and prenatal vitamins through nursing.

CHANGES DURING PREGNANCY

Breasts—Your breasts are likely to get bigger and feel tender and tingly because of the hormonal changes of pregnancy. The breasts start to make colostrum, a yellowish-clear liquid which contains sugar, fat, protein, minerals and water, in about the same proportions as milk. You may be able to squeeze some out as early as the fourth month of pregnancy, and later on, your breasts may leak a little. Be sure to keep your nipples clean and dry as possible, avoiding the use of soaps (which are drying and, often, irritating). Get a good bra if your breasts are so heavy they need support.

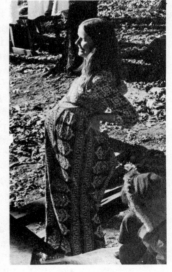

Complexion—If your complexion has been a problem before, there is a good chance it will clear up during pregnancy.

Weight gain—A normal weight gain in pregnancy usually involves at least 20 pounds. I always gained thirty-five pounds in a healthy pregnancy. Women who are underweight before pregnancy may gain 40-45 pounds, with healthy results, as long as all the basic nutritional requirements are being met. The optimum weight gain for each pregnancy depends on your metabolism, and your body size and type when not pregnant. If you are already underweight, you may find it easier to gain weight than usual.

Lovemaking—I have noticed that women who continue to make love during pregnancy (as long as they determine the pace and timing of the lovemaking) are less likely to have perineal tears at the birth of the baby. Another added benefit for couples who maintain some sort of intimate contact is that they are less likely to quarrel during pregnancy than those who swear off sex during pregnancy. Some couples especially enjoy sex at this time, since they are freed from worrying about getting pregnant. It is not unusual for men to be afraid of sexual contact with their pregnant wives, thinking that they may harm the baby. They can be reassured by knowing that there is no medical evidence that sexual intercourse during pregnancy is harmful. The only situations when intercourse may be unsafe are when miscarraige or premature labor threatens or when the water bag ruptures.

Some women prefer not to make love during pregnancy because of their increased size and because of the extra effort or imagination it may take. Try different positions than usual, especially if you are rarely on top or on your side. Pillows may help. Keep up your loving relationship as long as possible during pregnancy. This is a way your man can be as vibrationally close to your growing baby as possible, and he is much less likely to become jealous and child-like in his relationship with you as you approach the time of giving birth. If you are too tired for loving in the evenings, try taking an afternoon nap. In my experience, couples who keep sexual contact with each other during pregnancy are much less likely than others to stay pregnant long past the expected date of birth. The prostaglandins in semen seem to contribute to the ripening of the cervix necessary to go into labor.

Exercise — Exercise is quite important during pregnancy as it aids circulation, lessens constipation, strengthens muscles you will be using when you have the baby. Movement of some kind is best, better than just stretching or positioning yourself. I recommend the set of prenatal exercises given in *Essential Exercises for the Childbearing Year*, by Elizabeth Noble (Houghton Mifflin Company Boston, 1988). Walking is the best exercise you can possibly do. Try to walk as much as you can. Get in the habit of holding your belly in as you walk.

MINOR DISCOMFORTS OF PREGNANCY AND WHAT TO DO ABOUT THEM

Morning sickness occurs in about one half of pregnancies and is worse on an empty stomach. So do eat. Try eating a few crackers (avoid really salty ones) before getting out of bed in the morning, and eat one or two when you wake up to pee during the night. They seem to absorb extra stomach acid. Eat a high protein snack before going to bed at night, as protein takes longer to digest. Vitamin B6 tablets may allay morning sickness. They come in 30 or 50 mg. tablets. You may need about 100 mg. a day for the first few days, after which you may decrease the amount. Another remedy that helps many women is ginger tea or capsules (fill "00" capsules with dry ginger root powder), taken with a little food. Alfalfa tablets are stomach settlers, and they also help with heartburn and indigestion.

224

North Carolina midwife Lisa Goldstein also recommends that pregnant women eat half a fresh orange before going to bed at night and notes that orange juice, for some reason, does not have the same beneficial effect.

Constipation — This side effect of pregnancy is caused by the hormones of pregnancy that relax the smooth muscles of the digestive tract. Constipation is also caused by the pressure the baby puts on your intestines and in many women by the iron supplements they take. It is helped by eating lots of fresh fruits and vegetables. Eat bran muffins and prunes. Drink lots of water and get plenty of exercise. Alfalfa tablets prevent constipation in most women; add a couple of tablets a day until you notice good results.

Hemorrhoids sometimes occur during pregnancy, but they will usually disappear after the birth. Sit in a very hot tub or sitz bath and hold the hemorrhoid back with your fingers. Sometimes it will stay in place. You can also use astringents such as witch hazel soaked into a gauze pad or alum compresses to reduce swelling. You can use hemorrhoid cream or suppositories if they don't contain hydrocortisone. You may need a stool softener for a while; ask your druggist for one suitable for pregnancy. Don't strain when you shit.

Stretch marks are less likely to occur if you're not uptight. Put cream or lotion on your belly to keep the skin pliable and soft. Let your man or your girlfriend give you thorough stomach rubs. Let him squeeze you good, not to the point of pain, but just to the point where you relax to his touch.

Heartburn is very common in middle or late pregnancy. This very irritating condition is usually helped by eating 6-8 small meals a day instead of 2 or 3 large ones. Avoid drinking anything with your meals, as you want to salivate properly and you don't want to dilute your stomach acids. Alfalfa tablets taken after meals are often a great help, as is peppermint tea. Avoid taking antacids, except very occasionally, as they usually contain aluminum compounds and they may upset your body's calcium-magnesium balance.

Tiredness—You are likely to feel tired in the first couple of months. Your body is changing radically and getting used to being pregnant. Get plenty of rest. Nap in the afternoon if you feel like it. You will feel less tired and more energetic after your

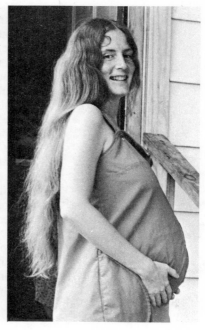

225

third month. Ask your midwife or doctor to check your hematocrit (iron level).

Bleeding gums are common in pregnancy and are caused by hormones changes. Brush your teeth and gums with a soft toothbrush, and you may use an oxygenating mouthwash. (Ask your druggist).

Backaches are caused by increased pressure and the weight of your growing belly. Stand straight and tall. Hold your stomach in some. Stick your tits out. Don't lean all your weight out with your stomach. Sleep on a firm mattress. Apply heat, such as a hot water bottle wrapped in a towel. Rubbing helps. Don't wear high heels. Walk a lot; exercise helps. There's also an exercise you can do where you lie on the floor with your arms out, and raise one leg slowly, then lower it, then raise the other one. There's another one called pelvic rock: get into position 8 shown on p. 240 (After Baby Exercises). Alternately arch your back like a cat, and curve it the other way as much as you can, with your head back.

Varicose veins are more common after several pregnancies or if you are overweight. This is what causes them: blood in the arteries keeps moving along because the heart pumps it directly. The veins, which return the blood, don't have much pressure and depend on one-way valves to keep the blood from backing up or pooling. With varicose veins, as the veins dilate, the valves are weakened and let the blood back up and pool. This puts more pressure on the vein, and more valves give way as the veins dilate. Do not sit or stand for long periods of time because gravity puts more pressure on the veins. Walk a lot. The muscular activity of your legs will help the veins return the blood and speed

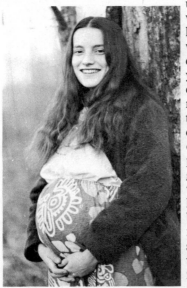

up circulation. When you do sit, elevate your legs about the level of your hips. Get a lot of exercise, control your weight, don't wear binding clothes, and elevate your legs often. Do not sit with your legs crossed at the knee. It puts direct pressure on major veins. Do not rub varicose veins — there may be a little clot in there which your body will disperse slowly. If a swollen vein is red or tender, see a doctor — it may be phlebitis. If you have varicose veins, or get them when you are pregnant, you will need to wear maternity support hose. Put them on while you're still in bed. Hold your leg high to let the blood flow out of it, and then put on the stocking. Vitamin E helps varicose veings. Take two 400 I.U. capsules a day for two weeks. Then take one 400 I.U. capsule daily.

Leg cramps are usually caused by poor circulation and by lactic acid and other acid and mineral by-products building up in your muscles. If you get a cramp, flex your foot upwards toward your knee. To prevent leg aches and cramps, ask your man or friend to rub out your legs often (provided that you don't have varicose veins), especially at night before bed. He should squeeze large handfuls of leg muscles firmly from the upper thighs, working down to your feet. Don't cross your legs when you sit, and be aware that a lack of calcium may cause leg cramps. Increase the amount you take by one half if you do suffer from cramps. A lack of B vitamins in your diet may cause leg cramps. Some women get relief from wearing support hose during pregnancy, but if you wear these, make sure that they don't fit too tightly around your belly and that the crotch is well ventilated, so that you don't develop an irritation.

Swelling of the legs is common in pregnancy. It is caused by water retention. Check with your midwife to make sure that any swelling you have is not a symptom of a complication of pregnancy. She will check your blood pressure and will likely want to know if you eat a lot of highly salted foods. Food additives such as monosodium glutamate, sodium nitrate and some artificial sweeteners may cause leg swelling. Avoid salty snack foods and diet drinks. Don't be afraid to drink water if you experience swelling in your feet and legs. Sit down and elevate your legs above hip level often during the day.

Shortness of breath is normal to some degree in late pregnancy. It occurs because the baby is so big that there's not much room for your lungs to expand. Besides this, your oxygen need increases during pregnancy. Mention this symptom to your midwife so she can rule out possible other, less normal, reasons for this condition.

Dizziness is common early in pregnancy. Muscles in the walls of the blood vessels relax from pregnancy hormones. When you stand up, there is more gravity to work against to get the blood up to the brain. Change positions slowly and stand up slowly, so your blood vessels have time to adjust. Eat six small meals a day rather than three large ones. Mention any dizziness to your midwife so she can rule out possible abnormal causes of it. Dizziness accompanied by high blood pressure and albumin in your pee is not normal.

Yeast. Normally, you have some bacteria called lactobacilli, and yeasts, called *Candida albicans* (monilia) in your puss. As the cells inside your puss slough off, sugar is released and the yeasts live on sugar. The lactobacilli change the sugar to lactic acid, which is a poor medium for most things to grow in, including yeast. But hormones in pregnancy alter the sugar in the cells and make it a more favorable environment for yeasts to grow in. So pregnant women are susceptible to yeast infections. At term, about 25% of ladies have some yeast infection. The only real cure for this is delivery, when the hormones and the sugar go back to normal. Another way to get a yeast infection is by losing your normal inhabitants of lactobacilli. This can happen because of sickness, regular douching, or taking antibiotics.

If you have itching and burning and mild-smelling curdy discharge, it's probably yeast. The discharge won't smell bad, but may be a little like bread dough. You can have burning when you pee, too.

You can cure an early case of yeast by douching with a vinegar solution of 2 T. vinegar (4-5% acetic acid) to a quart of warm water. Douches are okay in the first and second trimester of pregnancy if you be very gentle. Use a bag, not a bulb syringe. Hold the bag only about 18 inches above your puss and only insert the tip in about 3 inches. Douche once or twice a day for 5-10 days depending on the severity of the condition. If this doesn't seem to help or if you are too irritated from vinegar, use buttermilk or diluted yogurt twice a day for 7-10 days. Buttermilk and yogurt contain a lactobacillus which is similar to the lactobacillus you have in your puss. Douching with it will help restore the natural balance of yeasts and bacteria there. After you have washed and douched, you can put on some petroleum jelly or vitamin A & D ointment to protect and heal your outer parts. Don't wear underwear if you can do without it, especially nylon underwear, as it tends to hold the moisture down there and makes better growing conditions for the yeast. Don't make love while you have a yeast infection because it makes it worse by breaking up and spreading the yeast colonies.

Don't douche except to cure yeast. Your puss is set up to keep itself clean, and if you douche a lot, you upset its normal environment.

If these home remedies do not cure your yeast, or if you are in your third trimester, you should go to a women's clinic or doctor for a prescription.

Trichomonas are little protozoa that can cause a vaginal infection. The discharge is slightly foamy, profuse, smells bad, and you itch. If you have a bad-smelling discharge without itching, you probably have a bacterial infection. For trichomonas and bacterial infections, you need to see a doctor because the only medicines that will help these are under prescription.

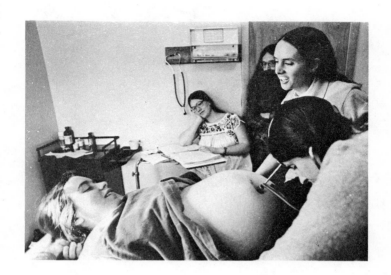

YOUR PRENATAL CARE

Besides all these ways of taking care of yourself, you need regular prenatal care from your midwife or your doctor. You should make:
— At least one visit in the first trimester;
— At least two visits in the 2nd, provided there are no complications;
— At least four visits in the last trimester. Weekly visits in the last month of pregnancy are advisable so your midwife or doctor can check the baby's position and presentation and keep track of the baby's size in relation to your pelvic size.

During these visits your midwife or physician will check your blood pressure and albumin (protein) in your urine to see if your kidneys are stressed. They will check for glucose (sugar) in your pee, which would indicate a diabetic or temporary diabetic state. They will also keep track of your blood-iron levels and your weight gain.

If your blood is Rh negative, they will have you tested periodically for antibodies. I do not favor the use of prenatal rhogam in pregnant Rh negative mothers, as I don't think the scientific evidence indicating its use is persuasive.

Even if you think you've had German measles (rubella) or that you were vaccinated against it, get a test to find out whether you are still immune. If you are not immune and are pregnant, you cannot have a vaccination, because the vaccination might harm your unborn child. For this reason it's best to check for rubella before you wish to become pregnant.

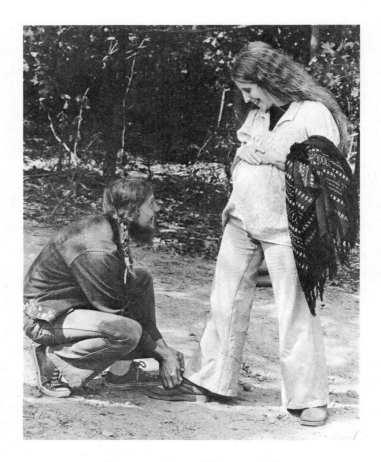

Preparing Yourself
for The Birth

ADVICE TO MEN ON THE CARE
AND FEEDING OF PREGNANT WOMEN

Be tantric (telepathic in the language of touch) *with your lady—be subtle enough in touch with her that when she tries to steer you, you feel it and follow her like a good horse follows a rider. Try to do it with her exactly as she directs on the most subtle planes. If you do that, she'll trust you and get you high. It's a tasty yoga—you have to work at it, but you can do it. It's actually fancier than just dancing by yourself. You feel somebody else and let them direct; and if you let them direct, they'll tell you what to do.*

                                                       —Stephen

Ina May: Fetch and tie her shoes when she can't bend anymore; rub her back, her legs, her belly; help her with the other kids when you can; and lift for her.

Give her lots of water — she'll drink more if you give it to her than if she has to waddle to the faucet. Play and talk with your baby while she is still inside. She can hear you and will recognize and enjoy your voice.

Realize that pregnancy is often an emotional time for a woman because of various hormone changes. Hormones are powerful substances that alter the consciousness and need to be understood as that. You can help her through her hormone changes by not being judgmental about how she might seem to be and by knowing that her state of mind can quickly be transformed by your being her loving buddy.

One of the most important things you can do for your mate is to let her know that she's still attractive to you, that she's still a turn-on. At the same time, remember not to put pressure on her to make love to you.

Being impatient about when your wife is going to have her baby is like somebody telling you to have an erection—right now.

—Stephen

Some Advice from a Father of Two Babies Born on the Farm

Dear folks,

The first thing I think of when she/we are pregnant is how much more I am aware that we are really One; that we have our agreement together with God to create a new life. I feel both happy and responsible for it. It is now time to turn into the very smart and patient knight in shining armor.

Help her out and let her get plenty of rest. Help her with the kids, the dishes, the laundry, the cleaning. It is a great job raising a bellyfull of baby. Stay real well-connected with her if she's emotional and don't get upset. Keep your body connection strong and make her feel good. She is going to get more lovely and psychedelic as the months go by, and it is a blessing to be in her presence. Don't hide your feelings from her and don't be embarrassed about them. Don't forget that she is the one that is carrying the weight.

At the birthing, don't get overly excited. It is a very here-and-now natural happening and what you're needed for is your kind attention and helpfulness. The ladies are doing the job, and they'll love your help if you're not overbearing.

Love to All,
Thomas

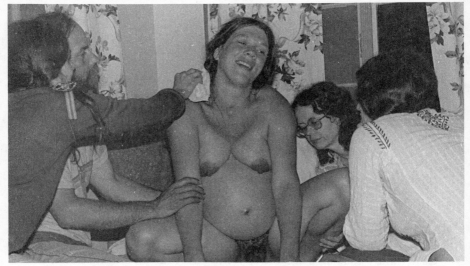

WHO SHOULD BE PRESENT AT YOUR BIRTHING?

The birthing energy flows smoothest when everyone present is part of the crew, helping the baby to its birth. If some of the other people present are spectators, or what we call "passengers," the birth can be slowed down by hours or can even be halted until some change takes place in the energy. This is because anyone whose presence is not an actual help is requiring the emotional support that should be going to the mother.

You may feel that you would like to have some close friend or relative be with you, as well as your husband. This is fine as long as the person you choose is someone you would feel all right with in life-and-death levels of tripping. Don't let anyone pressure you to let them attend your birthing.

We feel that it's a good idea to arrange for a close friend or relative to take care of your other children while you are in labor and for a few days after the baby is born. The baby being born needs your full, undivided attention, which can be hard to give if your other young children are present. The energy of a birthing is very high and intense.

Young children usually don't have disciplined enough attention habits to keep from interfering with the flow of energy of the birthing. Besides this, a child can easily mistake his mother's intensity during labor for discomfort, and worry about her, or think that she is in danger if he sees any blood.

We have had a few deliveries which were witnessed by a young child who woke up during the delivery and watched quietly, drawing no attention to himself. This felt so right at the time that we had no thought of interfering with the child's watching this sacred event.

You might have a teen-age daughter who you would like to have present at your birthing. This is okay, but you should keep in mind that you will be influencing her attitudes towards birth, so you should be very sure of both her and yourself.

232

WHAT HAPPENS DURING LABOR

During labor your uterine muscles contract at intervals and finally push out the baby. While this is happening, your cervix is thinning and opening. We call these regular bursts of energy "rushes." Labor progresses best if you pay attention to the expansion rather than to the contraction.

The first stage of labor begins when the rushes come ar regular intervals and start getting stronger. In the beginning they may feel something like menstrual cramps, but with more energy. The mucus plug in the cervix that has sealed off the uterus during pregnancy comes out. This blood and mucus is called the "bloody show." The rushes get longer and stronger as the cervix gets more dilated. The first stage of labor lasts until the cervix is fully dilated to approximately ten centimeters, a large enough opening for a full-term baby's head to pass through.

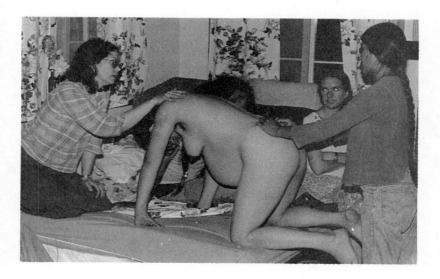

This usually takes from twelve to fifteen hours for a first baby (although I have known women who had 20 minute to half hour labors for their first babies) and less than that with later babies, but varies widely for different women and different situations.

When your cervix is nearly open, you are most apt to feel emotional, to feel that it is impossible to give birth, that you might rip in half or explode or that all your insides might come out if you allow your baby to move down the birth canal. This is a very scary feeling, and most women, when they are under the spell of this particular fear, are convinced that their bodies will be done great damage if they relax. It's important to remember that your brain can be quite unreliable at this

233

stage of labor. It is usually an amazing help to have someone remind you that you won't explode or tear in half at this point, but that person has to know what she's talking about and has to be convincing. The intense feeling usually passes when the second stage starts and a more active part of your work begins.

The second stage lasts from the time of full dilation until the baby is born. This may take from a few minutes to two or three hours. The combination of the uterus contracting and you pushing with your abdominal muscles gets the baby through your pelvic bones, down the birth canal, and out. The baby's head bones slide over each other a little, making the head temporarily smaller during its passage through the pelvic outlet. The urge to push is usually involuntary and powerful, but you have a tremendous amount of control during this time, too. On The Farm, the midwife serves as a guide to the woman on how to hold herself and how to breathe and whatever else may be relevant in order for her to get the most accomplished with her pushes and how to give birth slowly to avoid tearing.

The baby is crowning when the head start to emerge. It will usually come out facing downward and will spontaneously turn ninety degrees; then the body will be pushed out. When the head and the body are being born it is important to cooperate with your midwife so you can give birth to the head slowly.

Usually the baby will breathe spontaneously, but if not, your midwife or physician will give him assistance. At this point, the best place for your baby is on your belly or chest, to facilitate easy bonding and to keep both of you warm. Some babies open their eyes, wriggle their facial muscles and try to breathe even before their bodies have been born. The umbilical cord will be cut some time after the baby has begun breathing well.

The third stage of labor lasts from the time the baby is born until the placenta is delivered. In our practice this usually takes about 10-20 minutes. The rushes that facilitate this process are not so strong as those of the first or second stages of labor, and pushing out the placenta is generally pretty easy and comfortable—it has no bones.

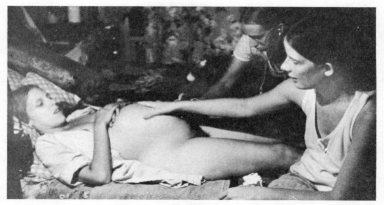

ADVICE FOR MOTHER AT THE TIME OF BIRTH

At a birthing, the mother is the main channel of life force. If she is co-operative and selfless and brave, it makes there be more energy for everyone, including her baby who is getting born.

Giving somebody some makes you and everyone else feel good. You don't have your baby out yet to cuddle and hold; so giving the midwives and your husband some is giving your baby some. If you are in a hospital, you can make there be more energy by finding someone you can connect and be friends with.

During a rush, keep your eyes open, and keep paying attention to those around you and to what's happening. If you feel afraid or if something is happening that makes you uptight, report it—the midwives can help sort it out until it feels good.

Don't complain, it makes things worse. If you usually complain, practice not doing it during pregnancy. It will build character.

Talk nice—it will keep your bottom loose so it can open up easier. It's okay to ask the midwives or your husband to do something for you, i.e., rub your legs or get a glass of water. Ask real nice and give folks some when they do something for you.

Be grateful that you're having a baby, and be grateful to your man who's helping you—it's an experience that you only do a few times in your life, so make the very most of it, and get your head in a place where you can get as high as possible.

Remember you have a real, live baby in there. Sometimes it's such an intense trip having a baby that you can forget what it's for!

Learn how to relax—it's something that requires attention. You may have to put out some effort to gather your attention together enough that you can relax.

Keep your sense of humor—it's a priceless gem which keeps you remembering where it's at. If you can't be a hero, you can at least be funny while being a chicken.

Remember your monkey knows how to do this really well. Your brain isn't very reliable as a guide of how to be during childbirth, but your monkey is.

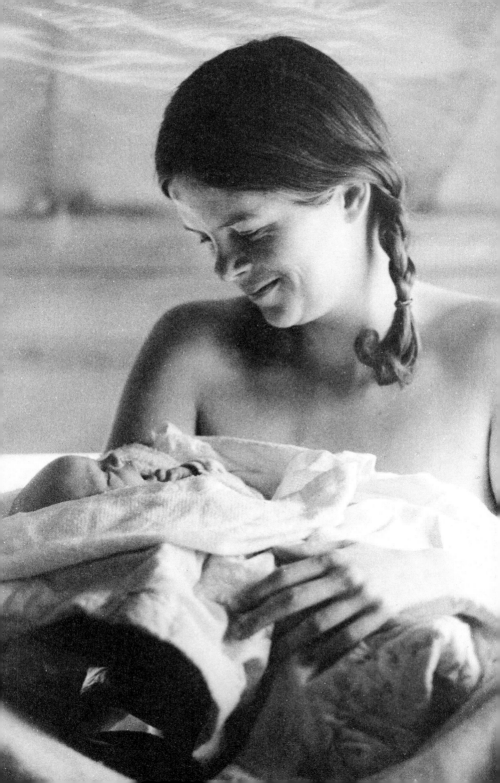

BONDING

Bonding is a phenomenon which has been understood from time immemorial by mothers, farmers, midwives, shepherds, and others familiar with the birthing process as it naturally occurs among mammals. Bonding is the original and immediate connection between mother and baby. It is the welding of the emotional and physical bonds between parent and infant which will ensure the continued maternal care necessary for the survival of the new infant. The period of time directly following birth is a time of extremely heightened sensitivity for both the mother and her infant. Deep psychic grooves are being cut in the consciousness of both which will drastically affect later behavior, especially in the mother's ability to care for her young.

Important research in this area has been done recently by Dr. Marshall Klaus,* Dr. John Kennell (both professors of pediatrics at Case Western Reserve University in Cleveland, Ohio), and others. This research has shown that interference with the normal bonding process has a great and sometimes drastic impact on the family. This exactly corroborates our own observations derived from delivering and caring for babies.

Klaus and Kennell's studies showed that ladies who had their babies with them immediately after birth, who were allowed skin-to-skin contact, undisturbed for a while, held their babies more competently, established more intimate contact with their babies, and had fewer problems with breast-feeding than mothers who were separated from their babies immediately following birth and rejoined later.

It seems that this mothering ability is greatly affected by how freely the mother is able to follow her own instinctual sense in the critical time just after birth, when changing hormone levels in her bloodstream following hereditary patterns evolved over millions and millions of years are preparing her physically and emotionally for the task of totally caring for her young as long as necessary.

We observe that there is a process of bonding between father and child as well. Fathers who have witnessed the birth of their children seem to form an especially close attachment to these children and, like their mates, have profound spiritual experiences at the birthings.

*Marshall H. Klaus and John H. Kennell, *Maternal-Infant Bonding: The Impact of Early Separation or Loss on Family Development* (St. Louis: C.V. Mosby Co., 1976).

TAKING CARE
OF YOURSELF
AFTER THE BIRTH

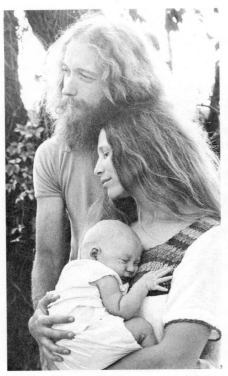

Check your uterus over the first couple of days after birth. It should feel hard, like a grapefruit. Very likely you'll continue to feel contractions over the next two or three days, especially while your baby is nursing. That's all normal—it's your uterus contracting itself back into shape and getting itself together. When you get these contractions, you might lose a tablespoon or two of fresh blood at a time. A few small clots might come out in the next couple of days too. If a clot bigger than an egg comes out, particularly if there is fresh heavier bleeding with it, check it right away with your doctor or midwife.

You will bleed like a normal heavy period for the first week or so after delivery. Then you'll continue to have a brownish or clear discharge for the next month or so. You need to wear sanitary napkins right after you have the baby. If you didn't tear, you can use tampons after the first week.

If you had stitches, keep them clean. Take a shower every day if possible, washing with an antiseptic soap. Pat your stitches, don't scrub them. Your bottom may be somewhat sore for the first week. It's good to lie down or recline a lot while the stitches are healing. Don't lift anything heavy, as this could tear the stitches out. Some soreness is to be expected while stitches are healing, but if they get more painful, or feel infected, have your husband look and see; and if there is any pus, call your doctor.

If you start to get a fever or feel achey or sick, call your midwife or doctor. It's fine to take it easy and be quiet and mellow with your baby at first, but you should feel healthy and well.

Your fluid intake should be around three to three and a half quarts daily. Continue taking your prenatal vitamins, iron and calcium supplements, while nursing. Have your hematocrit checked about six weeks following delivery. If it is 36 or higher, you can discontinue your iron supplement.

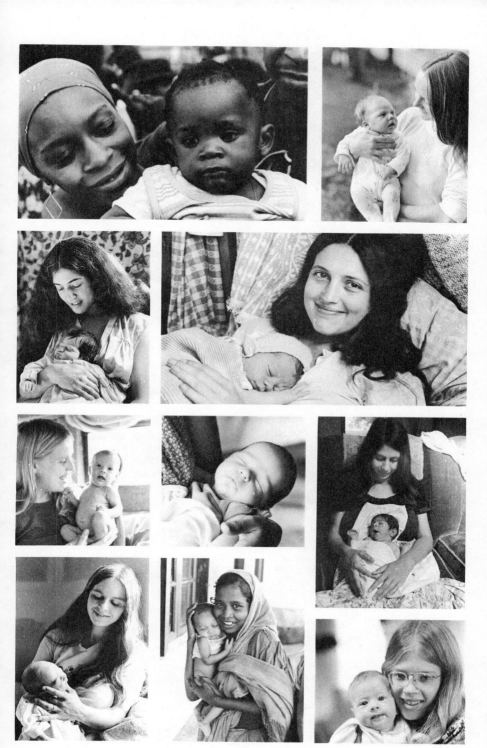

AFTER-BABY EXERCISES

After-Baby Exercises will restore your muscle tone after the baby is born. Start with the first exercise on the first day after the birth, and add a new exercise each day, in the order they are given. Do each exercise in sequences of 5, at least twice daily.

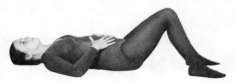

1. Breathe in through your nose, keep ribs as still as possible and expand abdominal wall upward. To exhale, blow air out through mouth slowly. Repeat.

2. Bend ankle up, pointing toes toward you; then point foot downward. Then make large slow circles with each foot, first clockwise, then counterclockwise.

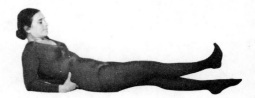

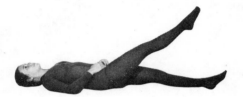

3. Bend knees up toward you and press feet into floor. Try to press the hollow at you waist into the floor and stretch neck. Hold, stretch for a few seconds, and relax.

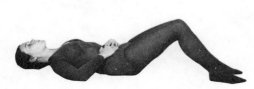

4. Contract the pelvic muscles, especially, the sphincter surrounding the urethra and vagina.

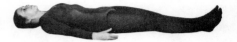

5. Roll pelvis back and contract abdominal and bottom muscles on outbreath. Hold for 3 sec. and relax.

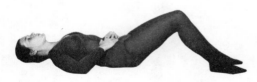

6. Flatten the lower back as you slowly slide your heels down.

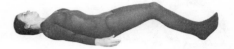

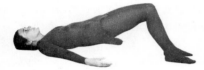

7. Raise hips so your knees and chest form a straight line. Contract your bottom muscles as you lift.

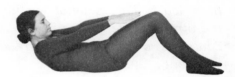

8. Lying on your back, bring chin to chest and lift head and shoulders as far as possible with you waist on the floor.

9. Lying on back, bring chin to chest and reach forward with outstretched arms to outside of left knee. Return and repeat movement to right knee.

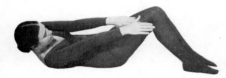

10. When you feel strong, do the same lift as for 8. and 9. with arms folded across chest. When these become easy, do the same with hands behind head.

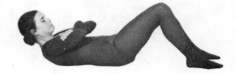

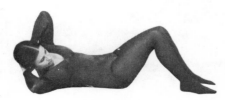

241

Children are our guides to the higher spiritual planes. They serve to remind us of what we may have lost or forgotten in our efforts to cooperate with our culture. They remind us that all human minds, young and old, are tuned to the same fundamental wavelength, and that we can all read minds — we just pretend that we can't, as we get older and find that our culture demands duplicity.

The child's state of consciousness is not to be rejected or replaced, but supplemented by the growing knowledge that you can't get what you want by force — physical or psychical. This is what we have to teach children, with the utmost patience we can muster, for the pain they may cause us is nothing to the revelation they offer at every moment.

— *Stephen*

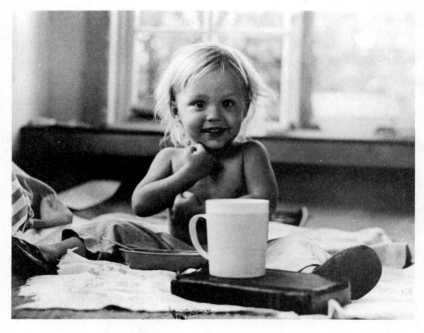

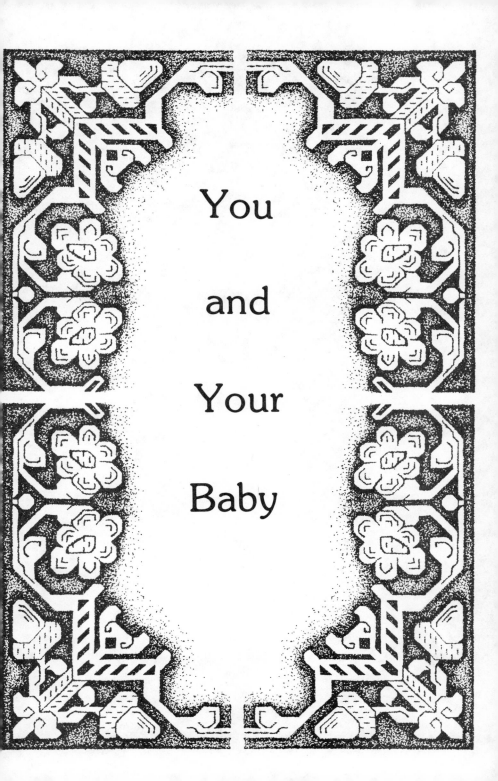

You

and

Your

Baby

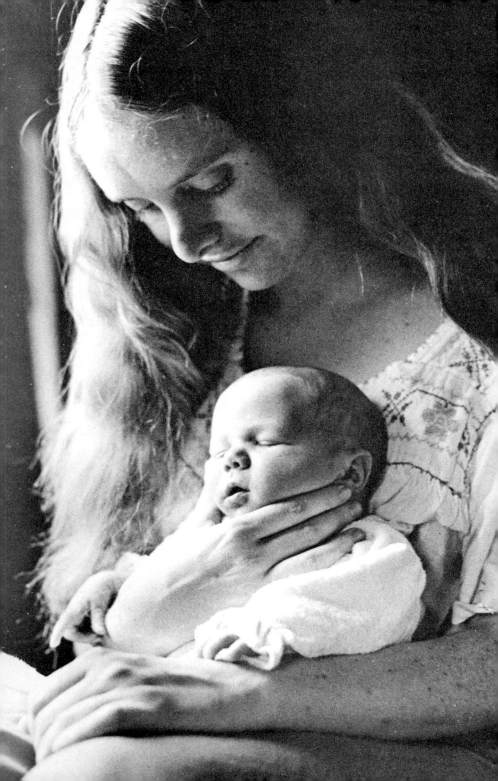

Touch Is The First
Language We Speak

Most mothers have talked touch with their unborn babies by poking and patting them when they kick inside their bellies. After the baby is born, the mother communicates something to him in every way she touches him. This is the way that babies get their information about the Universe that determines to a very large extent what kind of personality they will have as grown-ups. If the mother's touch is tentative and light and ginger [maybe she's afraid that the baby is so soft and new and delicate that she'll bruise him like a ripe peach], she's likely to find herself with an irritable baby who cries a lot. She's got to connect with him in order to give him some. What a mother communicates to her baby when she holds him with a good firm touch is that he can relax—she's not going to drop him—it's all covered.

Sometimes I'll see a mother breast-feeding her new baby and while the baby is sucking, she'll be rubbing her fingers back and forth on his leg, feeling how soft he is, cr maybe plucking at his toes, marvelling how tiny they are, and all the time she is fussing with his body she's not realizing that this is the same as tapping on someone's shoulder and trying to get their attention while they're trying to make love. I have cured several babies of colic by pointing out to the mother that the way she was handling the baby while he nursed made his stomach and intestines uptight and caused cramps. Once she learned how to get a nice firm grip on his thigh or his butt and let him know she was there without touch-talking irrelevant things to him while they made love, which is what breast-feeding is after all, then the baby would get over his bellyache.

—Ina May

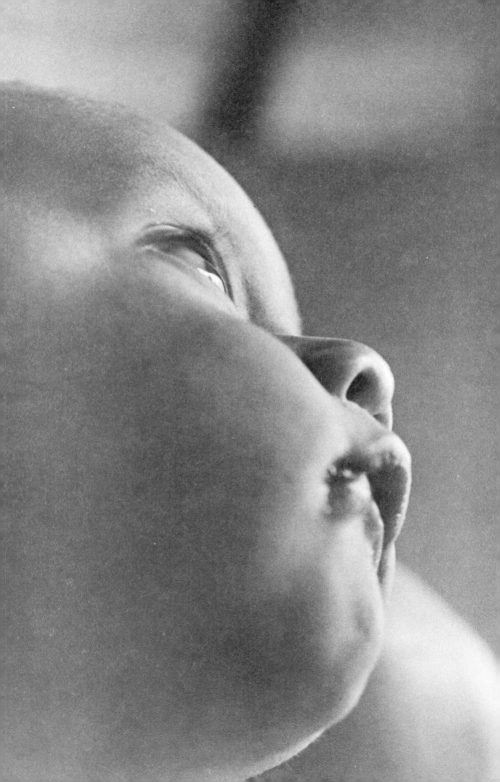

Taking Care of the Baby

The cord: The umbilical cord begins drying up soon after it's clamped and cut. In about 48 hours, your midwife or doctor will cut the cord clamp off. If the cord was tied off with string, it's not necessary to remove it. You should look at the baby's belly button frequently in the first 24 hours. Fold the baby's diaper low so it doesn't rub against his cord. Also, keep plastic pants low enough that they don't get around the cord and keep it from drying. Several times a day, put a few drops of alcohol or honey (both are drying agents) on the end of the cord where it was cut, and at the base where it meets the baby's body. Do this until it is completely healed. The cord keeps drying up until it falls off, which takes from a few days to over a week. It's common to see a tiny bit of blood around the belly button. A lot of times it's from the cord getting bumped. Just continue to put on alcohol or honey. That will dry it up and disinfect it. If the baby's navel gets infected, you will need to take him to the doctor. Here are the signs of infection: (1) redness around the navel; (2) oozing from the navel; (3) a bad-smelling navel.

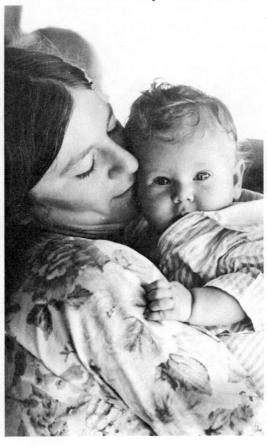

This is unlikely, but if there is active bleeding from the cord of more than a teaspoon *or* for longer than 10-15 minutes, you should call your doctor right away, or take the baby in to the nearest emergency room. If it's bleeding considerably and does not stop, you should put pressure against it with a sterile gauze pad to control the bleeding until you reach the hospital.

Fluids. Give your baby your breast right after birth and any time he is awake. Under ordinary circumstances, your baby will get all the fluids he needs from your breast. There are times, though, perhaps a very hot summer day when the baby loses additional fluids from sweating or in a room heated by a woodstove in the winter when your baby might need some sterile water given with a sterile (boiled for 20 minutes) eye-dropper or spoon. Pay attention to your baby's soft spot (fontanel). If it's depressed, you need to give your baby additional fluids.

Meconium is the sticky, greenish-black substance that is inside the baby's intestines while he is in the womb. A term baby will usually pass some within the first 24 hours, and a preemie within 48 hours. The baby should pee within 12-24 hours after birth, but he might take a little longer because the baby's fluid intake is small, or he may have peed during birth.

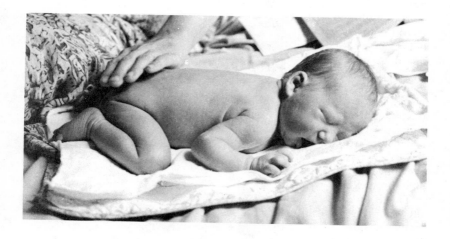

Sleeping the baby: The baby's crib should have a firm mattress. Tuck the sheet and blamkets in well, making sure there is plenty of room for him to breathe around his blankets. Especially at first, babies need a lot of sleep. Sometimes they may be awake all day, while another day they may sleep all day. Always sleep a baby on his stomach. That way, if he spits up or throws up he won't choke. If you get the urge to check the baby while he sleeps, do it. It's a natural urge and telepathic.

Jaundice: About two-thirds of all newborn babies get a little jaundiced. Jaundice is when the baby's skin turns a little yellow. This usually begins around the second or third day after birth, lasting up to a week or ten days after birth. The yellow color is caused by bilirubin in the skin. Bilirubin comes from the liver breaking down old or extra red blood cells and is usually excreted through the liver bile into the intestinal tract. But in the newborn, the liver is immature and overloaded so it does not get rid of it properly. This will pass. Give the baby as much water as he will take. Also, if the weather permits, take off as many of his clothes as possible and expose his skin to the sunlight for five minutes at a time (do not get him sunburned). This will take the yellow out. You can also lay him in the sunlight coming through a window.

Simple jaundice is not serious and usually disappears with no special treatment. If your baby looks pretty yellow to you in good light, see the midwife or doctor. If the palms and soles of his feet are yellow, see the doctor. If there is an accompanying fever, lethargy or lack of appetite, you need to see the doctor. He will do a bilirubin test, and if it is high, he will probably put him under a special lamp that does the same as the sunlight, only better. Quite high bilirubin can be harmful.

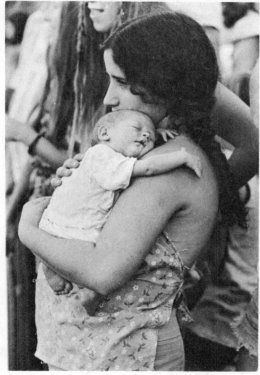

If jaundice appears at birth, or if it first appears after the fifth day, see the doctor.

Very rarely a baby may have "breast milk jaundice." This kind of jaundice usually develops from the fourth to the seventh day of life and peaks during the second or third week. It may continue for eight to ten weeks. With this type of jaundice, there is no need to stop breastfeeding. If the baby's bilirubin level is quite high, it may be necessary to discontinue breastfeeding for a couple of days to accelerate the drop in the bilirubin level. Express your milk during this time to keep your supply up, and begin breastfeeding again once the bilirubin has come to an acceptable level.

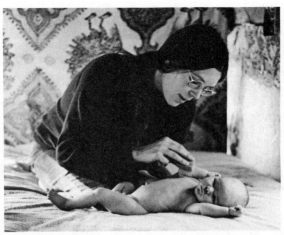

Washing the baby: Don't give the baby a full bath (immerse him in water) until his belly button is completely healed. Until then, warm water on a soft wash cloth works well to clean the baby off. Sometimes babies have skin that's dry, like parchment paper. You can use baby lotion for that. (Sometimes baby oil and lotion will clog up the pores and give the baby a rash, so you should watch for this.)

When you wash the baby, wash him really well, getting into all the creases and folds. Don't put Q-tips into his nose or ears. Wash behind the ears and under the arms. Get into the creases of the thighs and wash the crotch area well. Remember, the baby will be slippery, so get a good, firm hold on him.

You may notice in the first month that your baby's breasts look big. Full-term babies have large breasts from their mother's hormones; they may even have a little milk in them. Sometimes girl babies have a few drops of blood on their diapers. That's like a small menstrual period, also from their mother's hormones. Both of these manifestations will pass within a couple of weeks.

A newborn might have white spots scattered on his nose. This is common. His oil glands are beginning to function and are clogged. You don't need to do anything about them. They will go away. Washing them off with warm water is enough. Soap usually isn't necessary for a very young baby, but if you use it, just a teeny bit will do, and you should use a really mild kind. If a baby gets a pimple, or anything that looks a little infected, wash it and put some antibiotic ointment on it. If it doesn't get better, see your doctor.

Eyes: Sometimes babies' eyes will become goopy a day or two after birth. Your own breastmilk is a wonderful cleansing agent for this condition. We use an erythromycin (antibiotic) ointment to protect babies' eyes against infection after birth; state law used to require the use of silver nitrate, which killed bacteria but was very irritating to the eyes, causing them to become red and puffy.

Sometimes a baby has a red spot or two in his eye after birth, caused by a blood vessel that broke during delivery. It will clear up by itself.

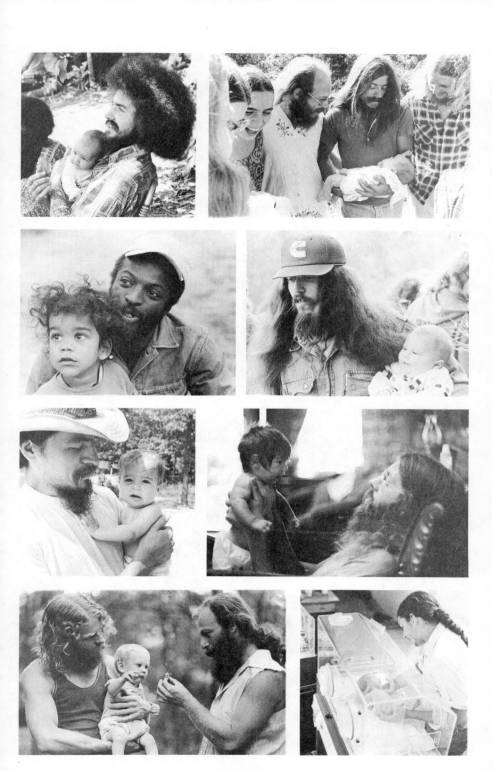

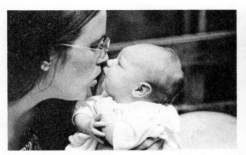
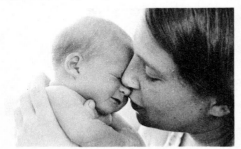
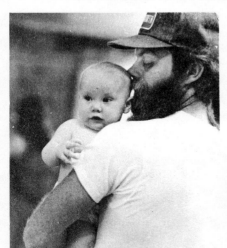
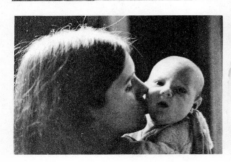
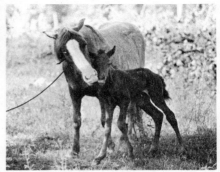
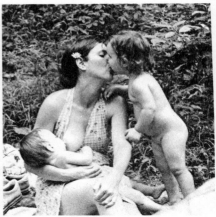
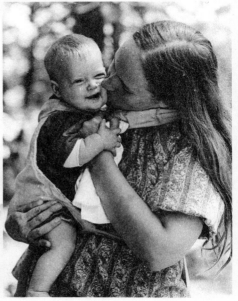

Man Does Not Live by Bread Alone

A nursing mother is really a Holy and sacred thing. If she'll really give her kid some and really let it go, she can become a tremendous generator of psychic energy. That energy is for the baby. They say, "Man does not live by bread alone." A kid that's been breast-fed for the first few months of his life is not making it on just the milk, he's making it on pure energy, which is being given to him in the form of — call it sexual if you like — vibrations. Those sexual love vibrations are a manifestation of Holy Spirit. When a child is nursing and soaks it up, it's good for the child and it makes him prosper and it makes him fatter, just as if it had put something material on him. You can come up to any lady who has a new baby and who's in love with that baby, and you can tune into it and it's just like those pictures called "Adoration of the Infant." To adore is to put your attention on somebody and become receptive to them, feel their vibrations in a telepathic and loving place, and it's the way you approach babies and Holy men and people like that. In religious art there are pictures of a bunch of people sitting around a baby and the baby has all these power lines coming out of his head and glows and has auras. You can see that on all new babies if you pay good enough attention and be pure in heart.

—Stephen

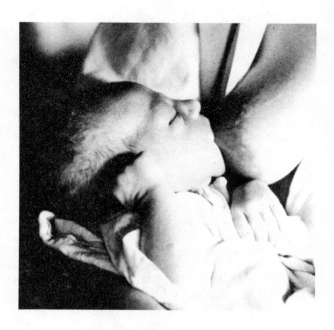

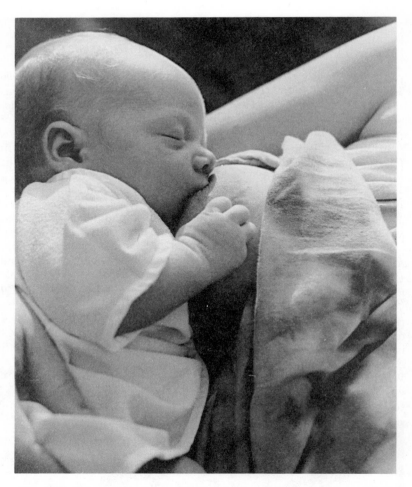

Breastfeeding: The best time to begin breastfeeding is immediately after your baby's birth. The quiet alert time, usually two or three hours, following birth is a time when the sucking instinct in the (undrugged) baby is quite strong. Your breast contains colostrum, which is beneficial both for its nutrients and the antibodies it contains, which give your baby immunities to invading bacteria.

When your milk comes in, usually two or three days after the birth, your breasts will become full, hard and heavy. Your baby's nuzzling, licking and sucking will tend to stimulate the release of oxytocin, which causes the let-down reflex, making the milk flow or squirt.

It is important to get your baby well latched on to your breast during the first few nursing sessions. Your main aim should be to get your nipple well centered inside the baby's mouth so it is held in a fixed position between the baby's tongue and palate. You don't want friction on your nipple caused by it being rubbed back and forth against the baby's palate or gums. Make sure that as much of the underside of your nipple is drawn into your baby's mouth as the upper side.

Don't be discouraged if your baby doesn't seem to know how to nurse immediately. Patience and persistence are required sometimes to get a successful latch-on.

Different babies have different styles of nursing. Some babies latch on the breast minutes after they're born and seem to be born hungry, while others aren't terribly interested until the milk comes in. Hold the baby so her head and body face yours. Stoke her cheek or her lower lip with your nipple and when she opens her mouth wide, draw her to you so she can easily reach your nipple. Some women need to pinch behind the nipple with their thumb and forefinger to make it stand out in an easily graspable mouthful. A little nipple soreness the first few days of nursing is normal. To avoid getting them more sore than that, make sure that your baby does not suck with her lips pursed, putting pressure on the end of your nipple. Sucking this way will only frustrate the baby, as it does not facilitate the flow of milk, and your nipple is likely to become sore from friction or from being gummed by your baby. When you want to take the baby off your breast before she is willing, put your finger right up by her mouth

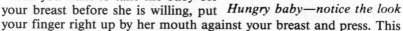

Hungry baby—notice the look

against your breast and press. This breaks the suction. It's important to take the baby off the breast any time you are feeling pain and to reposition the baby so she gets a better grasp on your breast.

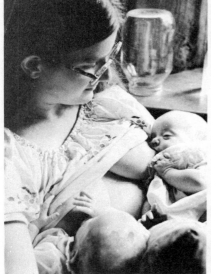

You may be amazed by how often your baby wants to feed. It is quite normal for a newborn to want to nurse every hour and a half or so. Babies don't understand feeding schedules, so nurse when your baby is interested.

Some women have the kind of breasts that leak and drip a lot; others don't. If you start nursing your baby on one breast and the other starts gushing, you can stop it by pressing your hand or a diaper firmly against your nipple.

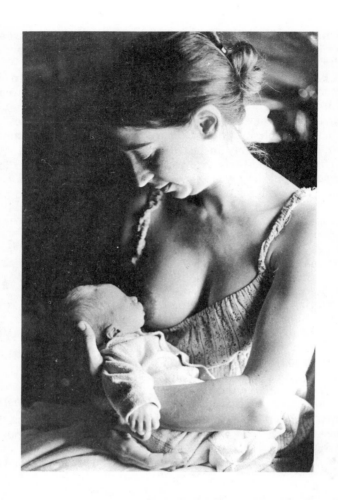

Burping: A good way to burp the baby is to hold him so he's sitting up straight, with your hand under his chin to support his head. Then run your fingers up his back, and that can bring the burp up. Or you can hold the baby to your chest and gently pat his back. If your baby doesn't burp after about five minutes, forget about it. A burp will eventually come up by itself. If the baby gets stomach aches or gas, try burping him longer and more often.

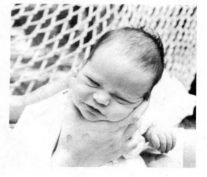

Spitting up and throwing up: Some babies just spit up once in a while but others spit up fairly often.

There's a difference between spitting up and throwing up. When a baby spits up, it comes out gently and sort of drools over him. It's just his stomach spilling over, and the amount isn't much. When he throws up, it comes out more forcibly and lands a distance away; it comes out with a spasm, and is most of the contents of his stomach. Every baby throws up occasionally, but if a baby throws up persistently, call your midwife or doctor.

Choking: If a baby spits up or throws up or starts to gag, sit him up straight *immediately*. This should be an automatic reflex. Don't worry about your clothes getting wet. There's a delicate balance between a baby's breathing equipment and his swallowing mechanism, and sometimes he gets confused between the two. If he is actually choking—that is, his airway is blocked—put his head lower than his body and whack him between the shoulder blades or squeeze his chest. If the baby really is not able to breathe, put your finger down into his throat to check for a foreign body and, if there is one, pull it out. The baby may need mouth-to-mouth resuscitation. Even an older baby or kid can choke while they're eating, so keep an eye on them.

Weight gain: Weigh your baby twice a week until he's regained his birth weight or weighs seven and a half pounds. After that, weigh him once a month until he's a year old. One way to make sure your breastfed baby is getting enough to eat is to notice how many wet diapers you get a day; there should be eight or more wet diapers per day.

Babies normally lose about 5% of their birth weight in their first few days. That figures up to about a half-pound or so. Then, when the mother's milk comes in, they start to gain. An ounce or more per day is an average gain. Babies tend to gain rapidly at first, and then slower as they get older. Larger ones gain faster than the smaller ones.

Babies gain at their own individual rates. As long as your baby is gaining, don't worry or compare him to the fattest baby around. Worrying makes uptight vibes and makes the baby lose his appetite. He knows how much he wants to eat, so don't force him to eat when he's not interested. (Except in the case of a preemie, who you might have to cajole to eat.) If it really seems to you that your baby isn't gaining as he should be, check with your midwife or doctor. Feed your baby all he wants, and squeeze and kiss him a lot and assume he's the size he's supposed to be. Remember: girl babies tend to be smaller than boys.

CHANGING DIAPERS

A mother's touch while she is changing her baby's diapers or while she is bathing him is a large determining factor in the formation of his personality. A baby can instantly tell if the person touching him is enjoying it or not.

Get right in there and enjoy changing diapers. There's nothing you can get on your hands that doesn't wash off with water. If you like cuddling him but touch him lightly and gingerly when you're changing him, he'll learn to think that his natural body functions are revolting, which can have a strong effect on his personality. If you enjoy cleaning all his cracks and folds, and like seeing a nice, clean, plump bottom, he'll grow up knowing his body is okay. I like to squeeze my kids' bottoms. They like it, too.

—Cara

Body and Mind
are One.
You affect your
baby's mind
by how you
handle his body.

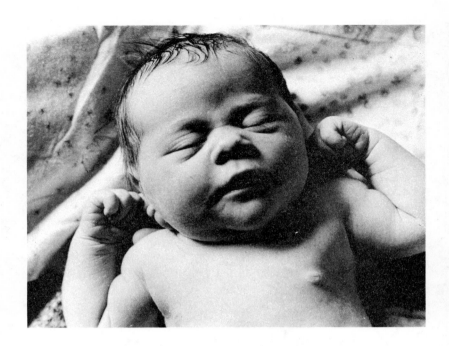

Diaper rash: Keeping a baby's bottom clean and changed will prevent most diaper rashes. Make sure you clean in all the cracks and creases. Apply a good baby oil after each change. Some diaper rashes are caused by the residues of harsh detergents or ammonia in the diapers. Bleach will remove ammonia, so a soak in bleach solution before washing is a good idea. Wash diapers with soap flakes, making sure to rinse them well. Bleach residue can be irritating, too. If the baby has a flat red rash, it's probably the same fungus as thrush. Paint it with 1% gentian violet. A bumpy red rash with water blisters on it is probably the ammonia burn mentioned above. Aloe vera gel or calendula cream are helpful for this type of rash. Sometimes babies get a combination of the two types of rash. If the weather permits, leave the diaper off your baby for awhile and sun her bottom. Avoid using disposable diapers with plastic liners or plastic pants over cloth diapers until the rash clears up. Try using two diapers for greater absorption.

Diarrhea: Some babies poop every two days while others do it six or seven times a day. But if your baby is going more than what seems normal to you, particularly if it smells bad (new, breastfed baby poop smells sweet), or if the baby has a fever or doesn't seem well, see your doctor.

Clothing, Fresh Air and Temperature: Newborn babies need to be kept warm, especially if they are small or premature. But babies who are a few weeks old and around eight pounds can maintain their body heat pretty well and shouldn't be way overdressed. Here's one way to judge if it's warm enough for your baby; his hands and feet can be a little cool, but if you put your finger along his neck or legs, or some other part of his body, it should be comfortably warm. Take your baby outside every day that weather permits. Sleep a baby where it's not too stuffy and there are no drafts.

Fever: If you think your baby is sick, or if he feels feverish to you, take his temperature. Use a rectal, or stubby, thermometer. Shake the thermometer down first, put a little petroleum jelly on the tip of it, and gently put it in the baby's rectum about an inch. The baby's temperature should be taken rectally, since this is the most accurate way. It measures the temperature inside the body, and that's the place that counts. You only need to leave it in for a couple of minutes to get an accurate reading. After you're done, read it carefully and wash it with soap and cool water.

A temperature from 97.5° to 99.5°F. is considered normal. If a baby has a fever in his first three months, check with your doctor. Often an older baby will get a fever of 101°F. and it will be gone by the next day; most likely it's a virus. But if the baby's fever is higher than that, or if it continues more than one day, call your doctor.

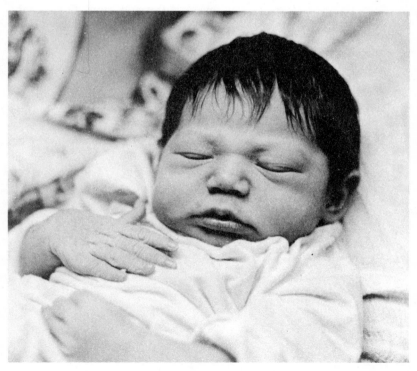

Snotty babies and colds: A baby can seem snorty and snotty, but sometimes it sounds worse than it is. A baby's nasal passages are narrow, so just a little snot can make a racket. A baby can catch a cold, though, and have a runny nose that makes it hard to breathe while he nurses or sleeps. You can suction out a baby's nose several times a day with a rubber syringe to clear it, but don't overdo it, because that in itself can be irritating. (For information on how to use the bulb syringe, see p. 357.) If a baby is otherwise healthy, being snotty isn't serious. You could mix 1 tsp. of salt in half a glass of water. Put 2-3 drops in each side of his nose, then suction out his nose. If he's still noisy, suction it out again in five minutes. The salt water helps thin the snot. Do this 2-3 times a day for 3 to 4 days. You wouldn't want to use it longer than this, as syringing can be irritating and cause more snot to be made. You could also try sleeping him in one of those little baby seats. You could ask your doctor to prescribe a cold preparation that would be suitable for a young baby if your baby seems bothered by the cold. It's not unusual for a baby to have a runny nose much of the winter months, but if he gets a fever or a persistent cough with it, call the doctor.

If he looks pretty sick and lethargic with a cold, even if he has no fever, get him checked out. A baby with a cold sleeps more; it's good for him. But if he sleeps all day, check with the doctor. Give a baby with a cold all the water he'll take; that will help loosen up the snot and keep him from getting dehydrated. A baby with a cold might not be as interested in food as usual.

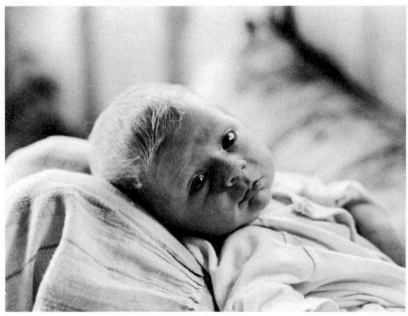

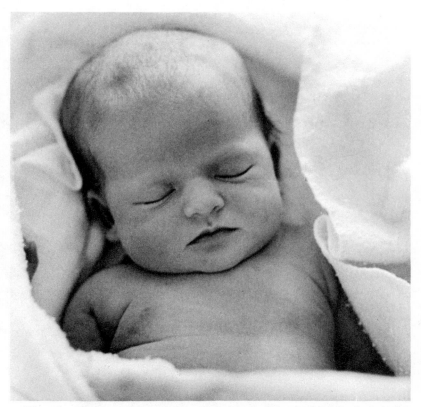

Thrush: If a mother has a yeast infection when she has the baby, the baby can pick it up in his mouth as he comes through the birth canal. It's called thrush, and is a pretty common fungus infection. The baby can also pick it up on his own. If your baby has it, you'll notice white spots in his mouth and on his tongue that look like milk curds but don't rub off. Sometimes a baby's whole tongue gets white. If your baby has thrush, paint his mouth with 1% gentian violet twice a day with cotton-tipped applicators until it's cleared up. Wash your nipples off with vinegar (and then rinse them) before you nurse the baby to prevent passing it back to him. (Vinegar creates an acid environment that thrush won't grow in.) Then give the baby some sterile water to rinse his mouth out, so there's nothing there to feed the yeasts.

Cradle cap: Cradle cap is very common. It's scaly patches on the scalp that look like a bad case of dandruff. Some doctors recommend Iodo-HC, an anti-fungus and hydrocortisone cream (needs a prescription). Others say to baby oil his scalp a few hours before shampooing and then scrub his head with a soft brush when you shampoo it. You need to have a doctor look at a case of cradle cap if it spreads or gets infected.

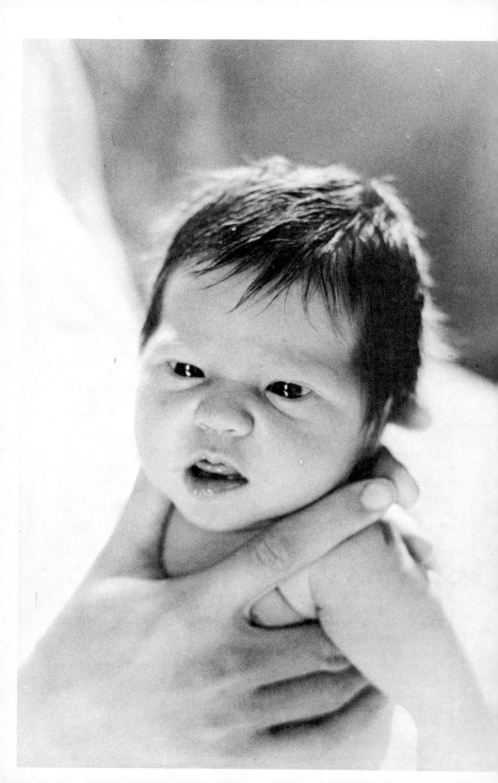

What To Do When Your New Baby Cries

Babies' cries mean many different things. They cry when they're hungry, when they're wet, when they want to be held, when they have a bellyache, when they want to be in a different position, when they need comforting. Don't be surprised if your new baby wants to be held all her waking hours. During her first nine months of existence, she was used to being surrounded by you. Your separation from each other by birth is only partial; she still needs your physical presence.

Sometimes there will be a conflict between your physical needs and those of your baby. Mothers have to make decisions constantly, so welcome to the club. If she is crying because she has just awakened and is hungry, pick her up if you're ready. But if you have to go to the toilet before you settle down to feed your baby, go ahead with good conscience. She won't starve in the meantime, and you need to set yourself up so you can be comfortable while nursing—your milk will flow better.

I preferred to change my kids' diapers before I fed them. Babies are like the rest of us—we'd prefer not to sit in a mess while we eat. Sometimes this won't be convenient, but generally it's a good practice. Take as much time as you need to do a good job of changing the diaper. Your hungry baby may not realize that your fixing up her bottom end will prevent discomfort later. If she is yelling frantically, tug on her leg gently and tell her why you're doing what you're doing, or lean down and gently whisper in her ear to stop crying. While you are changing the diaper, you can shush her and get her to quiet down before you nurse her. You can and should teach your baby to quiet down before you nurse her. She can't nurse well if she is crying—her stomach is too tight, her breathing will be out of rhythm and she will swallow air and get mad. If you make a practice of trying to stuff your nipple into your baby's crying mouth just to quiet her crying, both of you will learn a bad habit. Remember that you want to raise her so that you'll still like her when she's three or four years old. What you want to teach your child is that the way to get some (whatever that is) is to be sweet. She'll eat more at a time and will be able to digest it better.

If your baby hasn't stopped crying already, she'll probably do so when you bring her to nursing position. If she starts to get impatient, soothe her, and then put her to the breast.

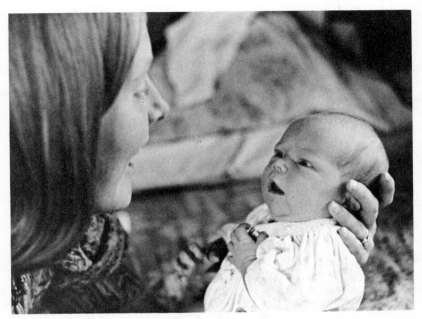

Deer babies react to a rustle in the brush or other external environment sounds or sights. A human baby responds to ruffles in the vibrations, more than the material plane. The human baby doesn't care what's going on in the material plane so long as the mother's vibrations are cool. The mother could be sitting on the carriage at a sawmill, nursing the baby, and if she's cool, the baby can be cool in that situation. But if the mother is uptight, or in an uptight situation, that can make the baby cry. That's what the baby really feels, and that is telepathic. That's why we feel that it's good for babies to be raised by their real mothers. We don't agree with the idea of the destruction of the family, that kids should be all desocialized by being raised by a whole bunch of folks. My real opinion about it is that it makes crazy kids. It's really good for kids to be raised by their biological mother who has certain interior psychedelics that her body manufactures to keep her stoned enough to match speeds with her kid, so she can be as stoned as her kid and relate with her kid. She's equipped to do that, but a lady who hasn't just had a baby isn't equipped the same way to do that. They are hormonal changes, and you get stoned on hormones; they get you heavy. So there is a relationship between a mother and her child that's realer than just conceptual, that is purely vibrational. The vibrations are really important and very real. If you take care of them, the rest of it will turn around and follow suit.

—Stephen

266

Circumcision

The Farm midwives neither recommend nor discourage circumcisions to new parents. If the family chooses, circumcision is done in a religious manner in the home or in the clinic, usually on the eighth day after birth, by one of the midwives, respecting the energy of the baby and his family. If circumcision is not done, retraction of the foreskin is not necessary. It's best to leave it alone. In one study, while only 4% of boys had foreskins you could pull back at birth, 90% of the boys' foreskins could be pulled all the way back by the age of three or four. Most two- and three-year-olds will mess with themselves enough to loosen up any adhesions. There are a very few babies whose foreskins are so tight at birth as to need manipulation. If the foreskin is loose and retractable, wash the baby daily (especially if you live in a hot, humid climate), and pull the foreskin back as far as it will easily go and wash with soap and water.

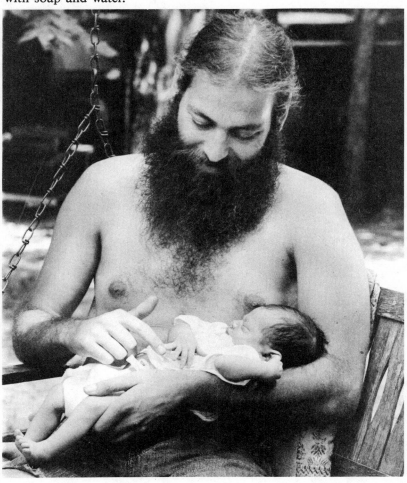

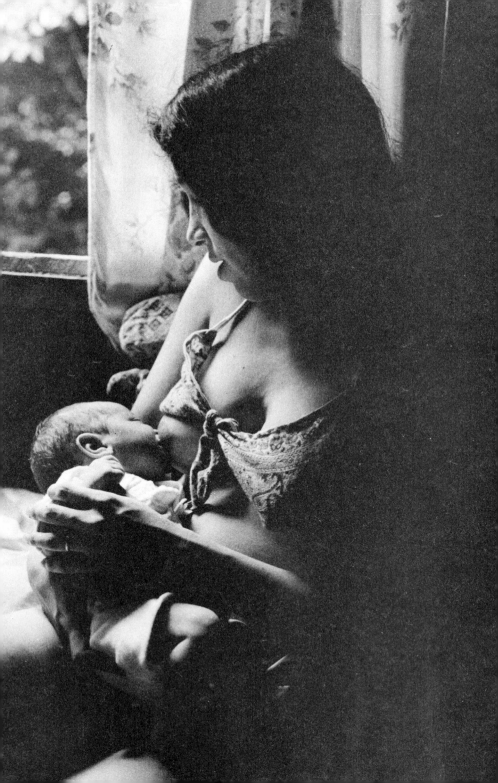

PROBLEMS OF NURSING

Sometimes mothers give up breastfeeding because of minor problems that arise, not knowing that there is usually a pretty easy solution. For instance, there are some mothers whose nipples are shaped in ways that make it more difficult to nurse their babies. These include women with inverted or flat nipples; the erectile tissue of the nipple does not gather into a convenient mouthful for the baby. I have had the greatest success in helping women with flat or inverted nipples when I have noticed the problem during pregnancy. I encourage the woman to have her mate help coax her nipples into a nice shape for the baby. As Caseaux, the famous French obstetrician of the 19th century, wrote: "Direct and repeated suction is, doubtless, the best means that can be employed."

Inverted Nipple

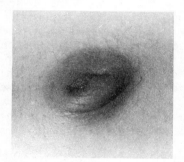 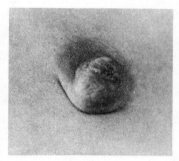

Before   *After*

Once the baby is born, the breasts may become painfully engorged. The breasts become swollen with milk, sometimes to the point that the baby can't easily grasp the nipple. It helps to soften the nipple if a little milk is manually expressed. If this is difficult to do, try getting into a warm shower before the next nursing session. Don't stop drinking fluids. Engorgement is preventable; it rarely takes place if the baby is suckled whenever possible.

Sore nipples occur when there has been friction or bruising damage to the nipple tissue. Again, prevention is the best course, and this lies in making sure the baby is correctly latched on to the breast, starting from the earliest nursing sessions. Your nipple should be centered in the baby's mouth, with as much of the underside of your nipple taken in as the upper side. This may be difficult for you to see. The baby's lips should look like those of the baby in the photo on the next page. When the baby has grasped your nipple in the right way, there is no friction, and his gums are no threat.

269

But let's say that your nipples are already sore and you need to know what to do. The first answer is to correct the baby's position at the breast in the manner described above, because your problem is that the baby is continuing to cause you damage either by friction or gumming. Chloe Fisher, senior Midwife from Oxford, England, has reported that she is able to correct 99% of problems with sore nipples by correctly positioning the baby at the breast. When the baby has correctly grasped the nipple, even one that is already traumatized, the mother is able to breastfeed comfortably.

Some women report that an ointment containing vitamins A and D was helpful. Sunning the nipples for 3-5 minutes can accelerate healing of a nipple that is sore to the point of cracking. It is important to note, though, that these steps alone will not correct a problem that is caused by malposition of the baby's mouth at the breast.

Breast infections sometimes develop during the nursing period. What keeps the breasts healthy during lactation is the regular flow of milk through the breasts. Warm sweet milk standing in the breast for too long a time makes an ideal culture for bacterial growth. In this instance, the negative effect is not directly on the baby, but rather on the mother. Early signs of a breast infection are the development of a hot area on the breast, soon followed by a reddened streak, and a fever. Other symptoms are flu-like: aching all over the body, chills and the shakes. The baby can safely continue nursing; there is no reason to wean because of a breast infection. It's much better for the milk to continue to flow through the inflamed area. The mother may need an antibiotic if the infection has progressed to the point that the baby's regular nursing does not correct the symptoms.

Breast infections are most apt to happen when the mother is travelling, over-tired, emotionally upset, grieving or separated from the baby for too long a time.

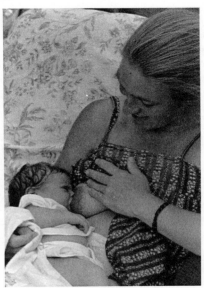

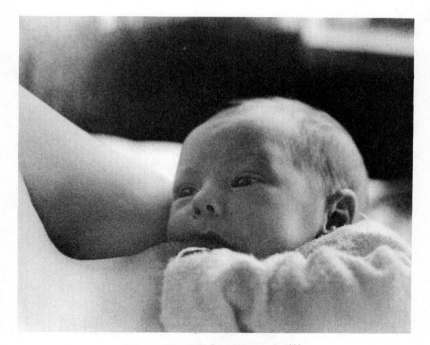

How To Make More Milk

It should be comforting to know that with the right diet and the right lifestyle and atmosphere, nearly every woman who wants to breastfeed her baby will be able to do so. Biologically, this is true. The experience of The Farm community lends a lot of credence to this statement, the women being drawn from all parts of the country, representing many social levels. During the early years of our community, our lifestyle did not include running water in most dwellings or electricity. No electricity meant no refrigeration, hence no infant formula, if it could be avoided. With almost no exception, the women of The Farm were able to fully breastfeed their babies until they reached a suitable weaning age, in most cases between one and one and a half years. This was appropriate for The Farm community but may vary according to local diet and custom.

Even premature babies were able to be breastfed, using the resources of the community to keep up the milk supply of the mothers while their babies were hospitalized. Friends and neighbors with nursing babies would stop by the home of the new mother, to let their babies nurse for a while, thus stimulating more milk production for her and boosting her confidence. In addition, she would pump milk and take it to the hospital to be given her baby.

271

The general rule to increase milk production is to slow your pace of life, increase the number of feeding sessions, eat well and get plenty of sleep. The frequency of feedings provides more effective stimulation to increased production than does the length of each session. Private feeding sessions are preferable to those in a busy, distracting atmosphere. If your stomach feels tense, take a deep breath and let it out slowly. There will be a twenty-four hour lag between the time you start programming your body to make more milk and the time it comes in.

Be sure to kiss and cuddle and play with your baby during these sessions. If she gets frustrated, stop for a play break for five or ten minutes, then put her back to the breast. Borage tea and red raspberry leaf tea may help to boost milk production.

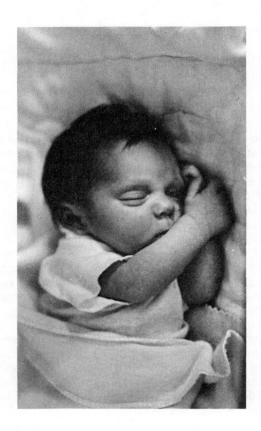

What To Do If Your Child Dies

There is no more helpless feeling than the one that comes when a child dies despite everyone's best efforts and prayers to keep him alive. It's a heart-breaker every time, and you don't ever get used to it. If you try to harden yourself and not feel the grief that naturally follows the death of someone who is part of your heart, you will repress that grief, and it will make you weird to do that. If you try to not feel the hurt in your mind and heart, it does not make the hurt disappear—your grief will manifest later in other ways. It's okay to cry. Grief has its own dignity. To feel it makes you telepathic with everyone else who has ever mourned, and it makes you more compassionate of others. Hold on tight to your family. Losing someone dear to you is one of the risks you take in loving anyone at all. If you keep your heart open, the rawness of the hurt will go away in time. This is how healing happens.

Don't be afraid to have another child.

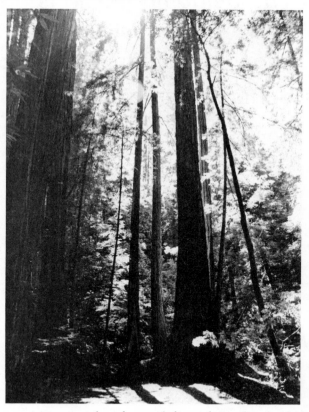

Helping out someone else who needs it, such as a lonely old person or a child who needs special care, is a good way to help your heart heal.

The Vow
of the Bodhisattva

*The deluding passions
are inexhaustible.
I vow to extinguish them all.
Sentient beings
are numberless.
I vow to save them all.
The truth is impossible
to expound.
I vow to expound it.
The way of the Buddha
is unattainable.
I vow to attain it.*

Instructions
to
Midwives

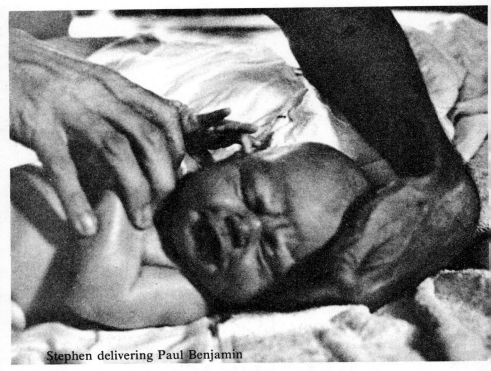
Stephen delivering Paul Benjamin

The Spiritual Midwife

The following discussion on spiritual energy is based on observations made at more than 1700 birthings. We have found that there are laws as constant as the laws of physics, electricity or astronomy, whose influence on the progress of the birthing cannot be ignored.

The midwife or doctor attending births must be flexible enough to discover the way these laws work and learn how to work within them. Pregnant and birthing mothers are elemental forces, in the same sense that gravity, thunderstorms, earthquakes, and hurricanes are elemental forces. In order to understand the laws of their energy flow, you have to love and respect them for their magnificence at the same time that you study them with the accuracy of a true scientist.

A midwife or obstetrician needs to understand about how the energy of childbirth flows—to not know is to be like a physicist who doesn't understand about gravity.

Every birth is Holy. I think that a midwife must be religious, because the energy she is dealing with is Holy. She needs to know that other people's energy is sacred.

Spiritual midwifery recognizes that each and every birth is the birth of the Christ child. The midwife's job is to do her best to bring both the mother and child through their passage alive and well and to see that the sacrament of birth is kept Holy. The Vow of the Midwife has to be that she will put out one hundred per cent of her energy to the mother and the child that she is delivering until she is certain that they have safely made the passage. This means that she must put the welfare of the mother and child first.

A spiritual midwife has an obligation to put out the same love to all children in her care, regardless of size, shape, color, or parentage. We are all One.

The kid in front of you is just the same as your kid. We are all One.

By religious, I mean that compassion must be a way of life for her. Her religion has to come forth in her practice, in the way she makes her day-to-day, her moment-to-moment decisions. It cannot be just theory. Truly caring for people cannot be a part-time job.

During a birthing there may be fantastic physical changes that you can't call anything but miraculous. This daily acquaintance with miracles—not in the sense that it would be devalued by its commonness, but that its sacredness be recognized—this familiarity with miracles has to be part of the tools of the midwife's trade. Great changes can be brought about with the passing of a few words between people or by the midwife's touching the woman or the baby in such a way that great physical changes happen.

For this touch to carry the power that it must, the midwife must keep herself in a state of grace. She has to take spiritual vows just the same as a yogi or a monk or a nun takes inner vows that deal with how they carry out every aspect of their life. So must a midwife do this if she is to have touch that has any potency. A person who lives by a code that is congruent with life in compassion and truth actually keys in and agrees with the millions-of-years-old biological process of childbirth.

If the midwife finds habits in herself where she does not always behave as if we are all One, she must change these habits and replace them with better ones. A midwife must constantly put out effort to stay compassionate, open and clear in her vision, for love and compassion and spiritual vision are the most important tools of her trade. She must know that she has free will and that she can change if she needs to. This is the spiritual discipline that she must maintain in order to be fit to do her work, just as an Olympic athlete must keep his physical and mental discipline to stay in top condition.

To one who understands the true body of *shakti,* or the female principle, it is obvious that she is very well-designed by God to be self-regulating. We are the perfect flower of eons of experiment—every single person alive has a perfectly unbroken line of ancestors who were able to have babies naturally, back for several millions of years. We are the hand-selected best at it. The spiritual midwife, therefore, is never without the real tools of her trade: she uses the millenia-old, God-given insights and intuition as her tools—in addition to, but often in place of, the hospital's technology, drugs, and equipment.

One of the midwife's most valuable tools is the same intimate knowledge of the subtle physiology of the human body that is the province of yoga. The spiritual midwife brings about states of consciousness in women that allow physical energy transformations of great power, great beauty and great utility.

> "Being a midwife is going to put you in danger of having your heart pierced—but that's okay, because when it does, a lot of love gets out that way. It will make you a better midwife."
> —Stephen

At birthings she must be able to guide a couple. She encourages and supports what feels good, and must be aware when a couple needs to talk something out. She must be able to teach a couple to give each other energy, if they need help. To do all this, she has to really know and love her husband, be his best friend and know how to give him some. If she has a solid, honest and loving relationship with her husband, she knows from her own experience what makes a good marriage, and her words will ring true.

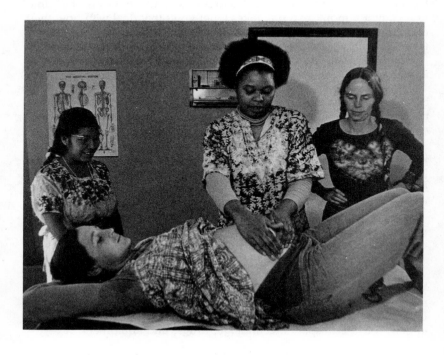

A midwife must be an avid student of physiology and medicine. She should read and study constantly in a never-ending quest for new information. She should never assume that she knows everything there is to know. A new piece of information she learned yesterday may be essential and life-saving tomorrow.

A midwife must have a deep love for other women. She knows that all women, including herself, are sometimes as elemental as the weather and the tides, and that they need each other's help and understanding. The true sisterhood of all women is not an abstract idea to her.

The trained midwife is entitled for fair compensation for her services. She may charge a fee or make a barter arrangement with the parents she serves.

In Zen Buddhism, they talk about your "original face." The Zen Master might say to a student: "Show me your original face." A midwife is an especially privileged person because she gets to see the original face of each child she helps to birth. The beauty and purity of the energy field that radiates from each child treated with proper respect is awesome and unforgettable.

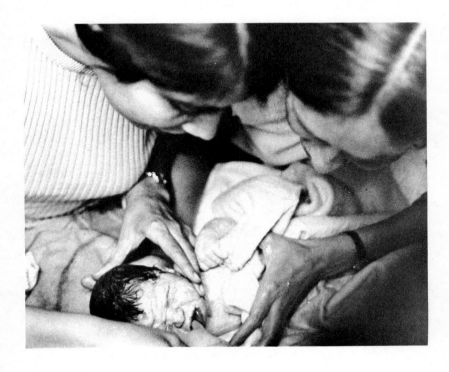

1. The Essential Anatomy of the Mother

THE FEMALE PELVIS

The pelvic girdle is a strong bony ring which supports, through the spinal column, the weight of the upper part of the body, and transmits this weight to the legs. It contains and protects the reproductive organs, as well as the intestines, bladder and rectum. The baby being born must pass through this bony ring, so you must understand pelvic anatomy in order to know everything you need to know to deliver babies.

The Pelvic Bones, Joints, and Ligaments

The pelvis is made up of four bones:
   The two hipbones (medical science calls these the "innominate" or
      unnamed bones),
   The sacrum, and
   The tailbone (in Latin, the "coccyx").

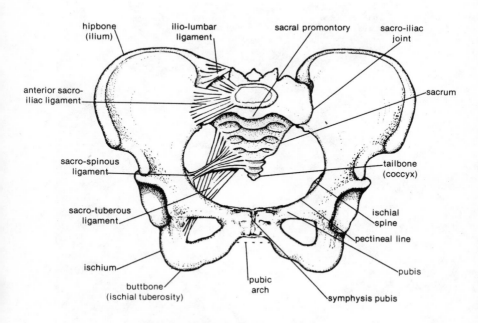

Fig. 1. Bones, Joints and Some Ligaments of the Pelvis.

The Hipbone

Each hipbone is made up of three bones: the ilium, the ischium, and the pubis. In a child, these three bones are separated by cartilage, but they fuse into one mass by the mid-twenties. The ilium is the upper wing-like part. Its crest is the upper curved border of the hipbone, felt just below the waist. The ilium also has a large curved inner surface. The ischium forms the lower behind part of the hipbone and consists of a body with two branches. The lower part of the ischium, the buttbone or "ischial tuberosity," is the part you sit on. These can be felt through the muscles of the buns, and the distance between them can be judged. Just above each buttbone and a little backwards and inwards is a sharp projection, the ischial spine. These can be felt from the inside, and it is important to note the distance between these in judging pelvic cavity size. The pubis is a small bone, having a body and two branches. The upper branch joins the ilium along the pectineal line, and the lower branch merges below with the lower branch of the ischium. The bodies of the two pubic bones meet at the symphysis pubis, forming the apex of the pubic arch.

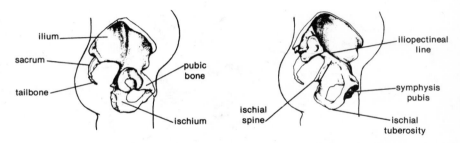

Fig. 2. Outer View of Right Hipbone. Fig. 3. Inner View of Left Hipbone.

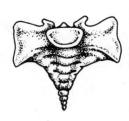

Fig. 4. The Sacrum and Tailbone.

The Sacrum

The sacrum lies between the two hipbones ("ilia"), and forms the back of the pelvis. It is a wedge-shaped bone composed of five fused vertebrae. The first of these five vertebrae is quite prominent on its inner surface which projects forward, and is called the sacral promontory. The sacral promontory is significant in determining the size of the pelvic inlet, and its prominence varies considerably in different women.

The Tailbone

The four small vertebrae, each smaller than the one above, located immediately below the sacrum, make up the tailbone, or "coccyx." The coccygeal vertebrae are fused to one another.

281

Sacro-Iliac Joint

A slightly movable joint between the sacrum and ilium.

Symphysis Pubis

A joint made up of cartilage located between the two pubic bones.

Sacro-Coccygeal Joint

This is a hinge joint between the sacrum and the tailbone, which allows the tailbone to move backwards a little as the baby's head passes by on its way out of the pelvis. Some women, following the birth of their children, don't feel quite right until enough pressure is put on their tailbone to push it back into its accustomed shape.

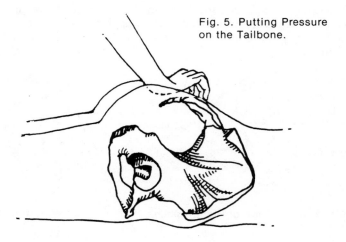

Fig. 5. Putting Pressure on the Tailbone.

It is important to know that powerful ligaments reinforce the pelvic girdle, the sacro-iliac joint and the symphysis pubis, giving the pelvis great strength and stability. There is always some limited movement of these bones, and this is greatly increased during pregnancy, as these ligaments are relaxed because of the hormones progesterone and relaxin and allow a fair amount of give when it's needed during birth.

The Pelvis As A Whole

The pelvis is divided by a bony ridge into a broad upper part and a smaller lower part. The upper division, called the false pelvis, is not important to the midwife, as it plays no part in the birth process. The lower division, the true pelvis, needs to be understood well by the midwife, because this is the part the baby's head must pass through

At the back of the true pelvis is the sacrum, at the sides are the butt-bones and at the front is the pubis. All of these bones are joined to form a pretty much unyielding ring of bone.

The true pelvis consists of three parts: 1) a brim or *inlet*, the first part the baby's head passes through; 2) a curved enclosure or *cavity*, which he passes through next; and 3) an *outlet*, which is the last bony part he must come through.

Fig. 6. True Pelvis.

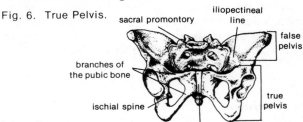

When measuring or estimating the dimensions of the true pelvis, it is useful to think of the pelvis as having planes — imaginary flat surfaces passing across it at different levels.

The Pelvic Inlet

The plane of the pelvic inlet is bounded:

1. In front, by the upper inner border of the symphysis pubis and the pubic bones;
2. On the sides, by the right and left iliopectineal lines;
3. In back, by the sacral promontory and by the alae (the wings or flared-out portions of the sacrum).

The Pelvic Cavity

The pelvic cavity is the middle section of the true pelvis, lying between the pelvic inlet and the pelvic outlet. It is a curved passageway, shallower in front (4.5 cm.), deeper in back (12 cm.), and bounded:

1. In front, by the pubic bones;
2. On the sides, by the buttbones and the ligaments which attach on one end to the sides of the sacrum and on the other to the ischial spines;
3. In back, by the hollow of the sacrum and the sacro-iliac joints.

The Pelvic Outlet

The pelvic outlet is the last bony passageway the baby passes through. It is bounded:

1. In front, by the pubic arch;
2. On the lower sides, by the buttbones and ligaments stretching between the sacrum and the buttbones;
3. In back, by the lower sacrum.

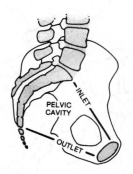

Fig. 7.
Divisions of the True Pelvis.

Essential Measurements

These are the most important measurements for the midwife to check when assessing the size of a mother's pelvis.

1. The Diagonal Conjugate

The diagonal conjugate extends from the underside of the pubic arch to the middle of the sacral promontory. This diameter is not the narrowest front-to-back diameter that the baby's head passes through, but it does help you to estimate (see Fig. 10) the obstetric conjugate, which is the smallest. The diagonal conjugate should measure about 12.5 cm.

2. The Obstetric Conjugate

The obstetric conjugate extends from the sacral promontory to the upper back side of the pubic symphysis, at the point where the pubis protrudes into the pelvic cavity. Because the sacral promontory and the inner side of the pubic symphysis both jut back a little into the pelvic cavity, this diameter is the smallest front-to-back diameter the baby's head must pass through. The obstetric conjugate can be estimated to be 1.5 cm. less than the diagonal conjugate. It should be about 11 cm. Remember you do have some leeway with this, depending on the size and preparedness of the mother and the size of the baby.

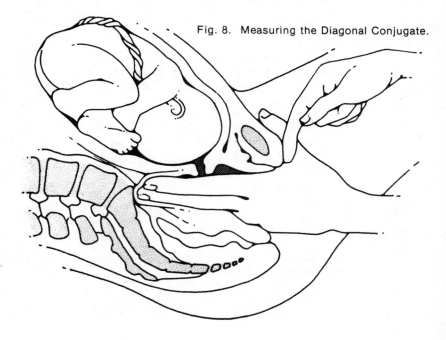

Fig. 8. Measuring the Diagonal Conjugate.

3. The Distance Between the Buttbones

This distance is sometimes called the bituberous diameter because of the buttbones being called the ischial tuberosities. This diameter should be 8 cm. or more, large enough for you to wedge your fist in between the bones when the mother is lying on her back with her legs bent at the knee and relaxed outwards.

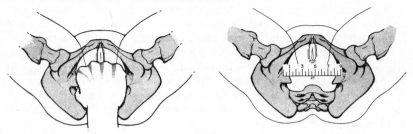

Fig. 9. Measuring the Distance between the Buttbones.

4. The Angle of the Pubic Arch

Estimate the angle of the pubic arch by tracing it with your fingers. Call it "wide" if it is greater than 90°, "medium" if it is 90°, and "narrow" if it is less than 90°.

5. The Distance Between the Ischial Spines

The ischial spines are the small protuberances on either side of the inner wall of the pelvis, located about halfway between the buttbones and the tailbone as you sweep your fingers around the inner curve of the pelvis. Feel them for sharpness and prominence, and estimate the distance between them. This will usually be greater than 10.5 cm.

6. The Distance Between the Pubic Bone and the Tip of the Sacrum [Obstetric Front-to-Back Diameter]

This distance is measured from the bottom inner edge of the pubic bone to the hinge joint between the sacrum and the tailbone. It should measure 11.5 cm. Note also the length and curve of the sacrum. (Refer to Figure 10.)

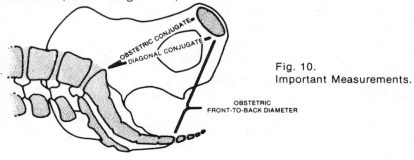

Fig. 10.
Important Measurements.

285

Most women's pelvises are large enough for them to give birth to the children they conceive. The experience of The Farm women should indicate that a random group of American women, approximately 1500 of them, did not have to have cesarean sections because of the size of the baby's head, except for four cases. Nine babies were helped into the world by forceps.

My conclusion after eighteen years' experience of helping mostly American women give birth is that the process of natural selection has worked well when it comes to the birthing process and the size of the baby's head to that of the maternal pelvis. We are not like the Boston Bull Terrier, a breed of dog which usually must be born by cesarean, since it has been bred over the centuries to have a large head size relative to its body size.

Occasionally you may find a woman whose pelvis is smaller or shallower than normal because of disease, accident or heredity. Rickets during childhood can affect pelvic size, so if you are attending births in an area where people are undernourished or where they don't get enough exposure to sunlight, watch for this. Dark-skinned people need more direct exposure to the sun's rays than do light-skinned people.

The main way to learn what size of baby head will come through what size of pelvis is to pay careful attention to your measurements during pelvic examinations. Experience is the best teacher. If you've trained yourself carefully, your own measurer-estimator works better than any pelvimetry equipment, including calipers, X-rays and ultrasonagraphy as pelvic size is a three dimensional measurement not always easily determined by two dimensional instruments.

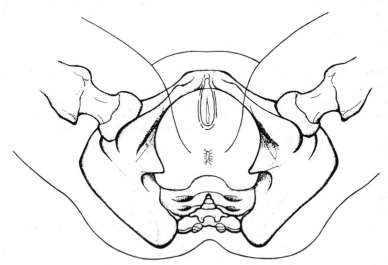

Fig. 11. The Outlet of the Pelvis Viewed from Below.

THE WOMB

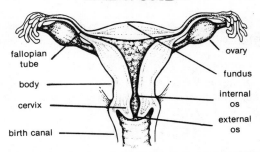

Fig. 12. The Uterus, Ovaries, Fallopian Tubes and Birth Canal.

The womb, or uterus, is a hollow organ located in the pelvic cavity and made primarily of muscle. You can think of it as having three divisions:

1. The *fundus* (the top of the uterus);
2. The *body* ("corpus"), which is the main part; and
3. The *cervix,* a narrow canal at the bottom of the uterus, with an opening above at the "internal os," into the inside of the uterus, and an opening below, the "external os," into the birth canal. The cervix is composed mainly of connective tissue with muscle fibers interspersed.

The womb is made up of three layers:

1. An outer layer, the *perimetrium,* which is peritoneal membrane, the same as that covering the abdominal organs and lining the abdominal cavity. This layer covers the uterus except at the sides.
2. A thick central layer made up of three layers of muscle fibers—the *myometrium.*

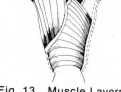

Fig. 13. Muscle Layers of the Myometrium of the Uterus.

3. An inner layer, the *endometrium,* the cyclically changing mucus lining of the womb. This lining is composed of many blood vessels, and has imbedded in it many tubular glands which reach down to the level of the myometrium.

The three levels of the myometrium are:

1. An outer layer of muscle fibers arranged longways;
2. A middle layer made up of interlacing muscle fibers and blood vessels;
3. An inner layer of circularly arranged muscle fibers.

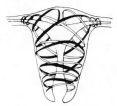

Fig. 14. Circular Arrangement of the Inner Muscle Layer of the Myometrium.

These three layers of muscle have the function of contracting to push the baby and placenta out of the uterus and the birth canal. The contractions of these muscles also serve to pinch off the blood vessels exposed when the placenta separates from the wall of the uterus.

287

Growth of the Uterus During Pregnancy

During pregnancy, the uterus grows from the size of a small pear (7.5 cm. long, 5 cm. wide, and 2.5 cm. thick) to the size of a big watermelon (28 cm. x 24 cm. x 21 cm.). The weight of the uterus increases from 60 grams to 1000 grams at the end of pregnancy. By the end of pregnancy, the uterus has changed from an almost solid organ to a thin-walled sac, muscular enough to push out ten or more pounds of baby and placenta.

Unusual Uteruses

The Septate Uterus
The septate uterus is one which has a septum of varying degrees of thickness dividing the inside of the uterus into two distinct parts.
The Double Uterus
Sometimes instead of one uterus, two form—each with its distinct cervix. When these occur, the birth canal can either be divided in two, or there can be two totally separate birth canals. (We have a lady on the Farm with a double uterus, who has given birth from both sides.)
The Forked Uterus
This type of uterus has just one cervix, but the fundus is divided into two parts.

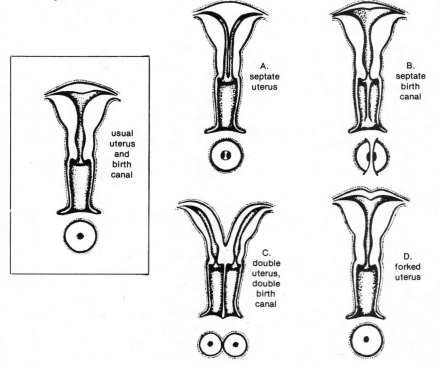

usual uterus and birth canal

A. septate uterus

B. septate birth canal

C. double uterus, double birth canal

D. forked uterus

Fig. 15. Unusual Uteruses.

THE PUSS

It is important for the midwife to know the structure and texture of the external genitals of women. I use the word "puss" rather than the Latin word "vagina" because I find it friendlier. I think midwives have to be friendly. You should use whatever word you find the most comfortable.

If you should find any of these words offensive to you, you should search your soul, because these are only words.

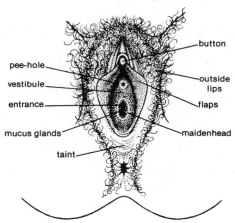

The Outside Lips [*Labia Majora*]

These are the two fat-padded folds of skin on either side of the opening to the puss.

The Flaps [*Labia Minora*]

These very stretchable folds of skin located between the outside lips vary a lot in size among different ladies. If a tear occurs during delivery, it is most likely to happen at the bottom of the lips (the "fourchette").

The Button [*Clitoris*]

This is a small, very sensitive structure of erectile tissue at the front junction of the flaps.

The Vestibule

The vestibule is the tissue you see when you spread the flaps. The pee-hole and the opening to the canal of the puss are located here.

The Pee-Hole [*I like this term because it's such good plain English — like fireplace.*]

This is a small opening below the button. The urethral canal is the tube extending upwards from here about 3.5 cm. to the neck of the bladder. There are two small ducts which open to the side and slightly behind the pee-hole. [*"Skene's ducts"—These are actually not Skene's; they're the woman's.*]

The Entrance [*Introitus*]

This lies between the flaps and below the pee-hole.

The Maidenhead [Hymen]

This is a thin membrane that partialy shuts off the entrance. This is torn with the first childbrith, if not with the first lovemaking.

The Taint [Perineum]

I call this the taint rather than using the Latin term—taint what's above, and taint what's below. This consists of a very stretchy group of muscles lying just pelow the puss.

The Mucus Glands ["Barhtolin's glands" in medical terminology—again, they're not really his.]

These are the two small mucus-secreting glands located on either side and slightly below the entrance to the puss. They lie between the flaps. They provide the mucus which helps to lubricate the canal.

The Birth Canal

The structure of the birth canal should be familiar to you. The canal consists of a lining of multifolded skin. This allows enormous stretchability. This canal leads from the outer part of the puss up to the uterus. The uterus lies above and behind the puss. The front wall of the birth canal is 7.5 cm., and the back wall is about 10 cm.

The area around the birth canal is supplied with blood through very small vessels, so even if there is a tear or an episiotomy during delviery there is not much blood loss. A tear to the upper part of the flaps or to the area right next to the button will be quite painful and can cause much more blood loss, so these should be prevented by doing a tiny episiotomy at the taint or by careful support of the taint while the baby's head is emerging.

Fig. 17.
The Pelvic Organs.

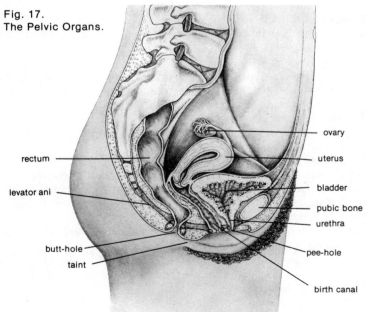

290

THE PELVIC FLOOR

The term **pelvic floor** refers to the arrangement of muscles, ligaments, and fascia (connective tissue) that forms a sort of diaphragm separating the pelvic cavity from the perineal area below. This arrangement of muscles and ligaments supports the pelvic organs, makes possible sphincter-like action for the tubes which pass through it—urethra, birth canal and rectum—and relaxes enough during labor to allow the passage of a term baby.

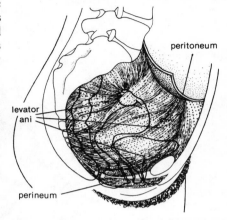

If these muscles are weakened and stretched through childbearing, involuntary contractions of the abdominal muscles as with coughing and sneezing can cause involuntary peeing. But the pelvic floor is amazingly elastic, and with proper exercise after childbirth, there is no reason for it to lose its integrity.

Fig. 18. Muscle Layers of the Pelvic Floor.

The pelvic floor has several layers. Starting from the top, there is:

The pelvic peritoneum. This peritoneal covering hangs over the uterus and fallopian tubes like cloth over a line. In front, it covers the top of the bladder, and in back, it forms a pouch behind the cervix, and then passes over the rectum. The peritoneal tissue covering the fallopian tubes is called the broad ligament. The broad ligaments are not really ligaments in the true sense of the word, as they do not support anything.

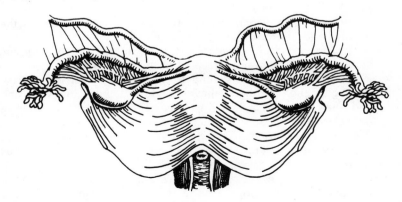

Fig. 19. The Pelvic Peritoneum.

291

The pelvic fascia. This is the connective tissue between the pelvic organs. It is the same tissue, in condensed form, that makes up the strong ligaments which support the uterus.

The ligaments supporting the uterus. These include the transverse cervical ligaments, the utero-sacral ligaments, the pubocervical ligaments, and the round ligaments.

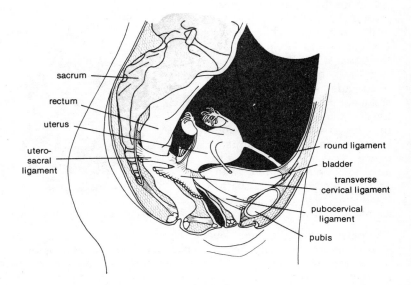

Fig. 20. Ligaments Supporting the Uterus.

The *transverse cervical ligaments* extend from the cervix and birth canal to the side walls of the pelvis. They provide the main support of the uterus.

The *utero-sacral ligaments* extend from the cervix, encircle the rectum, and attach to the front part of the sacrum.

The *pubocervical ligaments* extend from the cervix, running beneath the bladder and attaching to the pubic bones.

The *round ligaments* extend from the fundus of the uterus, passing through the inguinal canal and front abdominal wall, and end in the outer lips of the puss. They help to keep the uterus in its right position.

The deep muscle layer. The muscles of the deep muscle layer are described separately, but for all practical purposes form one continuous sheet of muscles which acts as a sling from the bony pelvis supporting the pelvic organs. These are called the *levator ani* muscles, and they provide the main strength of the pelvic floor. They originate from the back of the pubic bone over to the ischial spines, pass around the

292

opening of the puss, then around the butt-hole, fastening to the tailbone and lower sacrum. The levator ani muscles are divided into three individual muscles on each side (pubococcygeus, iliococcygeus, and ischiococcygeus).

The *pubococcygeus* itself has three divisions: the pubovaginalis, the puborectalis, and the pubococcygeus proper.

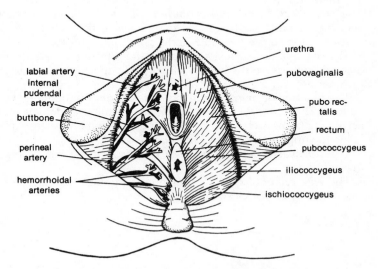

Fig. 21. Deep Muscle Layer and Blood Vessels.

The fibers of the *pubovaginalis muscle* contact and blend with the muscles of the urethral wall, and then make a loop around the birth canal (vagina). The ends of these muscles insert into the sides and back of the birth canal and into the central point of the taint (perineum). This muscle acts as support and sphincter for the birth canal, which in turn helps to support the uterus and its appendages, the bladder, the urethra, and the rectum.

The fibers of the *puborectalis muscle* form a loop around the butt-hole (with its internal and external anal sphincters) and the rectum. These fibers insert into the side and back walls of the anal canal between the internal and external sphincters and join with the muscle fibers of the sphincters.

The *pubococcygeus proper* are the muscle fibers which insert into the side margins of the coccyx at the back and at the front into the back side of the pubic bone. This muscle works in combination with the anal sphincter.

The *iliococcygeus* and *ischiococcygeus muscles* are less dynamic in childbirth than the muscles described above, but act with them to provide support for the pelvic organs.

293

The Perineum

The perineum is a diamond-shaped space just below the pelvic floor. It is bounded by:

> above, the pelvic floor—the levator ani muscles and coccygei;
> on the sides, the bones and ligaments of the pelvic outlet;
> below, the skin and fascia of the puss.

It is made up of:

The **superficial perineal muscles.** These muscles are relatively small, but do add some strength to the pelvic floor and add some sphincter action to the pee-hole, birth canal, and butt-hole.

The two *bulbocavernosus muscles* extend from the perineal body, around the puss, to the button (clitoris). They can squeeze together or open around the puss.

The two *ischiocavernosus muscles* pass from the buttbones to the button. The connective tissue, or fascia, from these muscles extends across the pubic arch to form the triangular ligament. This ligament helps to support the neck of the bladder.

The *transverse perineal muscles* pass from the perineal body to the buttbones.

The *external anal sphincter* surrounds the butt-hole and controls whether it opens or closes.

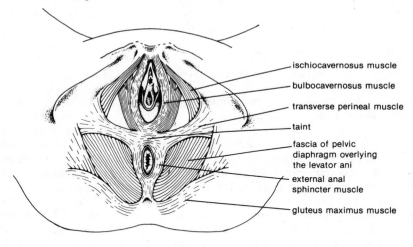

Fig. 22. The Superficial Perineal Muscles.

The **taint** (taint what's above; taint what's below) or **perineal body** is a wedge-shaped mass of muscular and connective tissue between the bottom part of the puss and the upper edge of the butt-hole. The taint is composed of the following muscles, which meet to form it: a) the external anal sphincter, b) superficial and deep transverse perineal muscles, and c) the bulbocavernosus muscle.

294

2. The Baby and Its Life-Support System

CONCEPTION AND THE GROWTH AND DEVELOPMENT OF THE BABY INSIDE THE WOMB

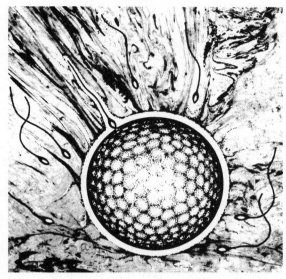

Conception or fertilization occurs when a sperm (the male sex cell) penetrates an egg (the female sex cell). This usually takes place in the fallopian tubes of the mother. Once fertilization takes place, none of the other 300,000,000 sperm cells that were deposited with the one that made it can enter the egg. As soon as the sperm and the egg unite, the inherited characteristics (such as sex, color of skin, hair and eyes) of the new baby are already determined.

After fertilization, the new baby (or zygote) divides and subdivides as it is swept through the tubes to the uterus. By the time the fertilized egg gets to the uterus four days after fertilization, it has subdivided into a small cluster of cells resembling a microscopic mulberry. Once in the uterus it burrows itself into the endometrium, the lining of the uterus.

By this time, the outside cells of the cluster have already started doing their job of nourishing the developing baby. They will grow to form the placenta. The baby starts to develop from the inner cells. Two weeks after conception, the 'baby' is made up of three layers of cells. The ectoderm, or outer layer, will develop into the nervous system, skin, hair, and nails. The mesoderm, or middle layer, will form connective tissue, urinary tract, bones, and muscles, and the endoderm, or inner layer, will form the lining of the intestinal tract, liver, and other organs.

By the *third week* after conception, the head end of the new baby (or embryo) can be distinguished from the tail end.

By the *fourth week,* * the baby has a rounded little body, with a head and trunk. During the fourth week, the spinal cord and the brain begin to take shape, and the back bones that will protect them begin to form. The face and throat begin to grow. The beginnings of eyes, ears, nose and mouth are present. The formation of most organs has begun—the stomach, the intestines, the liver and kidneys. The embryo has blood vessels, blood, and a heart, which starts to beat about the twenty-fifth day. Little buds that will become arms and legs form on the body. The baby's body is bent forward so much that its head almost touches its tail. By the end of the fourth week, the baby is one-fifth of an inch long from head to tail.

Fig. 23. The Baby at 4 Weeks.

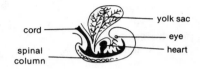

Fig. 23A. Enlarged View of Baby at 4 Weeks.

By the *sixth week,* the baby is about ½ inch long. The arms, legs, and face continue to develop. Fingers start to form in the beginning of the week, and a few days later the toes start forming. The arms and legs grow longer. The earliest reflexes are working. The baby has arms, elbows, fingers, toes and knees. He has footprints on his feet and palm prints on his hands. The brain already controls the functioning of the other organs. All the basic equipment is there; it just needs to develop and specialize. The tail is nearly gone. The arms are long enough so that the baby can touch his face, but they still can't touch each other. The skull is beginning to harden. There is a complete skeleton made of cartilage, which will later harden and turn to bone.

By *seven weeks,* the baby responds to touch—if you could touch his palm he would close his hand. If you could touch his eyelid, he would close it.

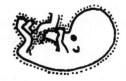

Fig. 24. The Baby at 8 Weeks.

*The average length of pregnancy is 266 days, or nine months, from conception to birth. Medical texts consider pregnancy to begin on the first day of the last menstrual period, about two weeks before conception. This makes pregnancy last 280 days, which is 40 weeks or ten lunar months. We are here considering pregnancy to begin at the time of conception.

By the *tenth week*, nails are starting to form on the stubby little fingers. Hair starts to grow on the head, the upper eyelids, and the eyebrows. You begin to be able to tell the boys from the girls. The kidneys secrete small amounts of urine.

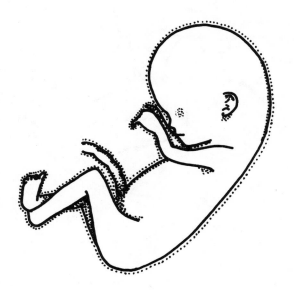

Fig. 25. The Baby at 12 Weeks.

By *twelve weeks*, the baby is three inches long from head to toe and weighs one ounce. His eyes are closed while they develop more. The baby starts to be quite active. He can move and bend his arms and legs, open and close his mouth and turn his head. He starts to be able to swallow and swallows amniotic fluid and pees a little once in a while.

At *fourteen weeks*, the baby completely fills up the uterus. Downy fuzz called lanugo begins to grow all over. The baby has fingerprints now. It's easy to tell the boys from the girls. There are even differences in the male and female pelvis. The baby's bones are beginning to harden, starting at the middle of each long bone and working towards both ends, a process that won't be complete until the baby is in his twenties. The mother may start to feel his movements now.

At *four months* of pregnancy, the baby is 7-8 inches long and weighs five ounces.

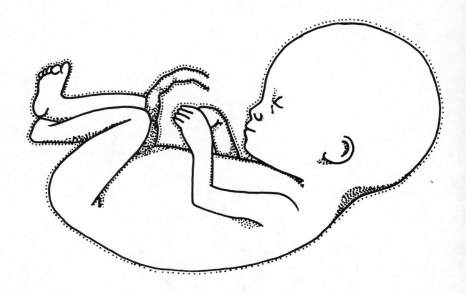

Fig. 26. The Baby at 4 Months.

At *five months* the baby is 10-11 inches long and weighs 1 pound. Hair starts to grow on the head. The skin is wrinkled and less transparent than before. The baby begins to store a little fat. There begins to be some vernix on the baby's skin. This is a thick, white cream which protects the skin. The baby starts to make primitive breathing movements. Some ladies can feel the baby hiccuping at about this time.

At *six months* the baby is 12-13 inches long and weighs 1½ pounds. His eyes are open again. If the baby is born at this stage, he will try to breathe and has a slim chance of survival.

At *seven months* the baby is 16 inches long and weighs 3-3½ pounds. From here on, the baby will gain about half a pound a week. He can suck now and may already have a thumb-sucking habit. He has a good chance of surviving if born now.

At *eight months,* the baby is about 18 inches long and weighs 6-7 pounds. He is getting fatter and less wrinkled. If born now he has an excellent chance of making it.

At *nine months,* the baby is about 20 inches long and weighs 7-7½ pounds. He is plump and smooth, usually with not much vernix on his skin. He is all ready to be born.

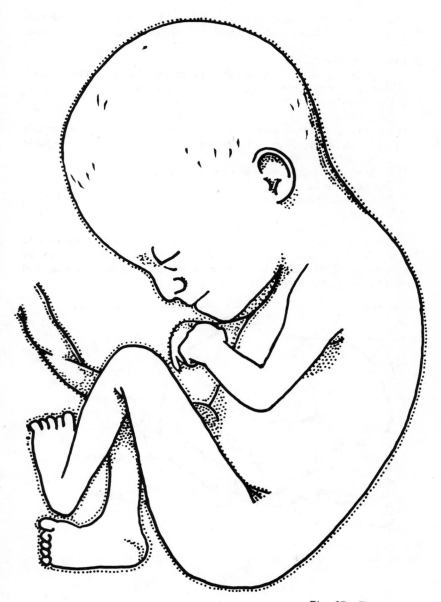

Fig. 27. The
Baby at 5 Months.

THE BABY'S HEAD

The baby's head is generally the largest and least compressible part that you have to deliver, so you need to understand how it is made.

Sections of the Skull

You can think of the skull as being made up of three sections:

The vault, containing the majority of the brain

The face

The base

The bones of the face and the base are united, hard, and therefore completely incompressible. The bones of the vault are compressible because of their movability.

The vault, or cranium, is made up of several bones:

The occipital bone

Two parietal bones

Two temporal bones

Two frontal bones

The seven bones of the vault are connected to each other and to the bones of the face and the base of the skull at the sutures by membranes. This makes possible a lot of molding and overlapping during labor, with no damage to the baby.

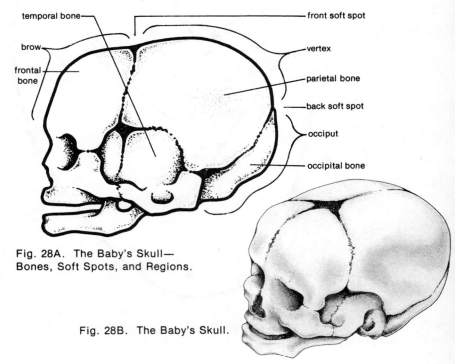

Fig. 28A. The Baby's Skull—
Bones, Soft Spots, and Regions.

Fig. 28B. The Baby's Skull.

300

Sutures of the Skull

There are four sutures of the vault. They are composed of soft, fibrous tissue. By knowing where they are, you can tell the position of the baby's head inside the mother. These are the four sutures:

The frontal suture, uniting the frontal bones;

The sagittal suture, uniting the parietal bones;

The lambdoidal suture, uniting the back edges of the parietal bones to the occipital bone; and

The coronal suture, uniting the frontal bones to the front edges of the parietal bones.

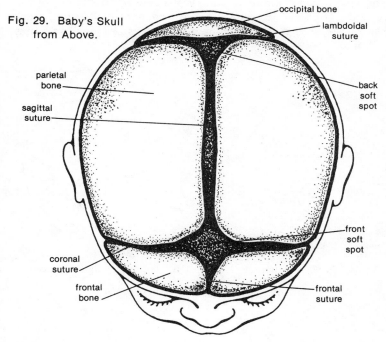

Fig. 29. Baby's Skull from Above.

Soft Spots [fontanels]

Soft spots are the membrane-filled spaces where the sutures intersect. You need to know two: the front and the back. Knowing these helps in determining the position of the baby.

The front, and larger, soft spot (the "bregma") remains open, diminishing in size, till the baby is 16-18 months old. It is diamond-shaped, 2 to 2½ cm. wide and 3 to 4 cm. long. You can feel it vaginally if the baby is lying with his face towards the mother's abdomen.

The back soft spot is much smaller, and is triangular-shaped. This soft spot closes at 6 to 8 weeks of age. You can usually feel the back soft spot vaginally in a vertex presentation.

Molding

Molding iş the change in the shape of the baby's skull that takes place when the moveable bones of the skull that are loosely joined by membranes slide over each other, reducing the circumference of the skull. When these bones overlap, the frontal and occipital bones pass under the parietal bones, and one of the parietal bones may slip over the other.

The actual volume of the skull does not change during molding. Compression of some of the circumferences of the baby's head is accompanied by expansion of other circumferences.

At the time of birth, the membrane is still between the bones of the sutures and soft spots. Eventually bone formation (ossification) takes place and there are no more membranous spaces between the bones of the skull.

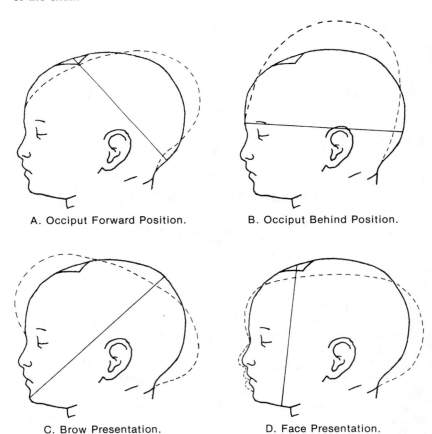

A. Occiput Forward Position.   B. Occiput Behind Position.

C. Brow Presentation.   D. Face Presentation.

Fig. 30. Molding of the Baby's Head.

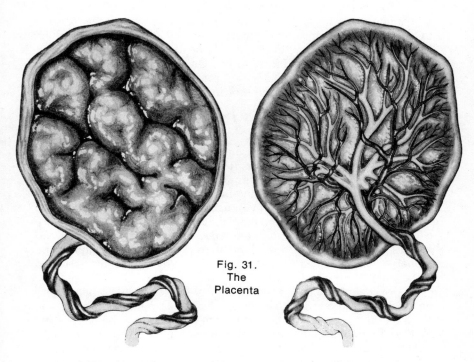

Fig. 31.
The
Placenta

A. Maternal Side.

B. Fetal Side.

THE PLACENTA

The placenta, at term, is a bluish-red, round, flat, meat-like organ, about 15-20 cm. in diameter, 3 cm. thick, and about 1/6 the weight of the baby. It serves the same function for the embryo and fetus in the womb as the kidneys, lungs and intestines do for us after birth. The placenta is made of tissue derived both from the mother and baby, juxtaposing but not mixing the blood streams of mother and child. Because maternal and fetal blood streams are so close, nutrients and oxygen from the mother's blood in the uterine arteries can move into the fetal blood, which has circulated through the baby and become depleted of these substances. Another part of the process is the movement of carbon dioxide and other waste products from the baby's blood into the maternal circulation. The entire surface area of the placenta, which is made up of great numbers of tiny villi, is estimated to be 15 yards. In multiple pregnancies there may be more than one placenta, depending upon how many fertilized eggs have been implanted in the uterus.

The placenta has two surfaces:

—the maternal surface is the rough, red, meaty-looking side, and is the side that is attached to the wall of the uterus during pregnancy;

—the fetal side is covered with a membrane and is white, smooth, and

303

shiny. The membranous covering is actually two membranes, the chorion and amnion, and these continue on past the outer edge of the placenta to form the water bag which contains the baby and the amniotic fluid. The umbilical cord arises from this side of the placenta.

The placenta has other functions besides that of providing a place for the interchange of nutrients and gases; it also synthesizes several nutrients for the baby and secretes several of the hormones of pregnancy.

Placental Circulation

While the baby does drink the amniotic fluid and pee in the womb, he doesn't breathe or digest food. The placenta does all this for him.

The baby's blood is pumped through his body by his heart, only two chambers of which function during the intrauterine period. In the adult heart, all four chambers function to maintain circulation. Blood from the veins of the entire body enters the right atrium and then the left ventricle, which then pumps blood to the lungs via the pulmonary trunk and arteries. Oxygenated blood from the lungs then passes through the pulmonary veins to the left atrium of the heart. What I have just described is the pulmonary circuit.

The oxygenated blood is pushed out of the left atrium when it contracts, moving into the left ventricle, which then pumps it through the aorta and the arteries which branch from it throughout the body. After moving through progressively smaller arteries into capillaries, it is finally picked up from the smallest veins, eventually pouring into larger and larger veins and returning to the right atrium through the superior and inferior vena cavae. This phase of circulation I have described in the paragraph is the systemic circuit. It is quite separate from the pulmonary circuit in the adult. The embryo and fetus, however, have three circuits within their circulation: the systemic, the yolk sac and the umbilical. No pulmonary circuit functions in the fetus, although the equipment, the pulmonary blood vessels as well as the lungs, is all formed, ready for service as soon as birth occurs. The circuit of the yolk sac functions only temporarily during prenatal life. The umbilical circuit, which includes one umbilical vein, two umbilical arteries, and the placenta, functions throughout the prenatal period up till the time of birth, when it is discarded.

Two devices in the fetal heart keep the oxygenated blood from flowing through the pulmonary circuit. At birth, the two devices, the foramen ovale and ductus arteriosus close, and the baby now switches to using just the pulmonary circuit and the systemic circuit, the adult pattern of circulation.

Some drugs, viruses and antibodies can cross the membranes that separate the mother's and baby's blood. Because of this, it is important for mothers to be sure they are taking no substances that can cross the placental barrier and have a harmful effect on the developing baby. Such substances are called teratogens.

304

Types of Placentas

Placenta with One or More Smaller Lobes

Most placentas are of the type shown in Figure 31. Sometimes, a placenta may have small lobes separated from the main body and attached to the main placenta by blood vessels. The danger with this type of placenta is that the smaller lobe can pretty easily become detached from the main body and be retained in the uterus after the rest has been expelled. This can cause post-partum hemorrhage and infection. If you ever see a tear or defect with torn blood vessels at the margin of the placenta or in the membranes, you probably are dealing with this type of placenta, and steps must be taken to empty the uterus completely.

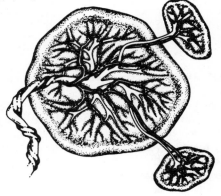

Fig. 32. Placenta with Additional Smaller Lobes.

Double Placenta

This is a placenta divided into two main lobes. It is quite uncommon. Examine for this type in the manner just described: that is, check for completeness of membranes.

There are a few other uncommon varieties of placentas which present no problems in delivery.

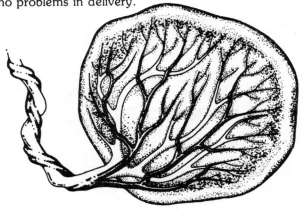

Fig. 33. Placenta with Marginal Insertion of Cord.

305

THE UMBILICAL CORD

The umbilical cord connects the placenta to the baby. It is filled with a whitish-gray, jelly-like substance which protects the umbilical vein and the two umbilical arteries from being compressed. Usually the cord is about 50 cm. long and 2 cm. thick.

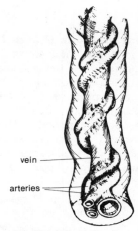

Occasionally there is only one artery in the cord instead of two, making the total of blood vessels in the cord two instead of three. This is the case in about 1% of cords, and about 15% of these are associated with congenital abnormalities of the baby.

Fig. 34. Umbilical Cord.

Abnormalities of the Cord

The cord can be very short, very long, very thick, or thin. A short cord can cause problems, but fortunately it is very rare. A too-long cord is more likely to become knotted, prolapsed or wound around the baby's neck or limbs. A very thick or very thin cord is harder to tie off than a normal cord, so this must be very carefully done and inspected to prevent hemorrhage. Very rarely a piece of the baby's intestine can protrude into the cord. You will probably never see this, but suspect it if the cord is swollen close to the navel. Occasionally the cord will be precariously fastened to the placenta and may tear loose in the third stage.

THE MEMBRANES

There are two fetal membranes: the *amnion*, the inner stronger membrane which secretes the amniotic fluid; and the *chorion*, the outer membrane, which lines the uterine cavity. It is continuous with the edge of the placenta. The two membranes lie next to each other and can be easily separated from each other.

THE AMNIOTIC FLUID

The amniotic fluid usually amounts to from one to one and a half liters at term. This liquid is secreted by the inner membrane of the water bag, the amnion. This fluid makes a nice shock absorber for the baby, allows the baby to move freely, helps the baby maintain its temperature and keeps the membranes from sticking onto the baby's skin.

306

3. Prenatal Care

A program of good prenatal care is essential for the physical and spiritual welfare of the mother and baby. If you are dealing with a couple, the father of the baby must also be included in this program so that he is well aware of the physiological and emotional changes his wife will be going through and how he can best support her during this special time. In some cultural situations, it is necessary for the midwife to prepare the entire family of the pregnant mother for the birthing. The midwife needs to see the pregnant couple on a regular basis in order to get to know them well. She must make sure that all of her couples are well-prepared for labor, giving birth, and accepting responsibility for a new life. If she is caring for several pregnant couples, it's a good idea for her to assemble them and have educational discussions with them all together. This way they share with each other the benefits of their common experience—be community for each other. Single women need extra support.

Prenatal checkups should be given monthly starting from the probable diagnosis of pregnancy up to the last two months. During the eighth month, the checkups should be done bi-weekly. By the last month the midwife should have screened out any women who would not be good candidates for home birth and turn them over to the care of someone else with better facilities for their care. The criteria for judging whether a home birth is safe or not are discussed on page 319.

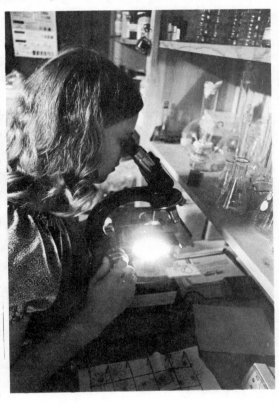

You need to have access to a good lab because there are certain tests it's a good idea to do in order to insure the safe care of the mother and baby. These will be discussed later in this chapter.

307

Basic Equipment for Prenatal Care

- fetoscope: (there are several types available).
- blood pressure cuff: (avoid the cheap ones or those with a pin-stop, as these may give inaccurate readings).
- stethoscope
- watch with second hand (if you use a digital watch, make sure seconds are indicated).
- speculum
- strips for testing for protein or glucose in urine (make sure these haven't passed their expiration date)
- sterile and non-sterile examination gloves
- tube of sterile lubricant
- tape measure
- betadine or some suitable antiseptic soap
- scales

These supplies should be available through a local medical supply house or from a mail order birth supply company. See Resources in Appendix B.

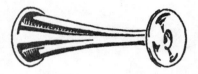

Fig. 35. Horn Fetoscope.
(British type)

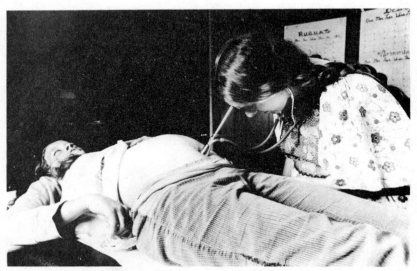

Listening to the baby's heartbeat with a standard American fetoscope.

308

THE FIRST CHECKUP

Get to know the mother (both parents if both are present) as well as you can. You are going to be very deeply involved with them, so a strong bond of trust and friendship is necessary. You have the responsibility of two lives in your hands. Notice how the parents feel about the coming baby and with each other. Help them talk with each other if you see that they need to. The first visit should include history-taking; a general physical examination as described below; and a pelvic examination to ascertain pregnancy and to determine pelvic measurements. You don't have to be rigid about the order in which you do any of these procedures. Sometimes a thorough stomach rub and a pelvic exam is the best way to begin. Sometimes it's best to get all your history taken first before you do a physical exam. You might even choose to postpone doing a pelvic exam for a week or two after your first meeting with a lady, so that you have a chance to win her trust first—particularly if she is a young, single lady.

It is important to keep thorough and accurate records of medical history and physical examinations of each person in your care. See page 465 for a sample form. These records are important both for your own reference and for intelligent communication with any doctor or midwife you might need to consult about any of your ladies.

History Taking

The Present Pregnancy
Find out the date of the first day of the last normal menstrual period. Of course, not all women keep records of their menstrual periods, so you must keep this in mind. You need to know whether her last period was a normal one, in keeping with the rest of her menstrual history. A scanty "period" is possible after conception because of bleeding at the time of when the fertilized egg (the blastocyst) implants itself into the uterine lining. The probable date of birth will be nine months and seven days after the first day of the last normal period.

Find out about menstrual history up to the last period. If the mother has long cycles, a history of missed periods, or an irregular cycle, your calculations of her due date may not be very accurate. Get her menstrual history in as much detail as you can. If you are not certain that the last period she reports is normal, note this on her prenatal chart so that you know there may be a possibility of mis-estimating her due date.

History of the present pregnancy also includes any complaints regarding the pregnancy by the mother in order that you may detect possible complications before they become serious.

Record any visual disturbances, headaches, fevers, unusual fatigue, nausea, vomiting, dizziness, shortness of breath, back pain, pain on urination, vaginal discharge or bleeding, leg cramps, backache, edema (noting where this occurs), infections, varicosities, breast changes, abdominal

pain, heartburn, variation in heart rhythm or rate, constipation, infections, accidents, medical treatments, medications or drugs taken, exposure
to radiation (including X-ray), ultrasonography, feelings about the pregnancy, sexual complaints, and the date the baby's first movements are
felt. Keep detailed notes on each woman under your care.

Previous Pregnancies

Find out about all of these, whether they resulted in a live, healthy
child or not. Find out about any miscarriages or abortions and at what
stage these occurred. Find out about probable causes and treatments.
Ask about all aspects of these pregnancies, deliveries, and the period
following—the length of pregnancies and labors, normal or compli-
cated, whether anesthesia or forceps were used, the birth weights of the
children, whether the mother hemorrhaged or not, and whether she
was able to breast-feed or not. Know the present health of any other
children.

Previous Medical History

Record important illnesses, all medications, blood transfusions,
allergies and drug sensitivities. Find out what contraceptive methods
the mother has previously used and if fertility studies have been done.

Record past surgical history, including all operations and serious
injuries. Give dates. Note especially surgery or injury to pelvis,
spine and abdomen.

Family History

Any woman who has relatives with diabetes or hypertension should
be watched carefully for the development of these conditions. The
presence of glucose in the mother's pee might mean she is diabetic
or in a diabetic state sometimes brought on by pregnancy. She should
be seen by a doctor. Find out if any near relative has tuberculosis,
as this disease is easily passed to newborns.

Other Things To Check

1. **Record blood pressure.** See p. 461 for instructions on how
   to do this.

2. **Record the mother's present weight.**
   Make sure she knows what to eat and in what amounts (see
   pp. 221-223), to properly nourish herself and her growing
   baby.

3. **Check her pee** with test strips for the presence of protein or glucose. Make sure your sticks haven't expired. The notice on the side
   of the bottle is relevant if the bottle has not yet been opened. Once
   the bottle is opened, the sticks can be trusted for accuracy for only

The Rh Factor

The Rh factor is a substance found on the red blood cells of most folks. 85% of people have this and are said to be Rh positive (Rh+). 15% don't and are Rh negative (Rh-).

This is of no importance in most situations except if, by chance, the blood of an Rh+ person gets into the bloodstream of an Rh- person. The Rh- person would develop antibodies in his blood to fight off the strange "invader." This would never happen except in a mismatched transfusion *or in the case of an Rh- woman pregnant by an Rh+ man.* Her unborn baby would often be Rh+ and under certain conditions, mainly during childbirth, their blood could mix. (Usually it doesn't.) This would cause the mother's blood to get sensitized and form antibodies against the substance in the baby's blood. These antibodies destroy the baby's red blood cells. This usually wouldn't harm a first baby because he would already be out by the time the antibodies were formed and they wouldn't get back into the baby's system. But the antibody response is stored in the body and the antibodies can pass from the mother's blood to the baby's blood through the placenta, and so could harm the blood of her next baby.

Fortunately, there is a way to control this. An Rh- mother with an Rh+ husband should have her blood checked for antibodies several times during pregnancy. Most likely, they will not show antibodies. Then, the day after birth, the Rh- mother will need a shot of *Rhogam* to prevent any antibodies from forming in case the blood did mix. Consult with your doctor on how to go about getting the *Rhogam* shot. This shot must be given within 72 hours after the birth in order to be effective. If the Rh- mother's baby is Rh- she will not need the shot because their blood would not be antagonistic.

If she has had several children, miscarriages, or abortions and has a high antibody count or for some other reason her antibodies are high, she will need to deliver in a hospital where they can induce labor early to get the baby out of a hostile environment, and transfuse it if necessary.

There is no complication from an Rh+ mother and an Rh- father. If the baby was Rh- like his dad, his blood would not have any extra substance in it to mobilize his mother's defenses.

4 months. Keep them away from humidity, and write the date of opening on the bottle. The pee you test should be fresh and unstirred, and its container should be clean before use. Dip the stick in the pee quickly, taking care not to stir. Wash your hands after completing the test.

4. ***Look for changes in the mother's breasts.*** They will probably be enlarged, tender and tingly, especially if this is a first baby. The nipples are likely to darken. The areola (the outer part of the nipple) in a pregnant lady usually begins to develop about fifteen little raised lumps called Montgomery's tubercles. You may be able to squeeze a little colostrum from the nipples.

5. ***Make sure the mother has an adequate supply of prenatal vitamins and iron.*** Ask your friendly local pharmacist to help you with this.

6. ***Examine the mother's puss, legs and feet for varicosities or edema.***

7. ***Check the mother's thyroid gland.*** This requires examining the mother's neck. The thyroid gland is a soft endocrine organ that sits on the lower and outer edges of the thyroid cartilage (Adam's apple). A normal gland is soft and smooth and it is not very easy to feel its margins. An enlarged gland can be seen and felt, especially while the mother is swallowing, since it will rise up in the neck when the thyroid cartilage moves.

The thyroid gland may be slightly enlarged in a normal pregnancy but should be checked by the doctor if it is especially large, or if lumps are found in it.

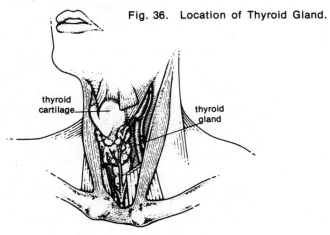

Fig. 36.   Location of Thyroid Gland.

thyroid cartilage

thyroid gland

8. ***If, for any reason***—general appearance, previous medical history, family history, or just intuition—you feel that the mother needs a more complete physical, consult with your doctor.

Pelvic Examination

Have the mother pee first. Put on an examination glove. It needn't be sterile unless there's an infection present. Be gentle and sensitive with the mother as you check her.

To check for pregnancy

Put two fingers inside the birth canal, under the cervix. Put the other hand on the lower abdomen. By pushing your two hands together you can feel if there is an enlarged uterus there. At six weeks of pregnancy, the uterus is larger than normal. By about eight weeks (ten weeks past the last period) it is about as big as a tennis ball.

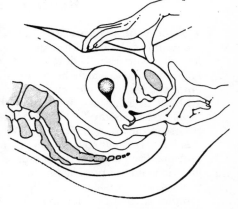

Other things to notice while in there are:

Cyanosis (bluish color) of birth canal—At six weeks (Chadwick's sign).

Soft cervix—Usually the cervix

Fig. 37. Checking for Pregnancy.

feels kind of hard, like the tip of your nose; when you're pregnant, at 4-5 weeks, it feels like your lips (Goodell's sign).

Softening of the junction between the cervix and the body of the uterus—at 5-6 weeks, you can compress it almost paper-thin with bimanual examination (Hegar's sign).

(Check the pelvic measurements—see p. 284 for how to do it.)

Pregnancy Tests

We don't usually do pregnancy tests, but sometimes for some reason it seems important to find out right away if a lady is pregnant. Then we do one in our lab.

Chorionic gonadotropin, a hormone secreted by the chorionic villi in early pregnancy, is excreted in the urine. This is what is tested for in the pregnancy tests. These tests are usually positive about 10-14 days after the first missed period, or at about one month of gestation, but you can get a false negative if the hormone is not being secreted yet. The percentage of error in these tests is about 5%. The hormone is secreted throughout pregnancy, but in smaller amounts later on. For these tests, early morning urine is used, since that makes the test most accurate—it's the most concentrated. You need about a tablespoon. It should be labeled and kept cool and taken to the lab as soon as possible.

313

SUBSEQUENT PRENATAL TESTS

Frequency • every four weeks during the first seven months
• every two weeks during the eighth month
• every week until the onset of labor

Routine Procedures

1. Record blood pressure, both systolic and diastolic, at each visit. If the mother's blood pressure gets too high, you should be in communication with your friendly doctor. The bottom number (diastolic) is the most important one to watch, because the top (systolic) changes a lot with your emotions, activity, etc. High blood pressure would be a reading over 130/90, or a diastolic rise of more than 30 mm. Hg. pressure above her usual blood pressure (or her blood pressure during the first two trimesters). So it's not just a high blood pressure to watch for but a blood pressure

that is high relative to the woman's normal pressure. High blood pressure is usually the first indication of pre-eclampsia. It should prompt you to watch carefully for other symptoms. Statistics for the 1700 births that have taken place under our care since 1971 show that the women who were complete vegetarians (their diet was based on the soybean, and they ate no dairy products) exhibited no hypertension, and pre-eclampsia among them was extremely rare (1 case out of a group of several hundred women). A cautionary note is needed for complete vegetarians, though: enough protein-rich foods such as dried beans, tofu, and nuts or nut butters must be eaten 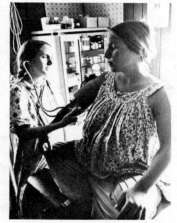 to maintain good health during pregnancy, and vitamin B12 must be supplemented.

2. Check the mother's weight. The mother's weight gain may be about 25-50 pounds during pregnancy. Some ladies, if they're underweight to begin with, can add forty or fifty pounds without it being an excessive burden to their system. This includes the weight of the baby, the placenta, amniotic fluid, some water retention and a little extra fat. Tell the mother to save some of her weight gain for the last couple of months when the baby will be growing rapidly, about half a pound per week. A weight gain of over four pounds a month for two months in a row might make you suspect twins. Be sure the mother is eating right, making especially sure that she is getting enough protein. You need to keep in mind that a lady may be ill-educated or too opinionated about nutrition to feed herself well.

Usually a weight gain of 25-35 pounds is about right during a pregnancy. With Kay Marie though, it felt best to me for her to gain more with each of her pregnancies. Before she got pregnant with her second son, she weighed only 87 pounds. (Her best weight was about 100.) Everyone was encouraging her to eat, but she wasn't able to gain any weight for a few weeks. Then she got pregnant, and recovered her appetite right away. She kept asking if it was okay to be gaining so much weight, but she looked very healthy and had no problems with her blood pressure or anything else. She just had a good appetite for the first time in a long time, and it felt like she was recovering weight that she needed. So I just kept saying, "Eat, Kay Marie, eat. Eat as much as you like." She weighed 135 when her baby was ready to be born—a total gain of 48 pounds—and looked good. (I had already seen how fast she lost weight and got her figure back while she was nursing, so I thought a bit of extra fat on her at birthing time would not hurt her any.) Her son weighed nine pounds, two ounces, at birth—about 1/10th of her pre-pregnant weight. It was an easy, mellow birthing, and everything went fine.

3. Check the mother's pee for the presence of protein and glucose. If there is excessive protein in the pee, check with a doctor. If you get a urine sample with more than a trace of protein, you'll need to check it again. The most accurate way to get a urine sample is what they call a clean voided mid-stream or a "clean catch." This way you don't get much contamination from the outside of the puss. Have the mother first wash off well with some good surgical soap and rinse well, then pee and catch some from the middle of her pee in a clean jar. (Use a sterile jar if you're going to have it tested for bacteria, if you think the lady has an infection.) Check with your doctor if the protein reading reaches +30. (The protein reading and the blood pressure reading give you a check on the mother's kidney function, which is quite important to both her and her baby's health during her pregnancy.) Again, glucose in the mother's pee can mean diabetes or a pre-diabetic state, so check with your friendly doctor if you find this.

If the mother's pee appears abnormal in any way, get a further urinalysis done.

4. Feel the mother's breasts. Pregnant tits need to be massaged and squeezed since they are in such a state of rapid change and development. Check the nipples, and if they are quite tender, have the mother or her husband massage them daily to toughen them.

315

5. *Measure the belly.* Measure from the top of the pubic bone to the fundus (top of the uterus). At twelve weeks, the fundus should be

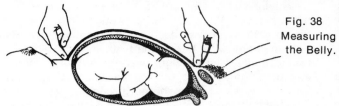

Fig. 38
Measuring
the Belly.

just above the pubic bone. At sixteen weeks, it should grow about one centimeter a week. After 20 weeks the fundal height from the pubis corresponds closely (within 2 centimeters) with the number of weeks of gestation. If it grows more, it may be twins. If it grows less, something such as high blood pressure or infection may be causing the baby to grow slowly.

Feel how high the mother's uterus is each time and check the growth of the baby.

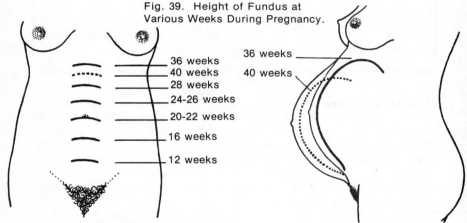

Fig. 39. Height of Fundus at Various Weeks During Pregnancy.

36 weeks
40 weeks
28 weeks
24-26 weeks
20-22 weeks
16 weeks
12 weeks

36 weeks
40 weeks

6. *Check fetal heart tones.*

The baby's heartbeat is usually audible from 20-24 weeks. It sounds something like a watch under a pillow. Early in pregnancy you can hear it in the middle just over the pubic bone. A baby's heart beats around 120-160 times per minute. When you first start hearing the heartbeat, it may

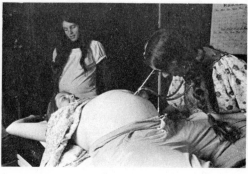

316

be as rapid as 150-160 beats per minute, and at term it's usually between 120-140 beats per minute.

7. Check the mother's arms and legs for edema or varicosities.
Seek further treatment if necessary. If you have a pregnant mother with edema, check her pee and blood pressure carefully. Pre-eclampsia is a dangerous disease, and it should not go unnoticed. Generalized swelling can be an indication of pre-eclampsia. If her swelling isn't severe and it's just in the ankles, and her blood pressure and urine tests are normal, don't worry. Have her keep her feet up as much as possible, and if she has a heavy salt intake, you might advise her to cut down to a normal intake. If she has any of the following symptoms: generalized swelling, pitting edema in her legs and arms, and facial swelling, you need to check for other symptoms of pre-eclampsia, such as high blood pressure and albumin in her pee. A diagnosis of pre-eclampsia is made when there are two of the symptoms associated with it.

8. Check the baby's presentation and position. See p. 325.

9. Check the mother's belly for amount of fluid. In cases of polyhydramnios (more than the usual amount of fluid), consult with your doctor, as this is, in some cases, accompanied by other unusual circumstances such as twins or certain congenital abnormalities, and it may predispose the mother to post-partum hemorrhage.

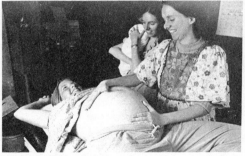

Other Things To Check

Find out from the mother when she feels the first movement of the baby. This is called quickening. It can be felt as early as twelve weeks, but is more usually felt at about 16-18 weeks. Ladies who have been pregnant before tend to notice the baby's movements earlier.

Internal exams should be done at each prenatal visit during the last six weeks of pregnancy. Check for the presentation, station, and position of the baby, as well as the degree of softening and thinning of the cervix. The ripe cervix will be quite thin and soft, and it may even be able to admit the tip of your finger in the last few days before the baby is born.

Screen for genital herpes (see p. 423) in the last two weeks before the due date. You will need to use a speculum and light to look into the mother's birth canal. If there are any active lesions in the birth canal or anywhere in the crotch, find out if they are herpes. If the mother has active herpes sores, a c-section is necessary.

Lab Work

Some labs can do hematocrits or hemoglobin counts separately, while others do these tests in conjuction with the complete blood count (CBC). You need to know the hematocrit (HCT) or hemoglobin (HGB) to assess if the mother has anemia and whether she is in need of any supplements to boost the oxygen-carrying capacity of her blood. HGB values should be about 11.0 and HCT should be at least 35. One of these tests should be done at 12 weeks and again at 28 weeks of pregnancy. A low hematocrit means that both mother and baby are suffering some measure of oxygen deprivation. The mother will tire easily, be more susceptible to illness, and the baby's growth may be adversely affected. Other symptoms of anemia are a fast pulse, dizziness upon standing, pale conjunctiva, and problems with breathing. Anemic women are more apt to hemorrhage after birth, and they don't tolerate blood loss as well as women who aren't anemic.

Some degree of "anemia" during pregnancy is normal, because of the normal dilution of the mother's blood that occurs due to the increase in her blood volume. During pregnancy, blood volume is increased by one third to a half, nature's protection to the mother in the event of hemorrhage.

There is a type of iron tablet consisting of ferrous peptonate, vitamin C and B-complex; the additions are there to aid assimilation. Ferrous sulfate is another possibility, although many women who take it complain of constipation and indigestion. In recent years, I have used alfalfa tablets and chlorophyll supplements for anemia in pregnancy, with excellent results. Hematocrits seem to improve more rapidly than with iron compounds, and there are fewer unpleasant side effects. Check at your local health food store.

A serology test for syphilis, such as the VDRL or RPR, should be done, along with a gonorrhea culture (GC). Syphilis can cause malformations, miscarriage, fetal death, prematurity or neonatal infection; gonorrhea can infect the baby's eyes at birth.

A Pap smear should be done along with the gonorrhea culture. This test is both economical and necessary, since it detects abnormal cells at the cervix. Pregnancy accelerates the growth of all cells, so detection of abnormal cells is important at this time. Repeat it at the six weeks postpartum visit. You will need a speculum and a cervical brush.

With the speculum in place and the cervix in view, gently roll the cervical brush within the os to collect the secretions. Roll the brush onto the labeled side of your slide in straight lines. Spray the slide generously with a fixative, working quickly and avoiding the movement of air or exposure to light.

While doing the speculum exam, check the cervix for inflammation or abnormal discharge. Common sexually transmitted disease such as gonorrhea and chlamydia may be detected this way. Both diseases have

How to Decide What Is Too High A Risk For Home Birth

While home birth is in many ways the most desirable for women who want natural childbirth, occasionally, for the safety of the mother or baby or both, it is preferable to have the baby in the hospital. What you can handle in a woman's home depends on your physical capabilities, medical back-up, accessibility to the nearest hospital, and each mother's history and condition.

Here are some situations which we feel would be too risky for a home birth:

- any mother with diabetes mellitus
- a hypertensive mother
- a mother who is in generally poor health, with malnutrition, severe anemia, lack of vitality
- a mother with Rh negative blood who has had a positive antibody test
- a mother with toxemic symptoms
- a mother with really severe polyhydramnios
- a mother with baby in a persistent transverse lie
- a mother with baby in breech presentation, unless you're experienced and skilled in handling breech births
- a mother with a baby presenting with its shoulder
- a mother with a baby of less than 35 weeks gestation
- a mother with a bad attitude—this includes people who don't like you and those with whom you feel you don't have the agreement to transport to the hospital if necessary

Women who develop complications still need your care and encouragement. This is just one of the reasons why midwives need to have good working relationships with backup physicians.

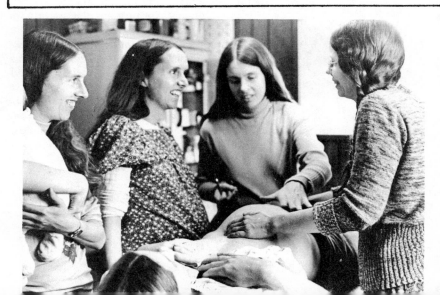

negative effects on babies, and mothers who are infected may not notice any symptoms, although their sexual partners may experience pain while peeing or have a discharge.

Chlamydia is now the most prevalent sexually transmitted disease in the United States, and nearly three quarters of the babies whose mothers are infected contract the disease while they are being born. Infection in the baby can cause conjunctivitis or pneumonia. This test is becoming routine in more and more areas of the country.

Any inflammation of the cervix must be followed up and diagnosed. Besides gonorrheal and chlamydial infections, there is a possibility of Group B streptococcus, a common vaginal infection that may pose danger to the baby. While few babies are infected during birth, even if their mothers suffer from the infection, the presence of this organism greatly increases the risk for the baby in the event of premature rupture of the membranes.

Not to be ignored is the test to determine the mother's blood type. Note it in her records. In the case of the Rh factor being negative, have an Indirect Coombs' test/antibody titre done to detect the presence of antibodies. Check antibodies at the beginning of pregnancy and every four weeks from the sixth month on. See p. 311. Most obstetricians in North America recommend prenatal Rhogam (the anti-antigen injection) for all Rh negative mothers at 28-30 weeks. There is some controversy over this practice, since this routine has not been followed and tested for very many years. Our practice for Rh negative mothers is to do antibody screening five or six times during pregnancy and to give Rhogam only when an Rh positive baby is born.

The rubella antibody titre indicates whether or not the mother has immunity to German measles. Exposure of the baby to rubella during the fetal period may result in vision, hearing or heart defects. A rubella titre of less than 1:10 indicates the mother should be given a rubella vac-

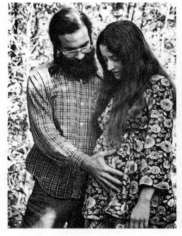

cine. The titre also detects current or past infection or immunization.

Urinalysis for protein, glucose and the presence of bacteria is standard during pregnancy. Pregnant women sometimes have asymptomatic bladder infections, which, if neglected, may travel to the kidneys.

The tuberculin test (PPD) may be necessary, particularly in crowded urban areas. Mothers infected with tuberculosis may not display symptoms.

PREPARING THE MOTHER
OR COUPLE FOR THE BIRTH

Good preparation of both parents is especially necessary if they are planning a natural birth at home. You need to make a judgment as to their emotional preparedness as early in the pregnancy as possible so that you have some time in which you can help them go through any changes they need to make.

Your objective is to have the couple or the lady (if she is single) happily anticipating the strong, mind-changing experience that is in front of them—loving and enjoying their baby all through the pregnancy.

Lots of times people make love without thinking very deeply about what they will do if they get pregnant. The optimum situation is when the pregnant couple is committed to staying with each other and caring for the new life they have created. But this isn't the only situation you will be presented with, life being what it is, so you need to have a good way with counseling couples through their changes. In the beginning, when you contract to deliver a baby for a couple, find out if they are truly committed to each other. The mother is less likely to be casual about her commitment than the baby's father because the pregnancy tends to be more real to her at this stage. If the father seems shaky in his commitment but seems to love the mother, you should be able to counsel them about how necessary it is that he be a solid base of support for her in the months ahead. Often as not, he just needs a reminder that he has some responsibility for this state of affairs too. Sometimes you will have a situation in which the man loses interest in the lady once she becomes pregnant. If he doesn't really love her and does not intend to stay with her and help her raise the child, it is best if he doesn't stay in a position where he's a drag on her and the baby's energy for a long time. Keep in mind that he may really love her and not be in the habit of letting her know that. Remember also that the birthing is an occasion that may radically change the father's outlook on things. Whatever the outcome, it is good to discuss the nature of the agreement the couple has with each other, so that you can assess whether they are good candidates for home birth. Home birth is not a good idea for a lady who does not have the strength of character to make and keep an agreement with another person. You need to be compassionate and telepathic enough with the lady that you know what she is feeling, and you need to have an agreement that the couple will contact you for help during the pregnancy if they are having trouble getting along.

Sometimes relations will be strained between a couple because the mother is not so eager to make love as the father. In cases like this we usually advise that the father be patient, not put pressure on the mother to make love to him, and let her initiate any lovemaking. We advise the mothers to be generous. Most ladies like to make love while they are pregnant if their husbands are not macho and rough with them.

321

This is one time of the mother's life when she doesn't have to worry about getting pregnant.

Sometimes a usually rational lady will become emotional and unpredictable while she is pregnant. If this is the case, you need to investigate and find out whether she is behaving this way out of fright about the birthing. You may be able to relieve her fears that she can give birth naturally by talking to her and listening to her. But there is no sense in trying to convince a lady to have a natural birth if she is already convinced that she wants anesthesia. That amounts to asking for trouble.

Sometimes a mother may not know during her pregnancy whether or not she intends to keep her child. Don't pressure her to decide this while she is pregnant. Going through the birthing will change her enough that you don't know how she will feel on the other side of the experience.

Note: It is up to you to teach the couples that come to you any ways in which they need to change their lifestyles or habits in order to ready themselves for the responsibility of a new infant. If they smoke cigarettes, you should get them to quit. The nicotine the mother's body absorbs from cigarette smoking causes the blood vessels in the placenta to constrict, so they carry less blood to the baby. So ladies who smoke tend to grow smaller babies. If they are dependent on any kind of narcotics, methedrine, cocaine, uppers, downers, or alcohol, you should get them to stop. Moderate to heavy use of alcohol during pregnancy greatly increases the chance of malformation of the baby. If the mother is addicted to narcotics, the baby too will be addicted. If she is dependent enough on any drug that it causes physical withdrawal symptoms to quit, you need to be in consultation with your friendly doctor about her.

Big Babies

If you have a mother whose baby is getting pretty big, you should check her blood sugar, as a big baby is sometimes an indication of diabetes in the mother. If there is any indication of diabetes in the mother, check with your doctor. None of our big babies were of diabetic mothers; some people just tend to have big babies. One mother had three babies: the first boy weighed 10 lb. 8 oz., the second boy weighed 9 lb. 8 oz., and her girl weighed 10 lb. 6 oz. We have delivered eight babies who weighed 10 pounds or more. The two biggest were 11 lb. 4 oz. and 11 lb. 2 oz. Both labors were relatively short. We make sure when we exclaim how big the baby is that the mother knows she has enough room to get the baby out. It's a reasonable thing for her to wonder about.

We usually tend on those deliveries to pay a lot of attention to the mother and make sure that we have a very good touch connection with her so that she's not inhibited about us being very close and intimate and loving with her as we handle her. Also, we make sure that she and her husband are really close, because if they've got a real loving trusting relationship their touch will be powerful, and the way they touch each other will tend to open her up more.

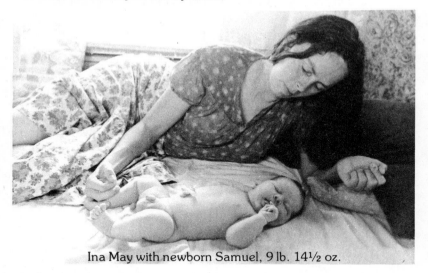

Ina May with newborn Samuel, 9 lb. 14½ oz.

When the Baby is Due

You need to pay especially close attention to how your couples are getting along during the final weeks of pregnancy. A quarreling or unhappy couple can waste away the energy that normally builds up to start off labor, enough to delay the birth of the baby longer than is safe.

Be prepared to intervene and smooth things out if you need to. Sometimes you may need to remind a couple that cuddling and being loving to each other is being loving to the baby. That also tends to build up the energy to the level that it needs to be before the birth can happen.

Inducing Labor

If labor still hasn't started, the membranes are still intact, and the baby will soon be too large to be a comfortable squeeze through the mother's pelvis, we let the mother know that lovemaking can be a good way to induce labor. Semen contains prostaglandins, which can contribute to the ripening of the cervix. Besides this, breast stimulation encourages the release of oxytocin in the mother, which, in turn, may cause uterine contractions.

Another way to get labor started is to induce with castor oil. After the mother has had breakfast, I have her take one tablespoon of castor oil with orange juice, followed by another tablespoon an hour later, and a final tablespoon an hour later. A warm bath is a good idea after all this, provided that the membranes aren't ruptured. I've had good success with this method of labor induction.

323

4. Determining the Relation of the Baby to the Mother's Pelvis

The midwife needs to know how the baby is lying inside the mother, as this can make a great deal of difference in the method of delivery that is ultimately chosen.

The Lie

The lie refers to the relationship of the long axis of the baby to the long axis of the mother while she is standing. It can be longitudinal, oblique, or transverse. A baby in an oblique lie will always turn to a longitudinal or a transverse one in time for or during labor. Over 99% of babies are in a longitudinal lie at term.

The transverse lie baby cannot be delivered naturally unless it can be turned.

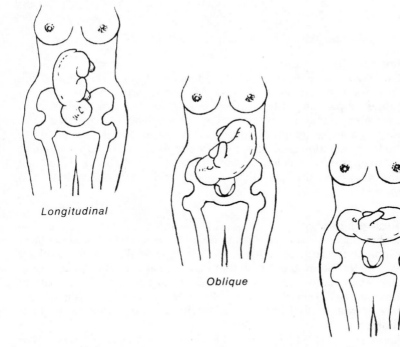

Longitudinal

Oblique

Transverse

Fig. 40. Lie of the Fetus.

The Presentation

The presentation refers to the part of the baby first entering the pelvic inlet on the way out. It can be 1) vertex, 2) breech, 3) shoulder, 4) face, or 5) brow, listed in order of occurrence. Vertex presentation occurs about 95% of the time.

Any transverse baby is considered to be a shoulder presentation, whether or not the shoulder actually is near the cervix. A shoulder presentation must be turned so that its head or its bottom presents first, or it must be delivered by cesarean section.

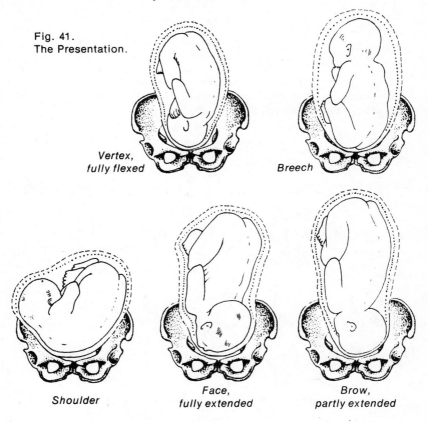

Fig. 41.
The Presentation.

Vertex,
fully flexed

Breech

Shoulder

Face,
fully extended

Brow,
partly extended

The *attitude* is the relationship of the baby's arms, legs, and head to his trunk. The baby's body can be fully flexed, poorly flexed, or extended to various degrees. The baby comes out best as a fully flexed, compact package, as in a vertex presentation. This makes for the presentation of the smallest diameter of the baby's head. If the head is only partly flexed, a larger diameter will have to come through the

325

pelvis and the birth canal, sometimes making labor longer. When the head is fully extended, the baby is presenting by face.

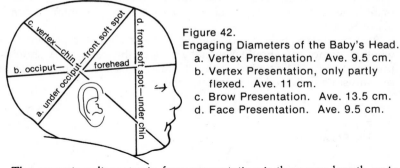

Figure 42.
Engaging Diameters of the Baby's Head.
  a. Vertex Presentation. Ave. 9.5 cm.
  b. Vertex Presentation, only partly flexed. Ave. 11 cm.
  c. Brow Presentation. Ave. 13.5 cm.
  d. Face Presentation. Ave. 9.5 cm.

The engaging diameter in face presentation is the same length as in a vertex but as the head makes its movements through the pelvis a larger diameter also will have to go through.

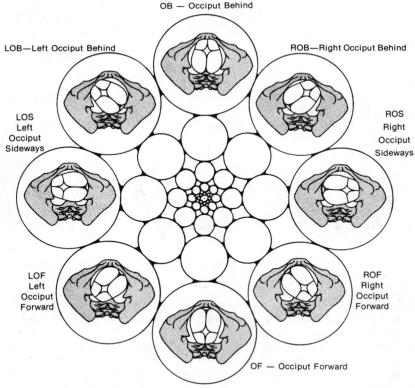

Fig. 43. Possible Positions of a Vertex Presentation—Viewed from Below.

In the designations of the baby's positions in the mother's pelvis, right and left refer to the mother's right and left sides.

The Position

The position is the relationship of the presenting part to the mother's right or left side, and the front or back of her pelvis. The part that determines the position in a vertex presentation is the back of the head (the occiput) and in a breech, the sacrum.

In a vertex presentation, the back side of the baby is usually lying towards the front of the mother. This is the most favorable position for his head to make the movements necessary to get through the pelvis and birth canal. When the baby's back is towards the mother's back (a fairly uncommon position), labor may take a little longer. In this case, either the head will turn so it is facing the back of the mother during labor (which is fairly likely), or the baby will come out with his face towards the mother's front. The baby comes out like this in about 1% of deliveries.

The Station

The station refers to the relationship between the presenting part and the ischial spines. When the presenting part is freely movable above the pelvic inlet, it is said to be floating.

When the baby's skull or his butt (in breech presentation) is at the level of the spines, the station is zero. Above the spines the station is minus one, minus two, on up to five, depending on how many centimeters above the spines the presenting part is. Below the spines, it is plus one, plus two, and so on. The baby's head is about plus four when it is crowning. In

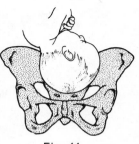

Fig. 44
Floating Head

a long or hard labor, swelling of the scalp may be mistaken for the skull and give a false impression of station.

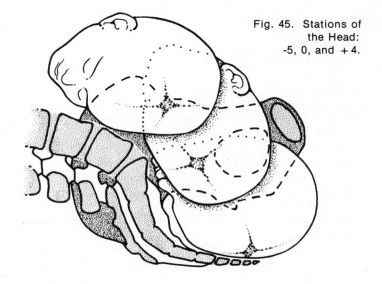

Fig. 45. Stations of the Head: -5, 0, and +4.

The baby's head (or bottom) is engaged when its widest part has passed through the pelvic inlet. In first-time mothers ("primigravidas"), engagement usually happens two or three weeks before the birth. In ladies who have had babies before ("multiparas"), engagement may happen at any time before or after labor begins. If a first-time mother's baby has not become engaged at term, check mother and baby out further to rule out any abnormal condition that might be the cause of this.

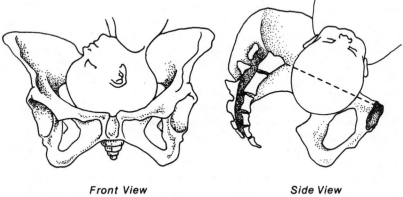

Front View   *Side View*

Fig. 46. Engagement of Baby's Head.

How To Feel Where The Baby Is

Have the mother lie on her back with her knees bent to relax her belly. Stand on the mother's right side if you are right-handed—her left side if you are left-handed.

1. Put both your hands flat on the mother's belly and feel the shape of the fundus of her uterus. Usually you will feel the baby's bottom here. If the baby's head is at the fundus, it will feel round, hard and movable in relation to the rest of the baby's body. If the baby's bottom is up, you will be able to feel its legs nearby. The bottom is not so hard, round or movable as the head.

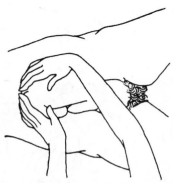

Fig. 47A. Feeling the Baby's Bottom in the Fundus.

328

2. Push the mother's uterus from side to side between your hands. You will usually be able to feel on one side a long smooth continuous object (the baby's back) and on the other, smaller irregularities (the baby's arms and legs).

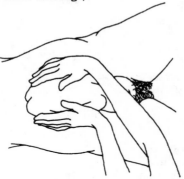

Fig. 47B. Feeling for Back and Legs.

3. When the mother's belly is well relaxed, you can feel for the presenting part of the baby.

Grasp the area just above the mother's pubic bone with the thumb and fingers of your hand, and see first if the head is there. If your touch is nice, you will be able to sink your fingers in quite deeply. If the head is there, try to move it back and forth. You may be able to feel the baby's neck as well.

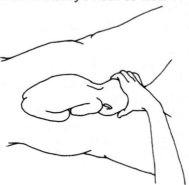

Fig. 47C. Feeling the Head.

4. Feel again the area just above the pubic bone, this time with the first three fingers of both hands. Push deeply in the direction of the birth canal, pushing the moveable skin of the belly down with the fingers. If the baby is head first, one hand will glide on down, over the nape of the baby's neck. The other one will be stopped on the baby's forehead, called the "cephalic prominence."

The cephalic prominence is felt when the baby's head is in flexion. It will be on the same side as the baby's small parts. Feeling a prominence on the same side as the back indicates a face presentation. If the baby's forehead feels like it is just under the skin, the baby might have his face towards the front of the mother.

You can also feel how far the baby has descended into the pelvis by noting the distance from the cephalic prominence to the pubic bone.

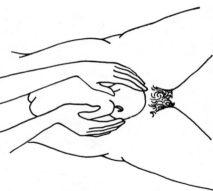

Fig. 47D. Feeling the Forehead.

When the baby's head is engaged you won't be able to feel the forehead because it will be down inside the pelvis. The head also will be less movable when it is engaged. Another way to determine engagement is by trying to feel the top of the baby's head. If the head is not engaged, your fingers can easily feel the lower part of the baby's head and will converge. When the head is engaged, your fingers will go over the nape of the neck and diverge as you reach the pubic bone.

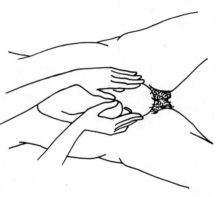

Fig. 47E. Determining Engagement; Head Engaged.

If you are doing a vaginal exam, you can also feel how far down the head is.

Beginning with the final month of pregnancy and at weekly intervals, recheck the mother's pelvic measurements and estimate by feel the size of the baby's head to make sure that it will fit through the mother's pelvis.

External Version

External version is turning the baby around from breech presentation or transverse lie to vertex presentation while it is still inside the womb. This is done by pushing on the mother's belly. It is best done at $7\frac{1}{2}$ to 8 months of pregnancy, though it can be done anytime up to the due date if the mother is very relaxed.

Before beginning:
1. Make sure that you are dealing with a single pregnancy.
2. Make sure that the baby is breech or transverse.
3. Make sure that there is enough amniotic fluid, and enough relaxation on the part of the mother, so that the baby is easily movable.

There are a few dangers to look out for:
1. There is some risk of premature separation of the placenta, so you shouldn't push hard to force the baby to turn.
2. There is some chance of accidents with the umbilical cord, so while you do the version you should listen to the baby's heart at times.

How to Turn the Baby
1. Have the mother lie down on her back with her knees flexed. Make sure her bladder is empty.
2. Rub the mother's belly for a while to relax her stomach muscles.
3. Check the baby's heart rate periodically while you are doing the turning.
4. Push the baby up towards the fundus as far as it will go.
5. Then turn the baby in the direction that it moves easiest. Don't force it. Keep the baby's head flexed. Be gentle. Use intermittent pressure. One hand can hold the gain from one step and the other hand be moving for the next step.
6. If the baby's heart rate changes greatly, or becomes irregular, wait a little while. If it doesn't go back up within 30 seconds or thereabouts, move the baby back and re-check. The cord may have become entangled.

Never try to turn the baby if:
- the mother has had deep uterine surgery—you don't want to rupture the scar;
- the mother has had vaginal bleeding (to prevent more bleeding from possible placental separation);
- the mother is Rh negative (to prevent trans-placental bleeding);
- the mother has very high blood pressure;
- the presenting part is engaged; or if
- the membranes have ruptured.

331

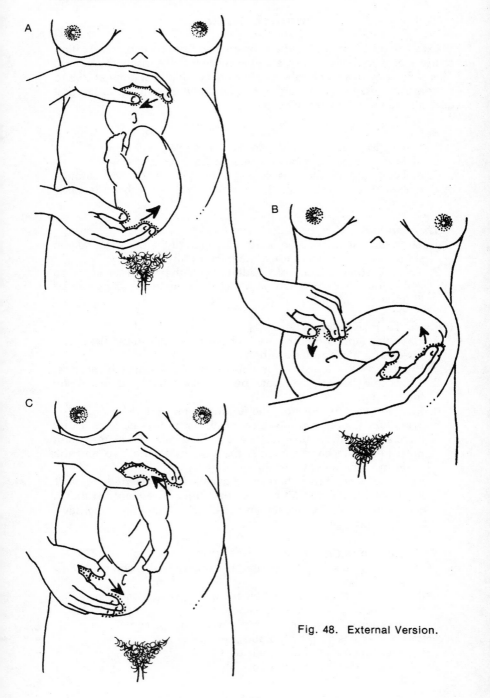

Fig. 48. External Version.

I tried to do an external version on a baby who was presenting breech at the beginning of the ninth month. It was the second baby for the mother, who was pretty nervous about the idea of a breech delivery. I had successfully turned a breech baby to a vertex presentation the day before and felt pretty confident that I could do another, but the mother's belly was pretty tense and I soon gave it up because I didn't like the feeling of forcing anything that didn't want to go easily. Meanwhile I saw the mother frequently and tried to relieve her worries about delivering breech by telling her about the breech deliveries we had already done. She became less nervous as time went on. Six days before she delivered, after spending the afternoon with her as she helped me compile our statistics, I decided to check her belly and possibly give it another try, so I asked her if I could check her. She laid down on the couch in our book company's office, and I began to feel around her belly. The baby's butt was down but not engaged; there was a moderate amount of amniotic fluid and the mother was very relaxed. I rubbed her belly and felt the baby and tried moving it in an arc first one way [which it didn't want to go] and then the other. The baby turned easily to transverse, so I decided to take it the rest of the way if I could. [All of this time I hadn't said anything about turning the baby because I didn't want to re-disappoint her if it couldn't be done.] As I turned the baby the rest of the way, I was pushing on the mother's side which was very ticklish to her and she started laughing. This relaxed her stomach muscles even more, and it was easy to get the baby's head in the right position. The mother was pleasantly surprised to hear what had happened, and after I checked the baby's heartbeat [which was fine], she walked one mile home in an effort to get the baby's head to settle further into her pelvis. An 8 lb. 4 oz. baby girl was born by vertex presentation six days later.

It's not so much the size of the baby as it is the relaxation of the mother which makes an external version possible.

—Ina May

5. The Physiology and Management of Normal Labor at Home

Labor is the work the mother's body does after approximately nine months of pregnancy to expel her passenger—the baby—and all parts of its life-support systems (the placenta, the membranes and amniotic fluid) from her womb, down the birth canal and into the world outside.

Normal labor results in a live baby born head-first within a reasonable amount of time (about 24 hours) by the natural efforts of the mother, with no injury to mother or baby. Many people, especially if they work in modern hospitals, tend to forget that the vast majority of labors are normal—the birthing process works very well by itself.

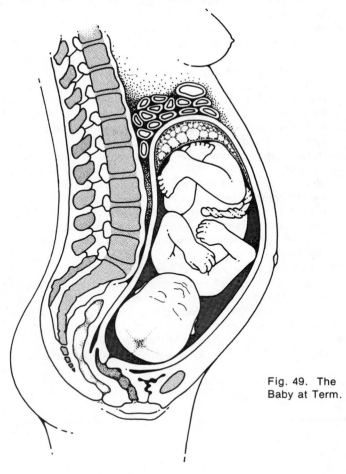

Fig. 49. The Baby at Term.

Signs of Impending Labor

1. The baby drops farther down into his mother's pelvic cavity about two or three weeks before delivery. The mother will feel increased pressure on her lower belly, will probably have to pee quite often, and may have some numbness in her legs. At the same time, she will have more room up around her lower ribs and her stomach. This phenomenon is called "lightening."
2. In first-time mothers, the baby's head becomes engaged two or three weeks before delivery.
3. There will be an increase in vaginal secretions. Mothers at term tend to be very juicy.
4. The mucus plug will be released by the cervix.
5. There will be some bloody show—pink-tinged mucus.
6. The cervix will be very soft to the touch, and it will be much thinner than it has been during pregnancy.
7. The mother's aura (energy field) becomes energized. You may see her glow sometimes.

How To Tell What Is True Labor

Many ladies go through a period of preparatory labor, sometimes called "false labor," before their true labor begins. I would call these irregular contractions of the muscles of the uterus or belly *preparatory labor* rather than false labor, because they do have a function other than to fool you—they keep the uterine and abdominal muscles toned up for the work that is ahead for them, and they begin the softening of the cervix which eventually results in the release of the mucus plug.

True labor is distinguished by the following:

1. Rushes occur at regular intervals with increasing intensity. I prefer to use the term *rushes,* as in rushes of energy, instead of *uterine contractions* because I think it gives both the mother and the midwife a better conceptual framework for dealing with the birthing energy.
2. The rushes increase in duration and happen closer together.
3. The uterus becomes very hard during the rushes.
4. The cervix begins to thin out and open up.
5. The presenting part descends.
6. It is impossible to sleep during true labor. (Sometimes true labor might proceed for several hours, then let up, so that the mother can rest. But when it begins again, she will no longer be able to sleep.)
7. The mother experiences a strong change in her state of consciousness. She becomes increasingly sensitive to other people's vibrations. The pupils of her eyes may become very dilated. She will probably feel best if the lights in the room are not too bright.

The Stages of Labor

First Stage

The first stage of labor lasts from the first rushes of true labor to the full dilation of the cervix (about 10 cm.). The uterus, especially its upper part, becomes very hard during the rushes, which occur at intervals. The mother may have to exert an ever-increasing amount of effort to relax during these spontaneous bursts of energy. The sensations which the mother experiences are hard to describe; they are often experienced as pain, but this is not always the case.

Some first-time mothers may not even recognize that they are in labor when they begin this stage; they may just think that they have a slight back-ache or gas.

This stage usually lasts about fifteen hours for a first baby and less than that if the mother has already had a baby. Sometimes this stage is complete in less than one hour.

Quite often the membranes rupture during this stage.

Second Stage

The second stage of labor lasts from the time of full dilation of the cervix until the birth of the baby. During this stage the rushes are accompanied by strong downward pushes of the uterine and abdominal muscles, and the baby's head descends through the pelvis. The presence of the baby's head in the soft tissue of the birth canal begins to stretch open the lips of the mother's puss, which then continues to stretch until the entire baby has passed through it. This stage can last from a couple of minutes to a few hours.

The Third Stage

During this stage of labor, the uterus continues to contract, reducing its size to just big enough to hold the placenta. Further contraction causes the placenta to separate from the wall of the uterus, and the placenta is then expelled, marking the end of this stage. The third stage of labor usually lasts about ten or fifteen minutes.

The Factors Concerned in Labor

There are several factors concerned in labor, which the midwife needs to take into consideration.

The first three are physical factors:

The Action of the Mother's Muscles

The muscular activity of labor involves both involuntary muscles (the uterine muscles), and voluntary muscles (the muscles of the belly and the thorax). The effectiveness of this muscular activity will depend somewhat on the mother's general physical condition.

The Birth Canal

Parts of the birth canal are hard (the bony pelvis), and parts of it are soft (the cervix and lower part of the uterus, the pelvic floor and the puss). The size of the hard part of the birth canal and the stretchability of the soft parts are both relevant.

The Contents of the Uterus

The contents of the uterus consist of the baby, the placenta, the cord, the amniotic fluid, and the membranes. The presentation and position of the baby, the size of the baby, and the amount of fluid affect the labor.

The last four factors are psychic rather than physical, and are of at least equal importance to the physical. The physical factors are what you are given; the psychic factors are what you can work with, because the psyche [or soul] is very changeable.

The Attitude of the Mother

The attitude of the mother cannot be over-estimated as a determining factor in the course of labor. A relaxed mother can have her baby much quicker and easier than one who is uptight.

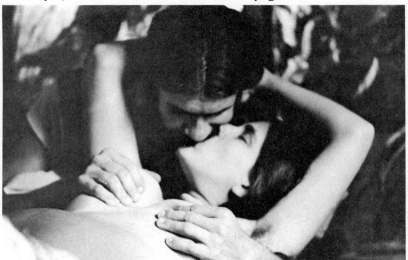

The Attitude of the Father if He is Present

The attitude of the father can be of equal importance to that of the mother. A loving and helpful husband is a great source of energy for his wife. By giving her his full attention and his physical strength (by smooching with her or by rubbing her breasts, her back or legs, etc.), he can greatly reduce the number of hours required for her labor. A compassionate husband is a priceless aid to labor and delivery.

The Attitude of Others Present at the Birthing

The attitude of anyone present at the birthing affects the course of the labor. If you are the midwife chiefly responsible for the welfare of the baby and the mother, you must make sure that the presence of everyone attending the birthing is beneficial.

Your Attitude

Your own attitude is a factor which you can't afford to ignore. If your own heart/mind are at peace, you can inspire the heart of the lady so that she knows that she can do it.

MANAGEMENT OF THE FIRST STAGE
THE OPENING-UP

When you first arrive at the mother's home after being notified that labor has possibly started, you need to make a judgment of the stage of labor, in case delivery is imminent. Usually the mother will be fairly early in the first stage.

Your Crew

It's best to have a trusted and trained friend there to assist you, two if possible. They should both be people you would like being around if you were the one having the baby. If you find on your way to a birthing that you have any disagreements in your heart with any members of your crew, work them out and resolve them first, or choose another crew that you feel in total agreement with, as any disagreement among the midwife crew can have a disadvantageous effect on the birthing.

Instruments and Equipment

Make sure you have all the instruments and equipment there with you. Lay everything out so that you know where it is, and cover it with a sterile sheet. Set up as soon as you feel the mother's in active labor. She might progress quickly. It's nice to be ready. (See p. 458 for a list of equipment and supplies.)

Make sure you have adequate light. It's helpful to bring a flashlight along for getting a good look at the mother's puss in the second stage.

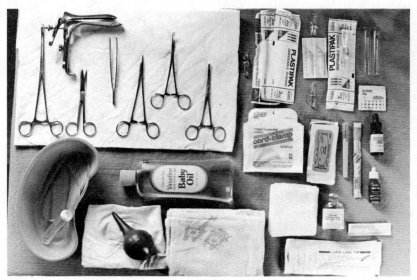

Records

Keep accurate records of the progress of the labor. Record the frequency, duration and intensity of the rushes. Record the dilation of the cervix, the station of the presenting part, and the rate of the baby's heartbeat. Make note of the time that the membranes rupture.

If the mother has had any history of high blood pressure, or other difficulties, keep a close check on her pulse and blood pressure. Her blood pressure will tend to rise a little during labor, especially towards the end of the first stage. A blood pressure of 140/90 is normal for a mother well into labor. Her pulse should stay below 100 per minute.

Washing Up

1. Scrub your hands carefully, up past your wrists, with a broad-spectrum antiseptic surgical soap. Make sure that your fingernails are cut close. Don't wear rings.
2. Then wash the mother's entire crotch area, including her pubic hair and the inside of her thighs, carefully with the same antiseptic soap. There is no need to shave the mother's pubic hair.

Examining to Determine Dilation and Position

Rectal vs. Vaginal Examination

Some believe that rectal examinations are safer than vaginal examination because of the danger of infection during a vaginal exam. If you had no sterile gloves and needed to check a mother's dilation during labor, it certainly would be safer to examine her rectally. Rectal examinations do have drawbacks though:

1. You can't be as accurate as you can in examining vaginally. It is much harder to feel the consistency and dilation of the cervix than in a vaginal exam.
2. It is also easy to mistake swelling on the baby's head for the skull, which can give you a wrong idea of how far down the baby's head is.
3. It is much more uncomfortable to the mother to be examined rectally than vaginally.
4. It is hard to detect a prolapsed cord by rectal exam.

There have been several studies recently which showed that there is no greater risk of infection with vaginal than with rectal examination. This has been borne out by our own experience on the Farm. We had no greater incidence of after-delivery infection after we switched to doing vaginal exams after our first year of midwifing.

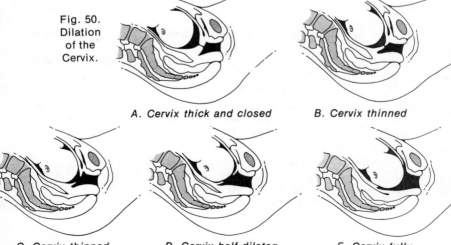

Fig. 50.
Dilation
of the
Cervix.

A. Cervix thick and closed

B. Cervix thinned

C. Cervix thinned and dilated 2-3 cm.

D. Cervix half dilated

E. Cervix fully dilated and pulled back.

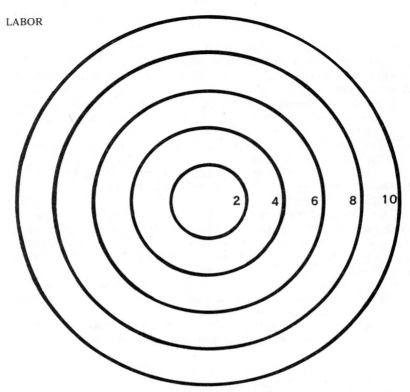

Fig. 51. Cervical Dilation 2-10 cm.
10 cm. is the size the cervix usually gets when it's fully dilated.

The Vaginal Exam

After washing the area around the mother's puss carefully with antiseptic soap, put on a sterile glove and gently insert your first two fingers.

•Check the cervix—

1. Is it hard or soft?
2. Is it thin and drawn back or thick and plenty of it before the baby's head?
3. Can you stretch it wider easily or is it resistant to being stretched?
4. How open is it? Estimate the diameter of the opening.

   Check the mother's dilation periodically, more or less often according to how fast she's progressing. Before you check her each time, wash her puss with antiseptic soap. Sometimes your fingers in there will help her dilate.

•Check for presentation—

1. What is coming first—the head, the bottom, the feet?
2. What is the station: if the top of the baby's head is level with the ischial spines, the station is 0. Above the spines, it is -1, -2, -3; below the spines, it is +1, +2, +3.

340

•Check for position—
1. Find the sagittal suture and the front and back soft spots. It's nice to know which way the baby is facing so that you can give the mother a more accurate idea of how hard she is going to have to work to get the baby out.

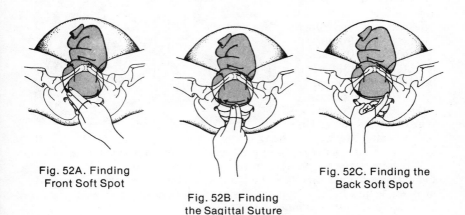

Fig. 52A. Finding
Front Soft Spot

Fig. 52B. Finding
the Sagittal Suture

Fig. 52C. Finding the
Back Soft Spot

•Check the condition of the water bag—
Sometimes you may feel forewaters coming in front of the baby's head. There is no need to rupture the membranes during the first stage. They may rupture spontaneously. If they do, check the fetal heart tone and do a vaginal exam to rule out prolapsed cord.

If dilation is almost complete, and the head is down far enough that there is no chance that the cord can slip past the baby's head through the cervix, there is no harm in carefully rupturing the membranes.

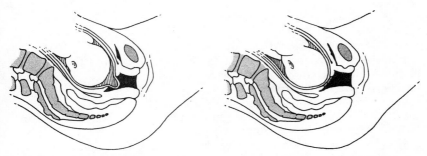

Fig. 53A. Water Bag
Protruding into Birth Canal.

Fig. 53B. No Forewaters.

341

Checking the Baby's Heartbeat

The baby's heartbeat should be checked and recorded every half-hour during the first stage. Always check if you have even a slight question in your mind about how the baby's doing. Then you can either dismiss the question or fix the situation.

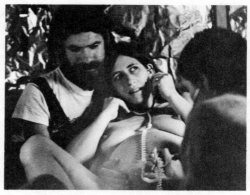

The normal heart rate is 120 to 160 beats per minute. The heart rate becomes slower at the onset, or sometimes the height, of a rush and returns to normal by 10-15 seconds after the rush. A heart rate of less than 100 or more than 160 beats per minute with the uterus at rest suggests that the baby is in trouble.

The baby's heart is somewhat harder to hear during a rush because the uterus is thicker, so check the heartbeat between rushes. A marked increase in the heart rate is the first sign of hypoxia, and also a sign of possible intrauterine infection of the baby.

The Enema

It is a good idea to give the mother an enema at some time during the first stage, for the following three reasons:

1. The mother is going to need all the room she has available inside to let the baby through, so it's best to clean out everything that you can.

2. Giving an enema during the first stage decreases the likelihood that some shit will be pushed out along with the baby's head—a time when you want a clean field of delivery.

3. An enema usually stimulates labor.

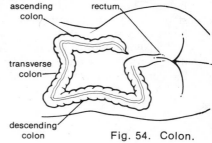

Fig. 54. Colon.

Use warm water, and have the mother lie on her left side, as this facilitates the action of the enema (the descending colon is on the left side).

Eating in the First Stage

Let the mother eat if she wants to. She may have to throw up later, but this won't hurt anything. It might even help dilate her cervix. The only instance where it would not be good for the mother to eat would be if there was a likelihood of her needing a heavy anesthesia (as in a cesarean) later.

Breathing in the First Stage

Breathing in the first stage is best if it is deep and slow. The practice

342

of panting during this stage tends to slow the labor and can cause hyperventilation in the mother, resulting in carbon dioxide depletion.

Sleeping in the First Stage

Let the mother sleep if she wants to. If she is able to sleep, she probably needs the rest and renewal of energy for the work that is ahead of her.

Position During the First Stage

Let the mother be in whatever position she likes, as long as it doesn't slow down her labor. She can walk or stand during this stage, and gravity will usually make the rushes stronger.

Keeping the Mother's Bladder Empty

Make sure that the mother pees every two hours or so during the first stage. You may need to remind her to do so. Find out the approximate amount passed if you are not catching it.

Visitors

If anyone comes to the door not realizing that the mother is in labor, explain the situation, and don't feel obliged to let in anyone who is extraneous to the situation. It could slow down the mother's labor for her to have to integrate another person's presence at this time.

Slow Progress During the First Stage

The mother's rushes may or may not cause her cervix to dilate at a steady rate. You don't have to have any pre-conceived notions about what is too long for the first stage. If the mother is replenishing her energy by eating and sleeping, rushes are light, the baby's head is not being tightly squeezed and the membranes are still intact, the first stage can stretch over three or four days and still be perfectly normal. Be sure to keep careful track of the baby's heartbeat.

Don't worry about slow progress if the baby's heartbeat and the vibrations are good. There should be no inhibitions or unspoken thoughts with strong emotional content. However, there is a certain type of laid-back lady, often overweight, who can make herself so comfortable during her labor that she doesn't do anything. This kind of lady needs some stimulation. She needs to do something or have something done to her that compels her entire attention. She might need a brisk rub or shake, or perhaps she needs to do the rubbing. Smooching with her man or taking a walk can also help to stimulate rushes. But don't ask her to do anything that you couldn't do yourself at this stage. If her rushes pick up when she starts some activity that you suggested, you will know that you are on the right track. If the mother has been in labor for several hours, is not dilated very much and is tired, let her sleep if she wants to. A soak in a tub of warm water can be very relaxing and pain-relieving. There is no risk of infection for women where membranes have not yet broken.

If the baby's head is high and the cervix isn't dilating well, recheck the mother's pelvic measurements and consider the size of the baby to make sure there's room. If the mother's pelvic measurements are adequate, make sure that you let her know that she has room enough. She needs to know this if she is to relax her full amount.

343

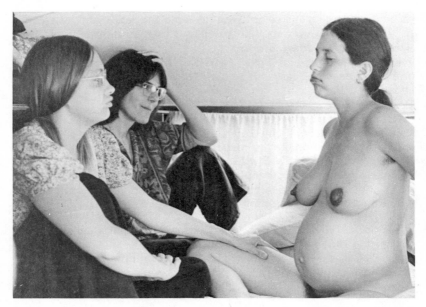

One way to help the mother open up is to have her blow through her lips. A loose mouth makes a loose bottom.

Managing the Energy

Make sure that you are in good touch with the mother. You should feel friendly and relaxed with each other; it should feel comfortable to look in each other's eyes. Be friendly and intimate in the way that you touch her. If there are any inhibitions, fears, or lack of communication between anyone present, especially the mother and her husband, you will need to talk these out and come to a resolution. (It is best for this kind of thing to have been taken care of during the prenatal period, but it does sometimes come up in the high energy of a birthing.)

Make sure that the husband is really attentive and compassionate with his wife. Let him know ways that he could be helping her if he hasn't noticed. Remember that your relationship with the husband must be impeccable in order not to cause any paranoia in the mother.

You may need to instruct the couple on how to talk to each other. They may not ordinarily be as considerate of each other as they need to be right now. You may need to help her instruct him how to touch and rub her, and vice versa. They may not ordinarily be as tantric (touch telepathic) as this occasion demands.

Since body and mind are One, sometimes you can fix the mind by working on the body, and you can fix the body by working on the mind.

344

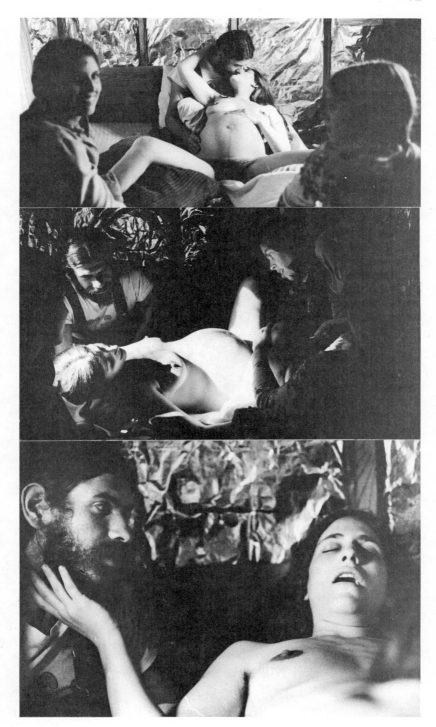

If the couple seems to be friendly but inhibited, instruct them how to be more downhome with each other. Have a good sense of humor yourself, and let them have a little time alone to try suggestions, but never go so far away that you can't be called if you're needed.

Don't be afraid to be silent for a while in order to get a good feeling of the vibrations. If there's no spirit or feeling of presence, something may be happening with the mother or the baby. Fix it until you feel it. The amount of spirit affects the health of the mother and baby.

Notice how your own body feels—if you have presence in your legs, in your bottom, if your stomach is tight. This is very likely what everyone is feeling. If it's good, enjoy it and have a good time. Sometimes it's an accurate thing to say, "It feels really nice in here now." Other times it might not feel just right and you may not be able to pinpoint why. In cases like this, mention how it feels to you. Someone else will probably have the rest of the pieces. In times like this, *Speak the truth and fear no man."*

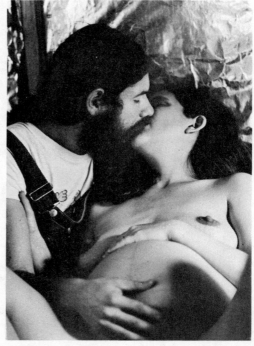

If progress is slow, ask the mother if there is anything in her heart that she doesn't feel at peace with.

Keep in mind that a watched pot never boils.

KEEP THE ENERGY HIGH: *Monitor the energy level and don't sit around feeling uncomfortable without saying anything. Not talking about what is really going on will make you dumb, and you need to be one hundred per cent alert and intelligent at a birthing. You can't fake it.*

Transition

Transition refers to the time of full dilation, just before the urge to push is felt by the mother. As the mother nears transition, prepare her for it. Tell her that you will need her to stay in good touch with you during transition and the second stage. Transition is an intense time during delivery. Some mothers go through transition very smoothly, and some will need your help. The mother may become emotional at this time when she wasn't emotional before and won't be later. Rational thought may leave her, and she may think for a moment that she can't do it. She may feel nauseous and throw up. Assure her that this is temporary and that her brains will return shortly—they are currently in her bottom. Transition lasts only a few moments, so don't take it too seriously, and help her through it. She should understand that she may have to exert *great pure effort* to keep herself together at the time of full dilation.

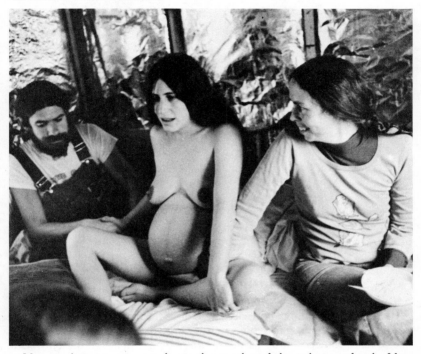

You can't come on preachy to the mother if she is being afraid. You have to be humorous, know exactly where she is at, and talk exactly to that state of consciousness. If you don't, she'll figure that you don't know what you are talking about or that it doesn't concern her and she'll tend to ignore you.

If the mother gets frightened during transition and wants to go to the hospital to get knocked out, don't assume that she won't change her mind. You can point out to her that taking the easy, less stoned way out of her delivery is not a very good preparation for being a parent, which requires a high level of consciousness. Remind her that she is her baby's environment—he has no other, and if she's afraid, she's making him feel that. She will probably change, if you really make her understand this. However, finally, if the lady insists she would rather be in a hospital, do not stand in her way.

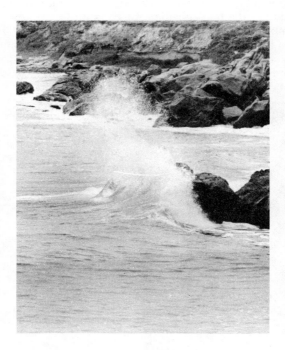

Laboring Mothers As Elemental Forces

The mother's state of consciousness goes through a very great change during the first stage of labor. This change in her consciousness must be taken into account by all the people helping her with the birth. She becomes less of an individual personality and more like an elemental force— like a tornado, a volcano, an earthquake, or a hurricane, with its own laws of behavior. This quality of women has been described as "a great, amorphous, gravity-tides thing, electro-chemical tropism, older and smarter than you, that always gets what it wants." You have to find out the laws of this tropism, whatever aspect of it you are faced with, and work within them, because you can't reason with an elemental force, and you can't predict what it will do. Don't expect a lady to be reasonable while she is having a baby. A lady who is usually very reasonable may find herself extremely emotional during her labor and have no particular thought content associated with the heavy emotions she is feeling. It is all right for her to be emotional as long as there is a sweet flavor to it.

348

One usually very reasonable lady that I know told me that during her labor she had felt on the edge of hysteria for hours — not that she had been afraid, but that she had felt like she might burst into laughter or tears for several hours at a stretch. She remembered having been surprised that I had considered this acceptable behavior for a lady doing natural childbirth. *It was acceptable — it was even nice — because she hadn't abandoned her principles that said to be kind and considerate of other people even when you are under emotional stress.* She had been very sweet.

The energy of labor causes the mother's body to become very soft — all the way through. This can be felt especially at the inside of her thighs. The change that takes place in her over-all texture is something like what happens to jello when you take it out of the refrigerator. As it warms up, it loses the more brittle quality it has when it is cold, and when jiggled, the warmer jello moves in larger waves.

Strong emotions go with this softening process. These become less personal-flavored and more elemental the deeper a lady goes into labor. Because she is so fluid and one emotion can so easily slide into another, the midwife needs to be a stable anchor for her. If the midwife resists the temptation to become flower-childy and flighty herself, she can keep the mother from drifting into being afraid or irritable or discouraged, and thus keep her from becoming rigid and brittle. If the mother is afraid, you are no longer talking to that particular person — you are talking to a tropism called fear. There is a teaching in Buddhism which says that **the antidote for fear is courage.** I find this to be a true teaching. You may feel the vibrations of fear off of the mother in your own heart, stomach, and legs — but you need not claim that fear for your own and react to it. You can be steady, tell her exactly what is going on, and inspire her with courage. The word *courage* comes from the Middle English word *corage,* which means heart, and heart is at least as contagious as fear. Remember that a humorous state of consciousness is a fluid and a flexible state. If you can remember your sense of humor at a heavy time, you may be able to help the mother remember hers. An amused lady stretches much better than a scared one.

Let her make a noise if she wants to — as long as it's sweet and comes out of an open throat. Give her a second-to-second feedback during her rushes approaching transition. Let her know what works as she is doing it. Be an enthusiastic cheerleader.

Ladies in strong labor can get amazingly beautiful. It's okay to let her know this sometimes — it can help a lady's morale to know that she is beautiful when she's sweaty and struggling.

MANAGEMENT OF THE SECOND STAGE
THE PUSHING OUT

When the mother's cervix is fully dilated, it is time for her to push the baby out.

The rushes of the second stage are very different from the rushes of the first stage. The muscles of the mother's chest and belly contract along with the uterus, pushing the baby down the birth canal. She no longer has to hold herself still on top of the tremendous waves of energy that soften and open her cervix. During the second stage, she becomes active and powerful and athletic. If it's her first baby, she probably works harder than she ever has, and she is rewarded by feeling the change in the baby's position and/or by the midwives telling her of the progress she is making.

The midwife's connection with the laboring lady is of utmost importance during this stage. She should have the mother's total confidence so that she can instruct her how and when to push.

Fig. 55.
Second Stage
of Labor.

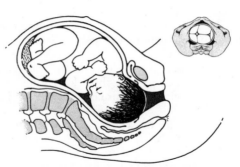

1. The baby is in left occiput sideways position (LOS). The mother's cervix is almost fully dilated, and the head is well flexed. The baby is ready now for descent and rotation.

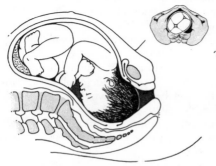

2. Dilation is complete now. The baby's head and body are beginning to rotate as the head is pushed down into the birth canal. The head turns when it meets the resistance of the pelvic floor. The head is now in left occiput forward position (LOF), and is well flexed.

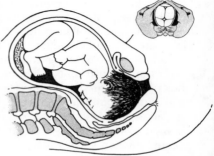

3. The process of internal rotation is now complete, as the baby's head has moved farther down the birth canal and has turned from left occiput forward position (LOF), to occiput forward position (OF). The head is beginning to extend.

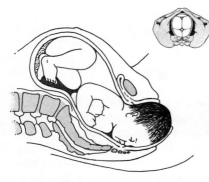
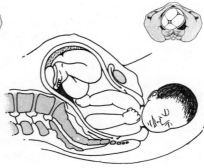

4. The baby's head is well extended and is beginning to crown. The mother's puss has begun to open.

5. The baby's head has been born, and its body has begun to rotate. When rotation is complete, the occiput will be directed toward the mother's left buttbone.

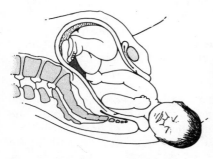
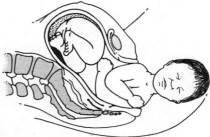

6. The forward shoulder has passed beneath the symphysis pubis and has been born.

7. The shoulder behind has begun to emerge and will be followed quickly by the rest of the baby's body.

Length of the Second Stage

This stage may only take a few minutes but sometimes takes as long as two or three hours or more. This is okay as long as there is a good strong feeling of presence and a good baby heartbeat. If you're having a long second stage, have the mother pee in between rushes.

Keeping the Mother's Bladder Empty

Make sure that her bladder is empty before the mother starts pushing. This will make room for the baby's head to pass through. Sometimes the mother won't have the urge to pee, and you will need to remind her. Emptying the bladder will also prevent its possible laceration during the second stage. If the mother can't empty her bladder and it is full, let your doctor know. She may need to be catheterized. The mother's lower abdomen should never look like this:

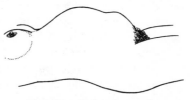

Fig. 56. Bulge Caused by Full Bladder.

351

When to Push

There is no need to have the mother push before she has the urge. It will come. You don't want her to wear herself out by pushing too early.

Pushing Too Early

Sometimes the mother's involuntary urge to bear down will be very strong before her cervix is fully dilated. If this happens, the front rim of the cervix can be pushed downward with the baby's head. This increases the chance of the cervix tearing and can contribute to uterine prolapse. Once the baby's head has started to move down, it's a good idea to do a sterile glove check inside to make sure that the baby's head has completely passed through the cervix. If there is some cervix back over the baby's head, gently push the rim of the cervix back over the baby's head during the next rush. If the mother needs to dilate more, have her refrain from pushing. If necessary, have her pant like a dog.

Wash your hands carefully for three or four minutes—five, if possible. Wash the mother's crotch area again, cleaning the taint in one sweep from her puss downwards across her butthole. If you need to make another swipe to clean her well, use a fresh sterile cloth with antiseptic soap, moving from her puss downwards. Her thighs should be washed 18 inches down on either side.

Pushing

Most mothers will be comfortable in the position pictured below. Make sure that the backbone, neck and head are lined up straight. She should have some firm support behind her (a wall or her husband, for instance), with pillows set in behind her for comfort and to make the

angle right. It's a good idea, when delivering a mother seated on a bed, to place a large plastic-covered beanbag seat under her bottom. Besides providing good support for her back, the beanbag elevates her bottom a few inches above the level of the bed, making for easier maneuvering during the birth of the head and shoulders. When the mother begins to push, she may involuntarily hold her breath when her uterus pushes the hardest. This is good—except when she involuntarily catches her breath, coach her to keep her breathing slow, light and shallow. While pushing her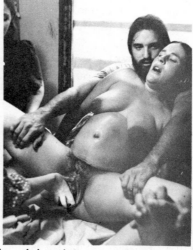
mouth should be slightly open and relaxed, her throat muscles loose. If she thinks she has to breathe forcibly and strain, she is more likely to tighten up the pelvic floor muscles and perineum. Emphasize slowness rather than deepness of breathing.

While the mother is pushing, have her keep her knees open wide, so that the baby will have plenty of room to move down. Have the mother keep her bottom firmly placed on the bed, especially during crowning rushes, as this will keep her muscles more relaxed than if she's lifting her bottom up. There are exceptions to this sometimes.

Tell the mother to keep her eyes open and her mouth loose and relaxed during a rush.

Give the mother moral support while she is pushing by letting her know when she gets off a good one and by telling her exactly how much progress she is making. On a first baby, or with a large-headed baby, it may take her some time to get the head through the outlet of her pelvis. Her bones will give a little, and the baby's head bones will mold (slide over each other) a little.

Some mothers do better moving the baby down while kneeling, squatting or standing, especially if the baby is large or it is her first labor. A standing lady can swing her pelvis around in different directions, and move the baby down in this way. You can have her sit down again once the baby's head has begun to crown. The semi-sitting position is best for delivering the baby's head, so that you can have eye contact with the mother and slow the delivery of the head.

Sometimes a mother will get impatient to see her baby and want to push continuously, but don't let her wear herself out by pushing when she is not having a rush. The energy of the rush will give her the energy to push with.

Hot Compresses

Sterile cloths dipped in comfortably warm sterile water or in warm olive, wheat germ, or baby oil may be applied to the mother's taint between rushes. This helps relaxation and may prevent a tear.

The Baby's Heartbeat

Check the baby's heartbeat every five minutes during this stage. It may be somewhat slower than in the first stage, but it should continue beating strong and steady.

If There Is Bleeding During the Second Stage

There may be a slight amount of bleeding during the second stage from broken capillaries, the separation of the membranes in the lower uterus from the uterine lining, or a slight nick in the cervix. This bleeding will usually be controlled by the pressure of the baby's head passing through. If second stage bleeding is excessive, take the mother to the hospital.

Rapid Second Stage

Ladies who have given birth before tend to have their babies very soon after full dilation. Always be prepared to act fast with them.

If the baby's head becomes visible in the birth canal after two or three good pushes, the baby will be born soon. You may even find it necessary to have the mother slow down the rushes while you and your assistants prepare for the birth. She can slow them down by panting during a rush—high and fast and light like a dog.

Encouraging the Mother

If the mother gets scared by the power of the rushes of the second stage, there are a few good lines you can tell her that will answer what she wants to know.

—"This may hurt, but everything's doing exactly what it's supposed to."

—"You've got plenty of room to stretch down here."

—"You're being really brave."

If you have let her know what to expect so that she is prepared for crowning, you should be able to calmly guide her through the climax of her birthing with her self-respect intact.

It's a good idea to let her know that nearly every mother, at some point in her labor, feels that it is going to be impossible to give birth. If she knows that this thought is likely to occur, she can take it less seriously when it comes. First-time mothers may need to know that many women have the thought that they may "explode" or "break in two" during transition or when pushing begins. This interpretation of the sensation of cervical stretching is frightening and usually increases the mother's discomfort, since it is nearly impossible to relax if you think you are exploding. The mother will be grateful to know that no damage is being done. It is important that you help her distinguish between the kind of pain which is damaging to the body and the pain of labor which comes from the resistance of the voluntary muscles of the body to the forces of labor.

If her legs go into a cramp, you can release the cramp by squeezing her calves, or by having her extend her legs and point her toes upward.

Preparing for the Birth

When you can see that birth is a few minutes away, slide a sterile sheet under the mother. Wash your hands and her puss again. Have your assistant wash her hands and be ready with the hemostats and scissors, in case you need to cut a cord or give the lady a snip; and the ear syringe, for suctioning out mucus from the baby's nose and throat. You should rupture the membranes when you see the water bag if it looks like the baby will be out soon.

Delivering the Head

Crowning is when the presenting part is visible at the opening and doesn't go back in between contractions. It is best to deliver the head slowly. When you see the head begin to push out of the mother's puss with each rush, use your hands to push against the head gently so that it comes out slowly and steadily. Don't let the head suddenly explode from the mother's puss. Coach the mother about how much and how hard to push. Support the mother's taint with your hand during rushes. It helps the mother to relax around her puss if you massage her there using a liberal amount of baby oil to lubricate the skin. Sometimes touching her very gently on or around her button (clitoris) will enable her to relax even more. I keep both hands right there and busy all the time while a crowning rush is happening, doing whatever seems most necessary. It's really important at the time of crowning that the mother doesn't complain at all, because how loose her mouth is will directly affect how much her puss will be able to stretch. Complaining goes along with rigidity. Instruct her to keep both her throat and her mouth

354

loose and relaxed. If the mother wants to know what she can do with her mouth to keep it loose she can laugh or sing or say "I love you."

A slow delivery of the head is most possible when there is a great deal of mind-contact between the midwife and the mother. You can have the mother "breathe the head out." Sometimes, while helping a mother through crowning, I feel like I'm outside a semi-trailer truck, directing the driver: "All right, bring it on a little now—Hold it for a few seconds now, okay, bring it on some more." You can get a very telepathic thing going with the mother, so that she can halt the progress of the head for sometimes just half a second, and while she holds back that tremendous force, the whole quality of her skin will change; she will relax and become more pliant and stretchy.

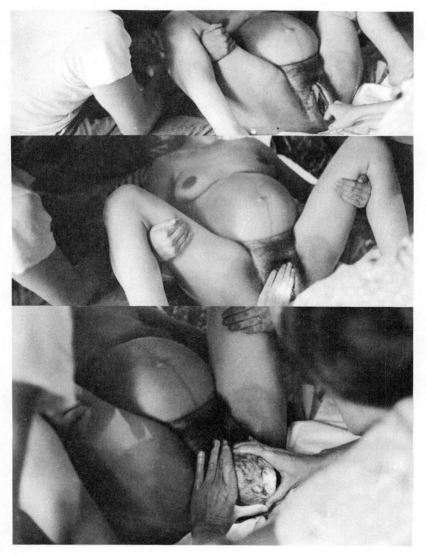

Episiotomy

When the head is crowning, the skin of the mother's puss will usually have time to stretch to accommodate it, but sometimes you may need to make a small cut (an episiotomy) to make more room. [*Even if a lady has already had an episiotomy with a previous baby, she can give birth without one. Scar tissue is stretchy.*] Do this with the sterile surgical scissors (the blunt/sharp kind with the blunt end inside so you don't hurt the baby's

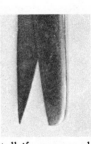

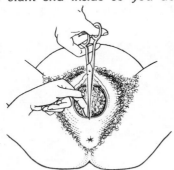

head.) You can tell if you need to do this, as the skin of the taint will turn white and look like it's going to tear. If the cut is made at the height of a rush when the skin is blanched white, the mother won't feel it. I like to make the cut straight down if I have to do one. If you make a cut of 1/8 inch you have added 1/4 inch to the circumference of the puss.

Fig. 57. Small Midline Episiotomy

Look for the Umbilical Cord Around the Baby's Neck

When the baby's head is born, feel to see if the umbilical cord is wrapped around the neck. About 2 percent of babies have the cord around their necks. If possible, try to slip the cord gently over the baby's upper shoulder.

Usually it will be possible to loosen the cord enough to deliver the body without cutting the cord. The baby's body can be born in a sort of somersaulting movement, while you keep the baby's neck close to his mother's crotch. Then unwrap the cord from around the baby's neck.

Another way to deal with this situation is to clamp the cord to the first notch on the clamps, with two clamps placed two inches apart, and then cut the cord between the clamps. Then unwrap the cord ends from around the baby's neck. Have the mother pant high and fast and light like a dog while you're doing this, so as to delay her next push.

You want the baby to come out quickly if you have to cut the cord before the shoulders are born. If you decide to cut the cord early, anticipate that the baby will be a little shocky. Keep it in mind that as soon as you cut the cord, the baby is on his own and is not getting any oxygen from his mother anymore.

The Rotation of the Shoulders

The head of the baby is usually born with the face down. The baby's head then rotates so that it's facing either the right or the left thigh of the mother just before its shoulders are delivered. The shoulders will rotate internally as they come through the birth canal.

Suctioning the Baby Before the Body is Born

When the baby's head turns towards one of the mother's thighs, your assistant should wipe any fluid off his nose and mouth with a sterile cloth. Then she should suction any mucus or fluid from his nose and throat with a sterile ear syringe, making sure to *squeeze the bulb first,* before placing the tip in the baby's mouth or nostrils. The baby's lungs could be injured if mucus was forced into his respiratory tract.

The right way to use the syringe is:

1. Squeeze the bulb and hold it squeezed.
2. Put the tip in the baby's mouth first, if possible.
3. Release it slowly, sucking in any mucus that is there.
4. Squeeze the top of the bulb syringe against a sterile cloth.
5. Repeat this action if necessary, always squeezing the bulb *before* placing it in the baby's mouth.
6. Repeat the above procedure, this time suctioning the baby's nostrils.

Make sure that you have removed all fluids from the baby's mouth and nose before delivery of the body. Routine suctioning of the baby at this point greatly reduces the chance that the baby will inhale fluid into his lungs with his first breath.

Delivery of the Shoulders

When the baby's head has finished turning, the shoulders have turned inside and are ready to be born. The upper shoulder usually delivers soon after the head. Sometimes the shoulder has difficulty coming through. You can help by gently moving the baby's head toward the floor. *Be gentle: use minimal force.* This will help the upper shoulder to come out. When the upper shoulder appears, help the lower shoulder to come out by applying gentle traction on the head toward the ceiling. Sometimes the lower shoulder will want to be the first one to come, so you will follow the above procedure in reverse order. Carefully hold and support the baby by the shoulder and head while the baby is delivered. Deliver the shoulders as slowly as needed to protect the taint. Be ready to hold the baby gently but firmly at all times. *Remember, the baby will be slippery.* Place the baby face down on the mother's thigh. Turn his head to face you.

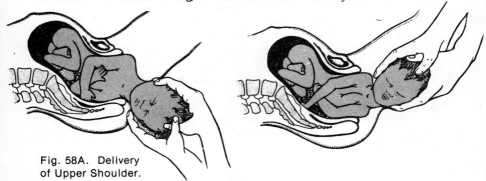

Fig. 58A. Delivery of Upper Shoulder.

If the Shoulders Seem to Be Stuck

If neither the anterior nor the posterior shoulder will budge with the mother's next pushes and she is in a seated or lying position, have her flip over so that she is on her hands and knees, with her bottom towards you. Apply traction to the baby's head, being careful not to press your fingers into the baby's neck. This position works very well to widen the pelvis in just the way that is required when the shoulders are stuck: instead of the mother's coccyx being pushed towards the symphysis pubis in the way it is in the seated position, there is no pressure on the coccyx and the baby's weight is pushing on the symphysis pubis, thereby widening the anterior

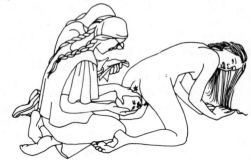

Fig. 59. Delivering Baby with Large Shoulders.

to posterior diameter a little. In addition, in the hands and knees position, gravity assists and favors the birth of the baby. I learned this technique from a Guatemalan midwife, who learned it from Mayan Indians. Since we midwives of The Farm began using it in 1976, we have never had a case of shoulder dystocia that we couldn't resolve with comparative ease. We have an excellent videotape of such a birth available through VideoFarm (see p. 2). It is important to note that the posterior arm (the one which will be uppermost when the mother is in the hands and knees position) will almost invariably be born first. If it doesn't come with gentle traction, locate the baby's posterior armpit, and, splinting your first two fingers across it, apply traction. In rare cases, it may be necessary to pull the baby's posterior arm out before the shoulders can be born.

I have seen other texts which mention the use of the knee-chest position to resolve shoulder dystocia. I would strongly advise against this position being used, since gravity is then working against you. The knee-chest position is most properly used when you don't want the baby to be born, as in transport for prolapse of the umbilical cord.

If the Water Bag is Covering the Baby's Head

The water bag usually breaks open during labor and fluid gushes out. If the bag doesn't break during labor, and you haven't had a chance to break it yourself, the baby may be born still enclosed in the membranes. If this happens you'll have to remove the water bag from the baby's nose and mouth so he can breathe.

Keeping the Baby Warm

Right away wrap a dry sterile and preferably warm receiving blanket around the baby. Change the blanket as needed to keep the baby from losing body heat.

358

Clearing the Baby's Airway

Act promptly. Put the baby on his mother's thigh, being careful not to put a lot of tension on the cord. The baby will usually be very slippery. Turn the head to face you.

If he isn't crying already, his airway may be blocked by thick mucus, so you or your assistant should thoroughly suction his mouth, and nose if needed,

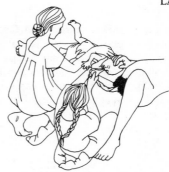

Fig. 60. Baby on Thigh.

with an ear bulb syringe. Rub your hand up the baby's spine. If the cord is long enough, and breathing is clear and regular, you can place the baby face down on the mother's belly and cover him with a sterile receiving blanket.

Let the baby cry for a while until he's good and pink. Crying is a good way for him to get his new breathing and circulatory systems going. If I have a silent baby, unless he is very pink and breathing deeply, I stimulate him a little until I get a good cry. **This is no time to be sentimental.**

[*If the baby needs more help starting, see* **Resuscitation,** *page 382.*]

Evaluating the Baby's Apgar Score

The Apgar score system was devised by Virginia Apgar so that everyone could have a standard way of evaluating and recording the condition of the baby. Check the baby's Apgar score one minute after birth and again at 5 minutes after birth. There are five things to check, and a score of 0, 1 or 2 points is given for each. A final score of 7-10 is fine, 4-6 is moderately depressed, and 0-3 is severely depressed.

Sign	0	1	2
Heart rate	Absent	Slow (below 100)	Above 100
Respiratory effort	Absent	Slow Irregular	Good Crying
Muscle tone	Limp	Some flexion of extremities	Active
Reflex irritability	No response	Grimace	Cry
Color	Blue Pale	Body pink, Extremities blue	Completely pink

Clamping and Cutting the Cord

You can clamp the umbilical cord after it has finished pulsating strongly. This will usually happen within five minutes. Don't "milk" the umbilical cord as there is a possibility that this can cause jaundice in the baby. You can use a plastic or a re-usable metal clamp or a sterile cotton shoe-lace carefully tied in a tight square knot.

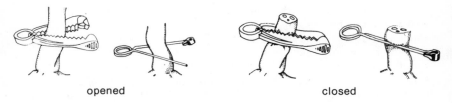

opened   closed

Fig. 62. Clamping the Cord.

A square knot is tied in this fashion: if you begin with the right strand crossing over the left for the first half of the knot, make the left strand cross over the right for the second half of the knot.

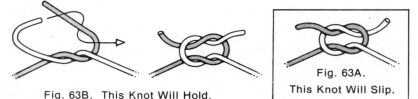

Fig. 63B. This Knot Will Hold.

Fig. 63A.
This Knot Will Slip.

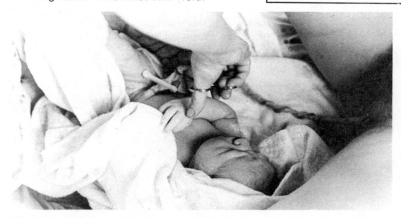

The clamp or knot should be placed one inch from the baby's navel. A large hemostat should be placed about three inches up the cord (towards the placenta) from the first clamp. Cut the cord between the clamps with blunt-end scissors. Watch the cord carefully to make sure there is no blood loss through the cord.

If you have a baby that you think might need emergency treatment or an exchange transfusion, put the first clamp about three inches away from the navel instead of one inch away.

With a sterile syringe, take a sample of blood from one of the vessels of the umbilical cord after it has been cut. You can put it in a sterile test tube and if you have to deal with a hospital about mother or baby, you may be able to use this for diagnostic tests and save the baby a poke or two.

A helper should take the baby to a clean, soft, well-lit place to clean and examine him (see p.366, "Tending to the Baby") while you stay with the mother to deliver the placenta. Keep the baby warm at all times! This is very important. Examine the cord stump to be sure that no blood is oozing and to see if there are three blood vessels in the cord. If there are only two, it would be wise to have the baby checked by a pediatrician, as this is sometimes associated with certain kinds of gastrointestinal tract, heart, and kidney abnormalities.

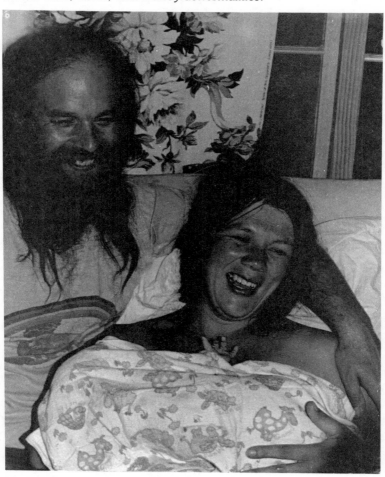

MANAGEMENT OF THE THIRD STAGE
DELIVERY OF THE PLACENTA

The Separation and Expulsion of the Placenta

The separation of the placenta from the uterine wall usually happens within five minutes after the baby's birth. The uterus gets smaller as it contracts and the placenta stays the same size. It eventually has to buckle up and so separates. Usually there's a small gush of dark red blood (about two to four tablespoons) from the mother's puss when the placenta separates. The placenta will usually come out shortly after this.

After the placenta has separated from the uterine wall, the contractions of the uterus push the placenta out through the cervix. It is then pushed the rest of the way out by the mother pushing with her belly muscles.

The placenta may come out neatly, with the baby's side first (Schultz separation), or messily, with the side that was attached to the uterus appearing first (Duncan separation). You will need to pay special attention to deliver the placenta without breaking off any of the membranes, leaving them inside the mother. This could cause more bleeding.

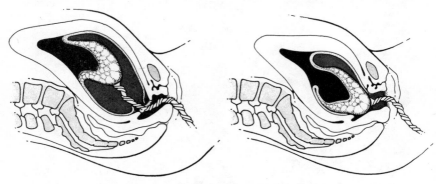

Fig. 64A. Schultz Separation of the Placenta.

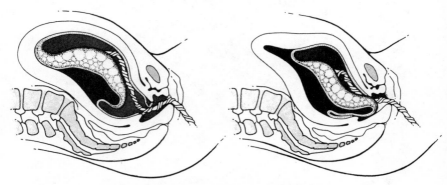

Fig. 64B. Duncan Separation of the Placenta.

Delivering the Placenta

Just after the baby is expelled from the mother's body, one of your assistants should feel the top of the uterus to make sure that it is keeping its tone. The husband or an assistant can be stimulating the mother's breasts and nipples, as this helps to stimulate uterine contractions. (Stimulation of the breasts causes a powerful endocrine hormone called oxytocin to be released. Oxytocin in turn stimulates uterine contractions.)

The rushes that will expel the placenta will be lighter than the rushes which birth the baby. These rushes feel to the mother very much like menstrual cramps.

To find out whether separation has taken place, push the uterus, which should feel like a firm mass about the size of a cantaloupe, up towards the mother's head. If the cord moves up into the mother's puss with it, the placenta is probably still attached to the wall of the uterus. If this is the case, *gently* massage the uterus and wait a few minutes for the placenta to separate.

When the mother feels a rush, have her try to push the placenta out. It will usually come right away.

You should deliver the placenta slowly. The weight of the placenta coming down helps the membranes to separate from the uterus. When the placenta is coming out, you can twist it around which will twist the membranes into a rope and that will make them stronger and less likely to tear.

Don't try to get the placenta out by pulling on the cord. It often helps in the delivery of the placenta if the mother is supported in a squatting position while she pushes it out. Have her lay right back down after the placenta comes out so you can check her for bleeding— this is a time it frequently happens. Have a bowl ready to put the placenta in as soon as you catch it. It can be buried later; it makes good garden fertilizer.

The thing to remember about delivery of the placenta is not to get impatient or uptight about it because that kind of vibration directly inhibits rushes. The midwives on the Farm have a saying, "The placenta always comes out."

Examining the Placenta

When the placenta is delivered, inspect it carefully to see if you've got the whole thing. Look at the membranes first and see if they look big enough to have held the baby inside. The placenta should be dark bluish-red and firm. All the little sections of the placenta should be there and should all fit together when you lay it flat. If either the placenta or the membranes seem to be missing a fair-sized piece, save the tissue and check with your doctor. Pieces left inside may cause post-partum hemorrhage or infection. If small pieces of the membranes or the placenta are left inside, they will usually come out with the discharge in the next couple of days. In this case, the mother may possibly have some trouble with bleeding. Check with your doctor—he may want to do a D & C.

Bleeding after Delivery of the Placenta

[For how to handle severe bleeding, see page 432.]

If there is bleeding from the mother's puss following delivery of the placenta, you need to find the cause. Act quickly. With your hands on the mother's belly, check her uterus to see if it is contracted and hard. If it is not, this relaxation of the uterus may be what is causing the bleeding, so you should massage the uterus into a contraction and keep massaging it if there is any tendency for it to lose its tone and relax.

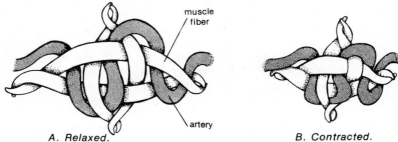

A. Relaxed.   B. Contracted.

Fig. 65. Interlaced Muscle Fibers and Blood Vessels of the Uterus.

When the muscles of the uterus are contracted, the blood vessels which are intertwined with them become constricted.

If the uterus was soft and relaxed at your first touch and has a tendency to go relaxed when not actively stimulated, give the mother an intramuscular injection of 10 units of pitocin in the thigh. (See page 463, Giving Injections.)

If the mother has no history of hypertension, you may give an injection of 0.2 mg. of methergine instead of pitocin.

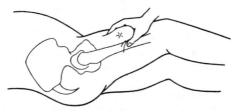

Fig. 66. Site of Intra-Muscular Injection.

If the uterus is quite hard and there is bleeding from the puss, check the birth canal for lacerations. Use a sterile gauze pad to wipe up the excess and see if you can spot the origin. There are some arteries about 1½ inches up into the birth canal and 1 inch beneath the mucosa which can bleed pretty heavily if torn.

If the bleeding does not stop at the source when you put pressure on it and you can see the pulsing of the blood flow, you are probably dealing with a torn artery. To stop the bleeding, you will need to pinch off

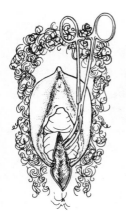

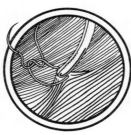

Fig. 67. Clamping and Sewing Off a Torn or Cut Artery.

the torn edges of the artery with hemostats and sew one or two stitches in the tissue just above the hemostats.

See Chapter 8 (p.377) for how to complete the repair of the laceration.

If there is no laceration causing the bleeding, the uterus is hard, and the placenta is complete, you should insert a sterile speculum into the birth canal and check for laceration of the cervix. The cervix can also be seen by clamping the upper edge of the cervix with a sponge forcep and gently lifting and pulling while your fingers are used to hold the puss open. If there is a laceration of the cervix, clamp it if you can with a sponge forcep, and take the mother to a hospital to have this repaired.

Fixing Up the Mother

After the placenta is delivered, check the mother's puss to see if she'll need any stitches, and do any stitching that's necessary. Then rinse her off with a sterile cloth and water. Wash around her puss first and then her legs and bottom. Put two sterile sanitary napkins on her and clean up everything so her surroundings are clean and pretty.

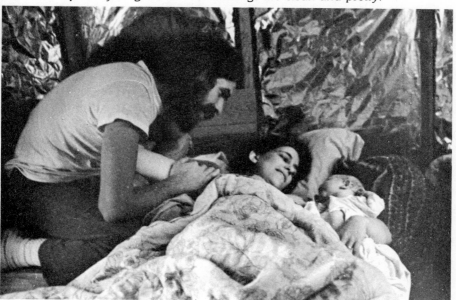

Brand-new babies are gorgeous. Being with a new baby, giving the baby your whole attention feels like giving your soul a drink of fresh pure water. New babies have strong, clear vibrations because their attention is not divided—whatever they do, they do it with their total attention. If you pay good attention to a new baby, the baby's serene intelligence will clean your mind for you.

6. Tending to the Baby

Your partner should do this while you deliver the placenta.

It's important to do a physical examination on a new baby, because there are some things you need to know about early—either because it's easier to fix early, or it just might be necessary for the baby's good health. Mostly this examination is just looking at everything carefully. Does his mouth look like a normal mouth? Does he have all his fingers and toes? If everything seems fine, you can divide the examination into two parts, so you don't have to disturb the baby too much when he's just born. The second part can be done when you visit the mother and baby the day after the birth.

Right After Birth

1. **Check his general appearance.**
2. **Check breathing:** He should breathe about 60-70 times a minute for the first couple of hours after birth, and then slow down to 40-60. The faster breathing for the first couple of hours serves to correct the normal metabolic imbalance that he has at birth. A newborn's respirations are frequently irregular, and they are easily altered by either internal or external stimuli. The baby's breathing should be fairly regular and it shouldn't look like he has to work hard to breathe. If he is making snoring or gurgling sounds, suction him out as much and as often as necessary to get his airways cleared out.

   Listen to the baby's chest sounds with a stethoscope. The breath sounds should be about equal on both sides and on the top and the bottom of each lung. (The best way to be able to tell this is to practice on your friends' and kids' chests.)

   Signs of RDS [Respiratory Distress Syndrome]:
   - *respiratory rate of more than 70 breaths per minute after two or three hours after birth*
   - *retracting—the chest drops down [is sucked in] right under the rib cage or between the ribs while the baby is breathing*
   - *grunting on exhalations*
   - *gasping for breath*
   - *flaring of nostrils while breathing*
   - *cyanosis [see #5 below]*

   If a baby shows any of these signs, check with your doctor or take him to the hospital.

366

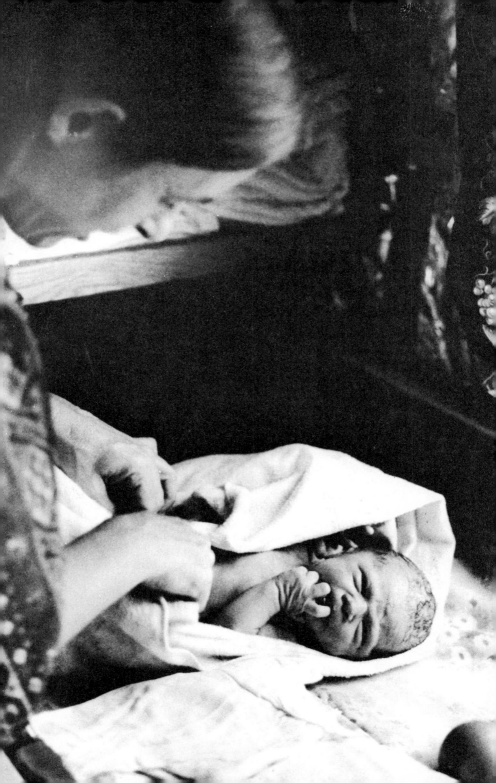

3. **Check the pulse.** When you use the stethoscope to listen to the breath sounds, also count the heartbeat and listen to the heart sounds. The normal newborn pulse rate is 120-160.

    If there are any unusual heart sounds or if the heart rate is outside the normal range, especially if it is under 100, call your doctor.

4. **Take the baby's temperature** at about five minutes. It should be 98-99.5°F. taken rectally. If it is below normal, you need to take special care to get it back up, by wrapping him in more blankets and/or making the room warmer. If his temperature hasn't started to rise by a half hour after this, you could try warming up a couple of blankets in the oven and wrapping him in them. If his temperature is still low and not coming up, you may want to check with your doctor.

5. **Check the baby's color,** especially at the lips and ears. For dark-skinned babies, check the fingernails and the mucus membranes inside the mouth and the lips for blue-ness (cyanosis).

6. **Evaluate the baby's Apgar score** at five minutes. (See p.359.)

> If any of the vital signs (pulse, temperature and respiration) or color are abnormal and the baby is otherwise doing well, note if the baby is dressed too warmly, or if he is crying, and recheck the vital signs in a half hour or so.

7. **Weigh the baby.**
8. **Check his muscle tone**—do all his extremities move alike?
9. **Check for scrapes, bruises, or other birth injuries.**
10. **Check for a good Moro reflex.** You check it like this: pick up the baby's arms without picking up his head, then let them go. The baby should extend his arms and fingers in an embracing motion.
11. **Clean the baby.** With a sterile, soft cloth, wipe off any water or blood, but leave the white cream (vernix) on the baby's skin. It is good for the skin and helps prevent infection. If the baby has any scrapes, keep them clean and dry, and watch them closely for infection.
12. **Fix the cord stump.** If you used a string instead of a clamp, trim the ends of the cord string. Use your sterile Q-tips to paint the cord with betadine solution, gentian violet or triple dye. Paint the base where it joins the abdomen and the place where it was cut.
13. **Dress the baby.** Put on a diaper and a kimono and wrap the baby in a receiving blanket with a corner over his head to keep it warm. If the room is very warm (80°F. or more) and free of drafts, you can leave the baby's kimono open in front so that he can have plenty of skin-to-skin contact with his mother. The mother can hold him close and warm him with her warmth. Add a light blanket to hold the heat in.

14. ***Put drops in the baby's eyes.*** It's important to put anti-bacterial drops in the baby's eyes some time during the first 2 or 3 hours. The mother can have a dormant gonorrhea infection and not even know it, and the baby can run into it on his way out. An infection of this kind may not be detected even on culturing. To protect the baby's eyes from the gonococci which can cause blindness, we use a special erythromycin preparation. Penicillin drops are used in some hospitals, and there is also the old stand-by silver nitrate drops. Silver nitrate drops are the easiest to obtain, but can burn a little. It is important to use one of these to prevent blindness from an undetected gononorrhea infection. You can wait a few hours to treat the baby's eyes if you don't want to interrupt the mother and the baby's first eye-to-eye contact.

Syringe out the baby's nose and mouth often to clean out mucus. You may need to do this several times in the first hour. If the mucus is plentiful and thick, it is good to give the baby sterilized water by mouth. Use a sterilized medicine dropper for this.

We put the baby to the breast as soon as we're sure that both he and the mother are okay. Babies and mothers are both happiest this way.

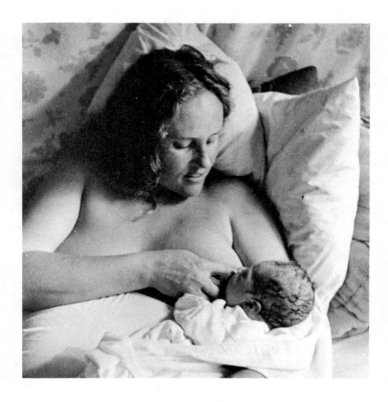

There is a distinction that midwives should have really well in their minds. We quit using the silver nitrate, not because it gave the baby unpleasant sensations for a minute, but because it actually caused a little tissue damage. You have to make a distinction between something that is a damaging thing and being sentimental. At first the infant's senses are wide open and they should be treated like living Buddhas, which is what they are. But you can't have a sentimental viewpoint or that will lead you into a sentimental viewpoint about ladies having babies too. "Oh, does that hurt, dear? Poor thing. Too bad, oh my." That's the attitude that giving anesthesia comes from.

— Stephen

You should always remain with the mother for at least an hour following the delivery. Check her uterus several times and make sure it's good and hard. See that she gets all that she wants to drink. Leave a lady you can trust to stay with the new parents and baby to keep the mother and baby quiet and well taken care of for a couple of days. Have her check the uterus every couple of hours for several hours. Before you leave, you should unwrap the baby and check the color of his extremities, ears, and lips, and check the umbilical tie. His ears and lips should be pink. If they're bluish, you should have a doctor look at him. Be sure that his cord stump is not oozing any blood.

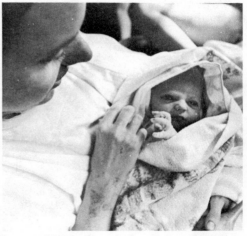

Instruct the mother to call you if he gets a fever, if her discharge smells bad, or if she has pain or tenderness in her abdomen. This could indicate a post-partum infection, and she would need antibiotics. Check with your doctor.

Before you leave, make sure the mother knows how to hold the baby, how to change diapers, etc. It's a good idea to help the new mother and baby get started nursing before you go. (Sometimes the baby isn't interested yet—that's okay.)

If the mother shows no interest in the baby (unlikely, but it does happen sometimes), stay with them until you are satisfied that the mother is *in love with* the baby. You can have a trusted friend help you at this time if necessary.

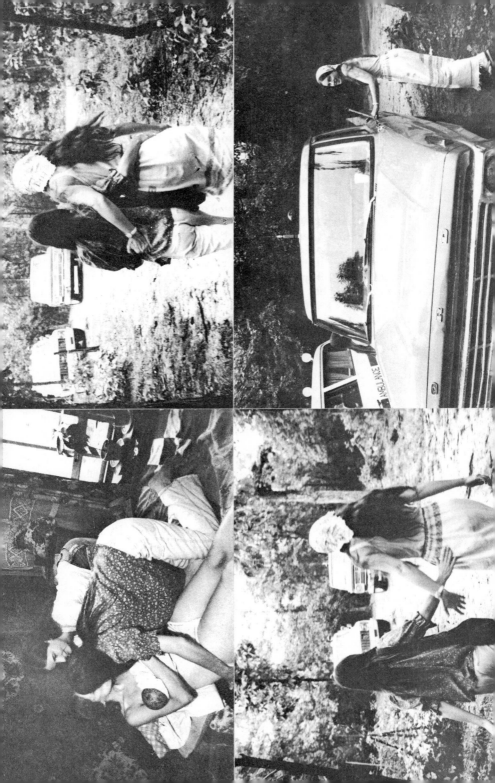

7. Follow-Up Care of the Mother and Newborn

Second Day Exam of the Baby

1. **Measure length.** The full-term newborn is 18-21 inches long.
2. **Recheck the weight.** It is common for the newborn to lose a few ounces before starting to gain. It usually takes anywhere from two days to a week for the baby to get back up to birth weight.
3. **Head:** Check the head circumference now and it will be more accurate, since the baby's head will have un-molded. The baby's head circumference should be around 35 cm. (14"). Check suture lines (the lines where the baby's head bones meet) and the shape of the head to make sure some of the suture lines haven't already hardened up. If they have, check with your doctor.

    Check the soft spots (fontanels). The front soft spot is diamond-shaped and is about 1" x 1" or so and the back one is triangular and may be closed at birth. If the soft spot is bulging when the baby is not crying, it means there is increased pressure in there, and you should take the baby in to the hospital right away. If it is sunken in, there isn't enough fluid, and the baby may be dehydrated, which means you might need to take him in, depending on how he is otherwise: if he's real sleepy, or just doesn't look good, you'd want to take him in.

    Check for cleft palate. A baby can have one that isn't obvious on the outside, and it may interfere with feeding. You can check it by putting a clean finger on the roof of the mouth and just feeling around.

    Check the baby's eyes. Sometimes there are small hemorrhages due to the pressure in the birth canal. This will start to clear up in a few days.
4. **Neck:** Check for masses.
5. **Chest:** Check shape. Check breath sounds with a stethoscope, and check the respirations for regularity and rate. By the second day, the baby's respirations should be 40-60 per minute.

    Check again for any signs of RDS (see p. 366). It usually will start within a few hours after birth but may come on gradually over a day or so.
6. **Abdomen:** Check for masses. Check first one side, then the other side. Put one hand under the baby for support on the side you are checking, and one hand on his belly. Gently press deeply into the baby's belly with the top hand. You should feel nothing much. It helps to practice on some bigger kids to get the hang of it. If the baby's crying, it will be difficult to make an accurate exam.

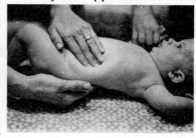

7. **Joints**: Check for congenital dislocation of the hip (see p. 438). This is one of the things that is usually pretty easy to fix if found early. Turn the baby on his belly. Check all the folds and creases in his legs and butt, and make sure they're symmetrical and that both legs are of equal length. Now lay the baby on his back and bend his knees. Holding the knees, rotate the thighs both inward and outward. On outward rotation, both knees will usually touch the table top. If the movement of the legs feels unequal, it is likely that the hip on the side that is harder to move is dislocated. If you feel or hear a click when you move the legs, it may or may not be a sign of dislocation. If you suspect a dislocation of the hip, have your doctor see the baby.

Make sure all the other joints move the right way, by moving them in their normal ways. The lower leg and feet may be curved in a little, from the position they were in when inside. If you can't take the baby's foot and straighten it out, he may have club foot, which should be checked out while the baby is very young.

8. **Bottom**: Make sure the pee hole is in the right place; see if the boy's testes are down (sometimes they don't come down until he's a year or so old). Check the butt-hole by sticking a thermometer in. Even if there's not a hole, the outside part still usually looks normal. Make sure the baby is peeing and shitting. His temperature should be 98-99°F. rectally (36.5-37.5°C.)

9. **Spine**: Make sure it looks normal.

10. **Reflexes**: Beside the Moro reflex you checked on the first examination, there are a number of other reflexes to check:

Grasp: The baby will grab onto your finger when you put it in his hand, and will try to grab your thumb with his toes when you put it under his toes.

Sucking: The baby is probably nursing; ask the mother.

Babinski: When you move your fingernail up the outside of the bottom of the baby's foot, his big toe will stick up and his toes may fan out.

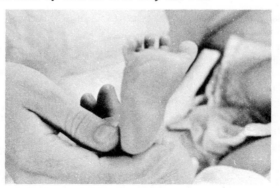

Step: The baby will move one foot in front of the other, like he's walking, when you hold him standing up on something.

11. **Pulse:** The baby's pulse should be between 130 and 160 when he's at rest, although it can go from 90, in a real relaxed sleep, to 180, when he's real active. Check for the wrist (radial) and femoral pulses. The radial pulse is on the inner side of the wrist, and the femoral pulse is felt in the groin.

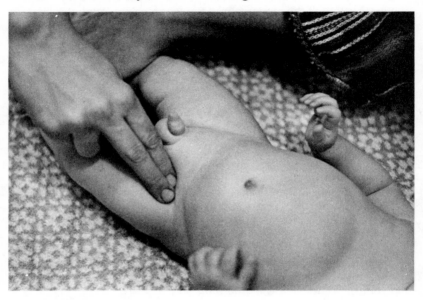

Care in the First Week

You or a trusted friend should visit the new parents and baby each day for the first week, longer if it is necessary, to make sure that they are getting off to a good start. Tell the mother to call you any time of the day or night if she has any questions at all.

In checking on the new baby in the first few days after birth, ask your doctor to check the baby if you notice or the mother reports any of the following:

- blueness (cyanosis) of the arms and legs
- difficulties in breathing
- fever or below normal temperature
- poor feeding
- projectile vomiting or any repeated vomiting other than normal spitting up
- jaundice in the first two days after birth
- anything about the baby that you or the mother don't feel comfortable about

374

Jaundice

Jaundice is the yellowness that comes from having deposits of bilirubin in the skin. About two thirds of all newborn babies get a little jaundiced. Simple jaundice usually begins around the second or third day after birth, lasting up to a week or ten days after birth. Bilirubin comes from the breaking down of old or extra blood cells and is usually excreted through the liver bile into the intestinal tract and a little bit by the kidneys. But in the newborn, there are a lot of extra red cells to break down and the liver is usually immature and over-loaded so it takes a few days to catch up. The baby with simple newborn jaundice is tan or orange-pink, eats well and is alert. Have the mother give the baby as much water as he will take. Also, if the weather permits, have her take off as many of his clothes as possible and expose his skin to the sunlight for five minutes at a time (caution her not to get him sunburned). Exposure to sunlight helps get rid of the bilirubin. (Sunlight is effective even if it is coming through a window.)

Simple jaundice is not serious and usually disappears with no special treatment. If the baby looks pretty yellow to you in good light, check with your doctor. If the palms and soles of the baby's feet are yellow, or if there is an accompanying fever, lethargy or lack of appetite, see your doctor. Most doctors like to put jaundiced babies under a bilirubin light (a special kind of light which produces the same results as sunlight) if the bilirubin level is about 15 mg/100 ml (which is about the level where you start seeing yellow in the palms and soles). If the bilirubin level gets too high for too long, it can be harmful to the baby.

If jaundice appears at birth, or on the first day, or if it first appears after the fifth day, see the doctor.

Breast Milk Jaundice

Sometimes a baby will develop "breast milk jaundice" in the second week. This is caused by a hormone in mother's milk which inhibits the enzymes needed for the breakdown and excretion of bilirubin. A doctor will need to determine if this is the cause. If the baby is otherwise prospering and his bilirubin count is not too high, let the mother continue nursing, making sure that she gives the baby as much water as he wants as well. If the baby has a high bilirubin count and doesn't seem to be doing well, check with your doctor.

Other Types of Jaundice

Jaundice can be a sign of other problems, such as infection, liver disease, Rh or ABO incompatibility. If the baby turns yellow within the first 24 hours, it may be from Rh or ABO incompatibility, and you should have him checked by your doctor. He may need a transfusion. If the baby isn't eating well, is sleeping more than usual for a newborn (is hard to rouse), or isn't looking good, have your doctor see him.

375

Some Other Things to Tell the Mother

Tell new mothers that it is possible to resume periods as early as four weeks after childbirth—*even while nursing.* A lady can ovulate two or three weeks after childbirth and get pregnant without ever having a period. (The first ovulation precedes the first period by two weeks.)

I recommend *A Cooperative Method of Natural Birth Control* by Margaret Nofziger, as a safe and effective method of birth control.

Make sure that the new parents are getting along well. Counsel them if they need it.

Encourage the mother, if she is completely well, to do after-baby exercises (p. 240) to get her body back into good shape. Tell her also to exercise the muscles of her taint and the muscles around her pee-hole by contracting and relaxing them alternately.

Six Week Check-Up

Six weeks or so after the mother delivers, she should be checked. Check her blood pressure, urine, hematocrit, weight, size and position of uterus, appearance of cervix, and condition of pelvic organs and perineum, especially if she was stitched. This is also a good time to do a Pap smear. Ask her how her bleeding is and check her baby.

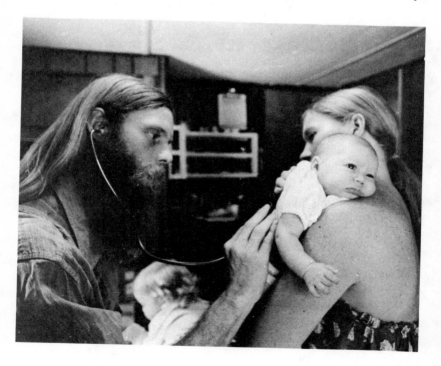

376

8. Injuries and Repairs of the Pelvic Floor

Tears [or Episiotomies] *of the Birth Canal and the Puss*
Tears of the taint can be divided into three categories:
1. First degree, involving tearing of the skin just below or inside the puss.
2. Second degree, involving the skin just below the puss, the taint, and the muscles of the taint (the perineal body).
3. Third degree, involving all of the above and the anal sphincter as well.

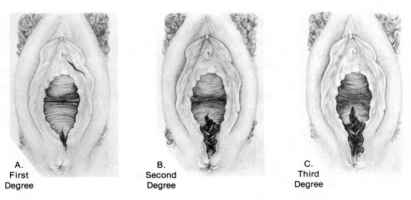

A.
First
Degree

B.
Second
Degree

C.
Third
Degree

Fig. 68. Tears of the Taint and Birth Canal.

Tears of the Lips
These tears are usually slight, but are fairly painful. Suture them if they are split enough that they will be uncomfortable during lovemaking after they are healed.

Episiotomies
The easiest type of episiotomy to repair and heal is the cut straight down from the bottom of the puss. This is much less painful to the mother during healing than an oblique cut. Slow delivery of the baby's head reduces the need for episiotomy and reduces the size the incision needs to be when one is necessary.

Repair of Midline Tear or Episiotomy
The midwife can repair first and second degree tears if she knows how to suture. Third degree tears, because of their extensiveness, are best repaired by a doctor, or at least with one in attendance.

You should wait to repair any tear or episiotomy until after the third stage is complete. They are repaired with dissolvible catgut sutures.
1. Clean the wound if there has been any contamination following the birth of the baby.

377

2. Infiltrate the edges of the cut with a local anesthetic such as xylocaine, just under the skin. You need to do this only on the edges of the taint, or the lips, as the edges of the mucosa of the birth canal are not sensitive to being stuck.

Figure 69. Injection of a Local Anesthetic.

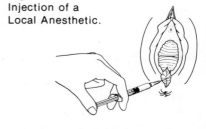

Use a medium, round Ferguson needle with 000 chromic catgut. You may occasionally want to use 00 or 0000 chromic, depending on the size of the tear. 0000 is finer; 00 is larger.

3. If you have a deep tear or cut, you will first have to put some deep sutures in. This will help in matching up the sides of the tear and in taking the tension off the sutures in the mucosal lining. Start by stitching the needle inside the wall of the tear and bringing the needle out in the bottom of the tear, then going back in near the same point at the bottom and bringing it up to the same place in the opposite wall. This can sometimes be done in one bite. Tie the stitch with three alternating knots, cutting the ends short. Use as many stitches as you need to pull a deep tear together.

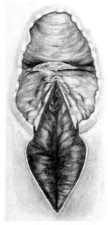

Fig. 70. Midline episiotomy ready to be sutured.

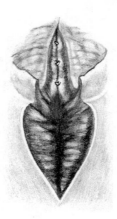

Fig. 71. Deep stitches uniting sides of cut.

4. Sew the mucus lining of the birth canal together. Begin at the top of the wound, taking the first bite a little above the apex. Tie this stitch, cutting the short end ¼" longer. Sew the edges with a continuous suture, matching them as well as possible, and taking care not to pull them tight and strangled. If you like, you can

use a lock (or blanket) stitch on the mucus lining. Each bite of the needle includes the mucus membrane of the birth canal and the tissue between the birth canal and rectum. This makes for better healing by eliminating dead space and reducing bleeding. Sew down to the skin edges. Use the hymenal ring as a landmark to get the tissues aligned. On the last one or two bites, make the stitches subcutaneous— do not come through the skin (the mucus lining). If there is no deep muscle tears of the taint, continue to step 6, using the same needle and suture. If there is a deep muscle tear, leave the end of the suture with the needle still on it because you'll use this again after repairing the deep muscle tear.

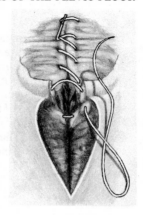

Fig. 72. Continuous stitches closing mucus lining.

5. Lay aside the continuous suture and make three or four stitches, each tied separately, drawing together the deep muscle and fascia of the taint. These stitches have to be of the right tension: if too tight, they will cut off the blood supply of the tissue; if too loose, the entrance will be too open.

6. Then, with the suture left from stitching the birth canal, stitch downward to bring together the next layer of muscle. Use a running stitch. Bring the needle out at the bottom point of the tear or cut.

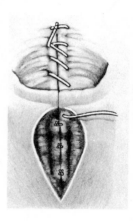

Fig. 73. Stitches drawing together deep muscles of the taint.

Fig. 74. Continuous stitches drawing together superficial muscle layer and fascia of the taint.

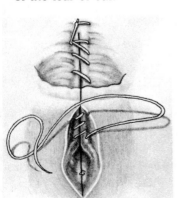

7. Lastly, close the incision using a continuous, subcutaneous stitch starting at the lower end. Take the first bite just under but not through the skin, going from side to side until the upper end of the wound is reached. Tie the end of this suture to a loop of itself when you reach the entrance to the birth canal.

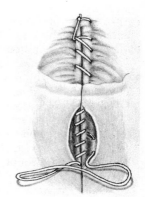

Fig. 75. Continuous stitches bringing together skin edges of the taint.

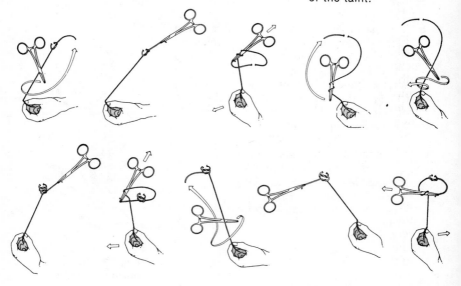

Fig. 76. Method of Tying Off Sutures While Maintaining Sterile Field.

Care of the Stitches

Instruct the mother in how to clean the stitched area and provide her with some mild antiseptic soap. She may use heat from an electric light bulb to reduce the swelling if necessary. Tell her to wipe from front to back after shitting. A daily shower is a good idea.

9. Asphyxia in the Newborn

The normal healthy baby should breathe within a half-minute to a minute after birth. Occasionally a baby does not breathe spontaneously or may start and stop breathing. This baby requires stimulation or additional help. While this situation may not occur often, you must, at each birth, *anticipate* that it may occur and be poised for quick action. You need to instantly recognize the baby with a problem with beginning breathing and treat him immediately.

Asphyxia can be mild or severe.

Mild Asphyxia

If asphyxia is mild, the baby may not cry, may breathe a little irregularly, and be a little blue with some but less than the usual amount of muscle tone. Your helper should note the exact time of birth and briefly listen to the baby's heartbeat with a stethoscope. If the heartbeat is greater than 100, there is no immediate danger. Keep the baby warm at all times. Be sure that the baby's airway is clear. He needs repeated suctioning with an ear syringe (which should have begun before the birth of his body), as long as there are any fluids or mucus that might obstruct his airway. Make sure that his head is lower than the rest of his body so that the fluid can drain from the chest and airway. Don't leave the syringe in his mouth for too long at a time as this can interfere with the rhythm of breathing. If the mucus obstructing the airway cannot be removed with the ear syringe you may need to use a DeLee infant suction set (see p. 461). You should be familiar with its use.

Often, a slightly asphyxiated baby will respond very well to stimulation by touch. Rub your fingertips up the baby's spine, starting at the base, and placing a fingertip on either side of the spine. You want to attract the baby's attention to his body. Be gentle, but try to get the baby to cry. Crying babies take nice deep breaths which expand the lungs and get oxygen into their systems rapidly. If the baby is breathing well and there is still thick mucus coating the baby's mouth, dip your fingers in sterile water and swab them around in the baby's mouth. Additional oxygen should be available for the mildly asphyxiated baby. This can be given at the rate of about 4 liters per minute with an infant face mask covering the baby's nose and mouth. A mildly asphyxiated baby will generally improve rapidly.

Severe Asphyxia

Asphyxia is severe if the baby is limp, blue or white, and if there is little or no response to stimulation (the Apgar score will be 4 or less). Keep the baby warm. Too hot or cold an environment will increase the baby's oxygen need, so keeping him warm is important. Do whatever is necessary to keep his temperature between 98° and 99.5°F.

Resuscitation

There are certain priorities to keep in mind while resuscitating a baby. These priorities are listed in order of importance:

A. *Maintain an open* **airway.**
B. *Maintain* **breathing.**
C. *Maintain* **circulation.**

A. Your first priority is to maintain an open airway.

Lay the baby at an angle of 30° from horizontal, with his head down and tipped back slightly. Tilting the head back draws the tongue out of the airway. In a baby, too much or too little of a tilt will close the airway, so you'll have to find the position that best allows the air to get through. A rolled-up towel placed under one shoulder will keep his chin from resting on his chest and will cause his head to roll a little to one side so any fluid that comes up will pool in his cheek rather than in the back of his throat.

Suck any fluids from the mouth and nose with an ear syringe. If the airway if not clear, use a DeLee infant suction set. See p. 461.

- *If the baby is breathing after you've cleared his airway, give him oxygen-enriched air with the infant face mask.*
- *If the baby still is not trying to breathe after 1-2 minutes, begin resuscitation.*

B. Your second priority is to get oxygen to the baby's lungs.

This is the time to use your portable oxygen kit. See page 459.

Resuscitation with an Infant Bag Mask

It is best to use a bag mask because you are able to see the baby easily while working on him. One with a built-in pressure cutoff is best because it protects the baby's lungs from being injured. Keeping the baby's head tilted back, place the mask over the baby's face with the point over the nose. Have an oxygen tube hooked up to the oxygen inlet and delivering 4-8 lpm. If the baby's color is pale white or blue, have the 100% adaptor attached. Using your thumb and first two fingers, squeeze the bag at a rate of 24 puffs per minute. This leaves enough time for exhalation between puffs. If there is not adequate ventilation, you can use more fingers, which will deliver more pressure. Be sure to make a good seal around the baby's mouth and nose with the bag mask. Watch the baby's chest and listen with a stethoscope to be sure that good air movement is happening.

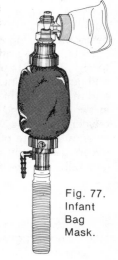

Fig. 77. Infant Bag Mask.

382

Mouth-to-Mouth Resuscitation

Put your mouth over the baby's nose and mouth and blow puffs of air into him from your mouth (not your lungs) at a rate of 24 puffs a minute. A newborn's lungs are fragile and can be injured by too much pressure. With this in mind, feel the chest inflate and the slight resistance to your breath when the lungs are full. You can increase the oxygen content of the air you give the baby by placing an oxygen tube in your mouth while breathing for him. Be sure to make a good seal around the baby's mouth and nose with your mouth. Watch the baby's chest and listen with a stethoscope to be sure that good air movement is happening.

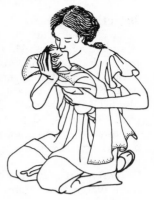

Fig. 78. Giving the Baby Mouth-to-Mouth Resuscitation.

C. Your third priority is to begin cardiac massage if the baby's pulse is less than 60 beats per minute.

You or your helper should find out the baby's heart rate. His heart will start to slow down if he hasn't been getting any oxygen for 1½-2 minutes. Listen with a stethoscope or feel the femoral or carotid artery. Combine resuscitation with cardiac massage if the heart rate is less than 60 beats per minute.

The baby should be on a firm surface. With your thumbs on the baby's breastbone (sternum) and your fingers around the baby's back, press down with your thumbs 2-3 cm. at a rate of twice a second. Give the baby a puff of air every fourth or fifth compression without interrupting the rhythm of the compressions. The breath must be given *between* compressions. This will take a bit of practice. Continue cardiac compression alternating 4 or 5 pushes with an inflation of the

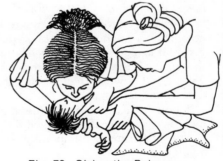

Fig. 79. Giving the Baby Cardio-Pulmonary Resuscitation.

lungs so that you puff into the baby's mouth at the same time that your thumbs are coming up. Do this until the heart is beating regularly at a normal rate.

Be sure that you are not giving cardiac massage to a heart that is already beating at a satisfactory rate. Even if the pulse rate is below 60 you may find that asynchronous compressions may make heart action less effective and could be damaging.

Cardio-pulmonary resuscitation continued for as long as 30 to 45 minutes has saved babies, without brain damage.

Injecting Caffeine

You can try an intra-muscular injection of 0.1 cc. of caffeine to stimulate a baby who is extremely lethargic because of asphyxia resulting from a long or hard passage in the second stage. Give the injection about 3-3½ minutes after the birth if the baby's respiratory efforts are weak or absent. One-tenth cc. is an extremely small amount of liquid. Use a TB syringe and 5/8" needle. TB syringes are very thin, with small gradations marked on the barrel. This injection sometimes will help (it has in my own experience) and this amount of caffeine will not harm a newborn. Give the injection in the front lateral part of the baby's mid-thigh.

Transport the baby to a hospital if there is no dramatic improvement within a few minutes of the baby's birth. Continue resuscitation if necessary until you arrive at the hospital.

If You Have to Take a Baby to the Hospital

When a baby's having trouble, check his vital signs—his temperature, pulse, and respirations—often, about every 15 minutes (more often if necessary), until he's stable. He is stable if his vital signs are staying about the same and he is holding his own. Once he's stable, check his vital signs about every half hour, to make sure he's staying stable. Do this on the way to the hospital, taking care not to chill the baby in the process.

Make notes, or at least make mental notes about how his color changes, whether or not his pulse feels strong and regular, if his breathing gets more or less labored, etc. Then when you get to the hospital, the doctor will know if the baby is getting better or worse, and how well he tolerated the trip. If you can, check the time when you leave.

If you have time, bring the mother's prenatal and birthing records with you. That will tell the doctor about the baby's past health, which may be important. Bring a sample of cord blood if you can.

Have someone call the hospital and tell them that you're coming, and who you're bringing, and what's the matter, as near as you can tell. It's good to figure out beforehand which is the quickest way to get to your hospital. If it's an emergency, have someone call the police or highway patrol; sometimes they'll clear the roads for you or give you an escort. You may be able to arrange to meet an ambulance on the way if you need one. For situations like these, it's nice to have a CB radio in your car. Channel 9 is the emergency channel. If at all possible, bring the father, and the mother too, if she is able to go. You or your helper can explain to them what's going on. It's good for them and the baby if they're there.

384

This seemed like an appropriate place for Tristan's story, which was written by his mother and father. Tristan was our first severely asphyxiated baby [required resuscitation and sometimes heart massage for 20 minutes] that we were able to care for at the Farm. He showed us that a severely asphyxiated baby showing the usual signs that these babies do in their first few days—lethargy, little or no sucking response, rapid breathing, convulsions, and less than normal reflexes—can make a full recovery. The above abnormalities are caused by the swelling of the brain that accompanies severe asphyxia, and normal newborn behavior will return as the swelling subsides. It is a great mistake to assume that these babies are permanently damaged in any way, so the parents of any such baby should not be led to think that their baby is not perfect. Keep in mind that any asphyxiated baby needs as much of his mother's touch as he can safely get, since the kind of necessary but intense handling that this kind of child is subjected to at birth is likely to leave him uptight.

Tristan's Story

Mick: 9 p.m., Tuesday.

I'm stepping outside for a minute and I look up and see the tail end of a shooting star. Staring up, there goes another, and another, in two different directions. Wow, that's three. Then the tail end of another one, and as I look up once more the biggest shoots right across the sky, leaving a green trail for a split second. Bright and clear, that's five shooting stars all over the one little patch of sky I can see through the trees, all in the space of a couple of minutes.

I'm leaving the house to go to bed out in the bus . . . "Sweet dreams everybody . . ." and Betsy, one of the ladies who lives in the house, says, "Sleep well, this could be the night."

Around 3:30 a.m. Wednesday the 6th, I wake up and Cathy's scrambling about, and then I realize the bed's all wet, and Betsy was right!

Cathy: Water bag leaking at 3:00 a.m. Reached down, hands all wet; what to do? Couldn't find matches to light the lamp, flashlight dim, dribbling and fumbling in the dark, feeling like a kid who'd wet the bed. . . .

Mary said to call back when contractions were five minutes apart and to try to get some sleep but I was too excited and a little uneasy—would I be brave enough? Would the birthing be the way I hoped?

Mick: By 4:15 a.m. Cathy's rushes were coming every five or six minutes, and they were pretty light. We were both a bit irritable because we couldn't get back to sleep! We called Mary again to let her know what was happening.

The contractions were coming along pretty easy, and by the time it was just getting light I finally realized that this was really it, and woke up. I put on some nice clean clothes and swept the bus and tidied things up.

Kathleen came over from the house to help out. We were feeling good, and a little bit apprehensive. The birthing kit arrived around 7 a.m. with oxygen bottles and bags and sterile things and scales, and I wondered who we were going to be weighing, and hoped we weren't going to need all those emergency things.

The rushes began coming on stronger, and by 7:30 we were *coping.* Kathleen told Cathy to look into my eyes, and that was a whole different thing. With each rush, we started to breathe together, and looking into each other it was like we could use the power of the contractions as a source of strength, and just ride through them.

Cathy: As the rushes came on, I felt in control between contractions but lolled over like a wounded elephant when one hit me. I was only a few centimeters dilated and I wondered how I was going to handle the later rushes because I was already feeling a little ragged around the edges.

Then one of the ladies helping said it helped to look into someone's eyes. On the next rush I looked into hers and was astonished by how intimate and powerful it felt. Then I latched onto Mick: I fell into his eyes and didn't come out. He felt so strong and pure and loving I fell in love with him all over again. He steered me through every rush breath by breath. He would smile and bring light into my soul. If he had to leave for a few minutes, my rushes would stop completely until he came back.

It was hot in the bus, in the high 90's, and I remembered a pound of margarine I'd seen on a kitchen counter melting in the sun. I felt like that, oozing in every direction. Twice Mick and the ladies helped me outside the bus and threw cold water on me. I was rushing and sizzling, feeling totally *electric!*

Mick: By noon it must've been around 100°, and Cathy was 3 centimeters dilated, and at 2 p.m., something like 4 centimeters. Things seemed to be going along real slow, and it was very hot in the bus. Mary said everything was fine and regular—like clockwork—no sudden speed-ups or slow-downs, just one rush, then another, real steady. A couple of times between rushes, we went out and poured cold water on Cathy, and we had all the windows and doors open in the bus. Every so often we cooled Cathy down with the fine mist of a plant sprayer.

It was all so strong and intense. I remembered the thing about the whole Universe moving over to make way for a new baby and understood. Outside the bus were the trees and the birds, and *everything* looked so clear and vibrant. Wasps and bugs flew in and around, and we could just vibe them out, and away. At one point a wasp came buzzing up to the back door and Mary just put up her hand like a traffic cop, and he turned around and buzzed off.

During the hottest part of the afternoon, a breeze blew up during each rush, and it seemed to die away in between. As each rush started I would think about the breeze, and along it came, right on cue, unfailingly.

There was something real, strong and Holy in the air. As I looked into Cathy's eyes it seemed like they were bottomless pools, and I could draw this energy out of them. There was a lot of energy going back and forth between us—just like A.C., the same current, vibrating—and it felt like we could just groove on indefinitely, like there was this infinite supply of strength and energy that we could draw on. It was hard work, and hot, just like when you put a big electrical charge through a thin wire, the wire gets hot. But we were nowhere near overloaded!

Cathy: The books had all described "transition" as the most difficult part of labor but I was never aware of any "stages." I only knew that things became deeper, stronger, more intense and that finally I had to squeeze Mick's hand with each rush. Colors were richer and I could see the smallest details of things.

I was almost fully dilated and Kay Marie and Mary arrived. I was glad we'd all be seeing the baby soon. But then time stretched out. Mick went to hook up the bus battery for the inside lights and I said, Oh, we won't need those, it's the middle of the afternoon. Later I looked out and was surprised to see it was getting dark. I was pushing hard but nothing seemed to be happening; the baby's head wasn't moving down past my pelvic bones. Making bullmoose noises helped out but I wondered if I was being too melodramatic, flopping back between pushes, hardly smiling at anyone anymore.

Mick: Eventually night came and it cooled down and Cathy started to push. She was working so incredibly hard, and I couldn't share the load any more. It blew my mind how hard she worked, turning all kinds of red, purple, straining colors on every push. Kay Marie was like the conductor, "Push now . . . stop . . . pant . . . push . . . harder, harder," then there's all this fast action with clamps and surgical instruments and stuff that I didn't want to see.

Cathy: Finally on one push Kay Marie said, "Can you push a little more? A little more?" and the baby's head slid down and out in one push—a dramatic crowning! I squealed and almost blew it, but Kay Marie told me firmly to do just what she said. His cord was tight around his neck so they had me push hard to get him out quickly. His cut cord was blue and purple and green and he lay on his side between my legs, luminous and perfect—not breathing. Time stopped. Kay Marie and Mary were working *hard* on him, suctioning him, giving him oxygen and mouth-to-mouth and still he wasn't breathing. Next to me, Mick was nearly delirious with joy and fear. I held him tight but felt as if I'd floated off and was watching from somewhere far away. Somehow I hadn't expected the baby to be so complete and perfect. He looked like an angel or otherworldly being and I didn't know if we'd get to keep him. I felt sad thinking of my parents and friends and all the folks who were waiting for him. I thought he's the one we've been waiting for so long!

Mick: His cord was wrapped tightly around his neck, and they had to cut it, and then he came out at 8:30 p.m. looking beautiful and perfect and translucent. I couldn't believe all those psychedelic colors. The cord was a beautiful greenish blue, and he was all transparent, pale greens, blues, pinks. He was just luminous and glowing, but he wasn't breathing. There was this tiny person lying still and tranquil and glowing, while everyone worked like crazy to get him to breathe. Diane was holding the flashlight on him, and he seemed to me big—like a giant lying flat on his back, with broad shoulders, deep chest, and clenched fists, just lying there with his eyes closed, waiting for some-body to breathe life into him. His heart would go, and stop, and he'd breathe once, lightly, and stop.

By this time, I'd started to lose it and get emotional. Cathy was so calm and just said, "Don't worry baby, he'll be okay, he's so beautiful." And there was all sorts of action going on all around us.

Cathy: The bus filled up with Jeffrey, EMTs, midwives, helpers, all focused on the tiny still baby on the rubber sheet. I'm not sure how or when he began breathing on his own. Later they said it took twenty minutes, but to us it seemed an eternity.

He was whisked off to the nursery for babies needing special care. Ina May arrived and hopped on the bed next to us. I agreed with everything she said although I can't remember anything we talked about. I only remember looking in her eyes and feeling warmed. We went to the nursery. The baby was in an incubator, bright eyes peeping out over a little green oxygen mask. My heart went out to him lying there in the glare of lights. Later I scrubbed up and put my hand into the incubator. He grabbed my fingers and held on tight, looking right into my eyes—a small, very sentient being.

Mick: Tristan was in an incubator with a little green oxygen mask on. He looked like a little frog/spaceman caricature. His head was so soft and translucent, and the bones seemed to move with each change of expression. At one point he opened his eyes, and I looked into them and thought, "Wow, I've been looking into those eyes all day." The same pools of strength, so pure and clear. I just thought to him, "Well, hi there, little buddy, this is it. If you want to stay here you've got to breathe, and take care of yourself, and work hard at doing it. You had a hard time, but here we all are." And he looked back at me, "Yeah, I know, I'm doing the best I can. It is hard work." And he closed his eyes again and I loved him so much and I knew he was going to be okay. Cathy said he gave us a fright like that to make us realize just what a precious gift he was. She was so strong and brave and knew all the time that he was going to be all right. It must have been around 11 p.m. by this time, and we just fell asleep, exhausted.

Cathy: It seemed like the next days were a continuation of the birthing: he went through so many changes and it was a few days before we could hold him and ten days before we got to take him home. He'd been on an IV for a few days and completely forgot how to suck. We had to coax him to suck on a bottle, pulling on his arms and legs, singing, talking to him, making noises and faces, and then give him a feeding tube or syringe to make up the rest of the feeding. He never did learn to nurse, but I got to nurse other babies for two months to keep my milk up so we could try him out when and if he learned to suck well. Another lady (Jean) with an older baby would let her milk build up and try to nurse him. This reassured me because I knew that we'd tried to get him to nurse and that it was not because I was too attached or my vibrations were strange. I also learned from watching Jean, who'd already had three babies, do her patient, gentle but firm yoga with him. She helped teach me not to take him too seriously despite what he'd been through.

When you give birth, you are really opened up from being the passageway for another soul into the world. And the baby is still linked to you, affected by your moods and feelings, so you are both very opened up, vulnerable to what is around you. We were enormously grateful that the baby was kept on the Farm in the nursery instead of being sent to the hospital as most "hard starters" before were. The Farm folks kept things tight technically but never forgot about the spiritual side of things.

Every baby and every birthing is special and I often wondered why his was special in that way. I guess it was because he wanted us to know what a precious gift he was. And we must have needed an extra heavy lesson about love and spirit, which we got, day by day, from him and from the many selfless people who took care of him. I know no one ever touched him who didn't love him, and I can think of at least a dozen folks to whom we owe a little piece of our hearts. Tristan now is a brighteyed strong boy, still a wonder and a mystery to us, still a teacher to us, the one we got to keep.

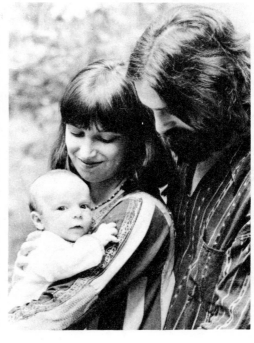

10. Breech Presentation and Delivery

A breech presentation is that when the baby's bottom or legs are the first part to emerge from the womb. Breech presentations at the onset of labor occur in three to four percent of pregnancies. There is a slightly higher risk for the baby in breech presentation than in the vertex, but this is not so great as to rule out delivery at home—provided that the midwife is knowledgeable and experienced, with a doctor backing her up, and that the mother is extremely well prepared for natural childbirth. If you have any alternative, you should not attempt to deliver a breech baby at home unless you have already been taught by someone skilled and have had some supervised experience in breech deliveries. Have a doctor present at the delivery, if possible.

Types

There are three major types of breech deliveries: the complete, the incomplete or frank, and the footling.

Complete: the thighs and knees are both flexed, as in the so-called "fetal position."

Incomplete, or frank: The baby is in a jack-knifed position—both feet touch the head.

Footling: One or both feet present first. This is rare. Even more rarely, the knees may come first.

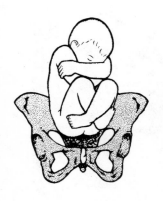 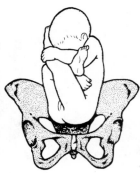 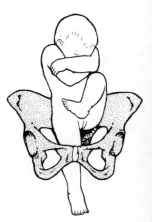

| Fig. 80A. Complete Breech | Fig. 80B. Incomplete or Frank Breech | Fig. 80C. Footling Breech |

Positions

There are eight possible positions of breech presentation. These are designated by the relationship of the baby's tailbone to his mother's pelvis. "Right" and "left" in these designations refer to the mother's right and left sides, not the baby's.

Tailbone forward	TF	Tailbone behind	TB
Left tailbone forward	LTF	Right tailbone forward	RTF
Left tailbone sideways	LTS	Right tailbone sideways	RTS
Left tailbone behind	LTB	Right tailbone behind	RTB

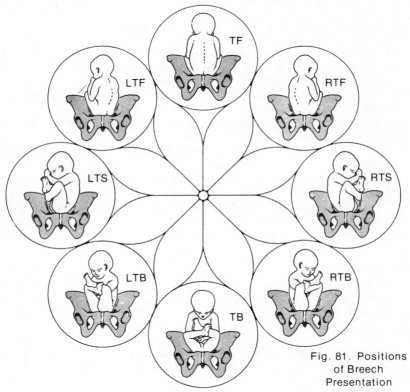

Fig. 81. Positions
of Breech
Presentation

The same designations using Latin terminology are as follows:

Sacrum anterior	SA
Left sacrum anterior (forward)	LSA
Left sacrum transverse	LST
Left sacrum posterior (backward)	LSP
Sacrum posterior (this is very rare—see p. 406)	SP
Right sacrum anterior	RSA
Right sacrum transverse	RST
Right sacrum posterior	RSP

391

Possible Causes for Breech Presentations

- Small or premature baby
- Lots of amniotic fluid
- Multiple pregnancy
- Placenta previa
- Contracted pelvis
- Uterine tumors
- Hydrocephalus (see p. 436)
- Large baby

Diagnosis

See page 328, "How to Feel Where the Baby Is."

Things to Watch Out For During Labor and Delivery

1. Prolapse of the cord is a greater possibility in a breech presentation since the bottom and legs leave gaps through which the cord can be washed down. (Prolapse of the cord occurs in four to five percent of breech deliveries, ten times its usual frequency.)

2. In a breech, the body is outside by the time the head comes through the cervix and the unyielding pelvic outlet, so with a large baby head, the cord can be squashed on its passage through the pelvis, causing hypoxia in the baby.

3. In a breech delivery, the after-coming head is usually larger than everything that has come out before. Sometimes the cervix may not open fully enough to allow the head to pass through.

4. In a breech delivery, the head has less time in which to mold to the most advantageous shape for delivery. Sometimes it may be necessary to get the baby's head out quickly in order to avoid asphyxia, but it must be done gently to prevent intracranial hemorrhage or fractures.

Version

Version means rotating the baby's position by placing hands on the mother's belly and moving the baby. This technique is discussed on p. 331.

The Tilt Position for Turning a Breech

Starting the eighth month on, have the mother spend 10 minutes twice a day lying on her back on the floor, with knees flexed and feet on the floor, and three good-sized pillows placed under her bottom, or better yet, have her lie on a tilted board. It's an awkward position but in one study, 89% of the babies spontaneously truned to vertex position without version. Do only if the baby is already in breech position.

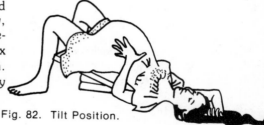

Fig. 82. Tilt Position.

Mechanism of Labor of a Breech in Right Tailbone Forward Position

There are three mechanisms of labor in a breech delivery, involving first the bottom and legs, then the shoulders and arms, and finally the head.

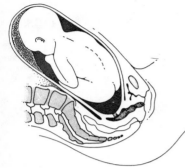

Fig. 83A. Beginning of labor of a breech presentation with baby in right tailbone forward position. The cervix is beginning to dilate and the baby's hips are floating.

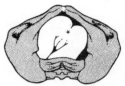

Fig. 83B. View from Below.

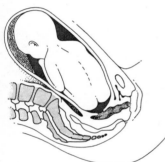

Fig. 84A. The baby's hips have moved farther down and have begun internal rotation. The cervix is thinner and continuing to dilate.

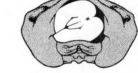

Fig. 84B. View from Below.

Birth of the Bottom and Legs

Descent: The baby's bottom engages when the widest part of the baby's hips (the "bitrochanteric diameter") has passed the pelvic inlet, moving down into the pelvic cavity. Dilation and descent may take longer than in a vertex presentation, as the bottom is not as efficient a dilator as the head.

Internal Rotation of the Bottom: The forward hip arrives at the pelvic floor and rotates forward 45° so that the baby is at the right tailbone sideways position (RTS).

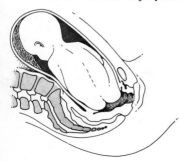

Fig. 85A. The bottom is engaged and dilation is almost complete. The baby has rotated to right tailbone sideways position.

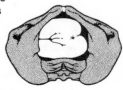

Fig. 85B. View from Below.

Flexion of the Trunk: The baby's body bends sideways at the waist to allow continued descent of the bottom down the curved birth canal. The forward hip leads.

Birth of the Bottom: The forward bun passes under the pubic bone (symphysis pubis), followed by the back bun passing over the taint.

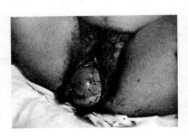

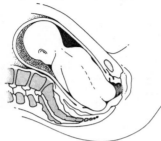

Fig. 86. The baby's bottom is descending.

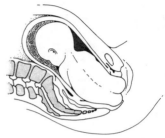

Fig. 87. The front bun is born.

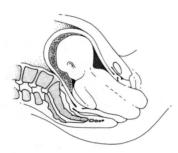

Fig. 88. Both buns have come out.

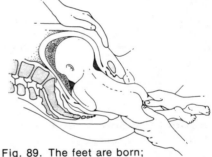

Fig. 89. The feet are born; shoulders are engaging.

Birth of the Shoulders and Arms

Internal Rotation of the Shoulders: While the bottom and legs are being born, the shoulders descend and rotate so that the forward shoulder is behind the pubic bone.

Birth of the Shoulders: The shoulders come out—first one, then the other. The back shoulder comes out over the taint, as the baby's body is lifted upward. The baby is then lowered, and the forward shoulder and arm slip out under the pubic bone. Or the baby can be lowered first, bringing the forward shoulder and arm out first.

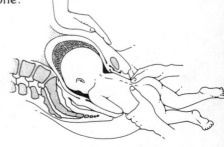

Fig. 90. The shoulders are descending and rotating.

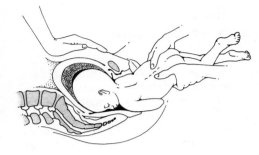

Fig. 91. The back
shoulder emerges first.

Fig. 92. The front
shoulder has just
emerged.

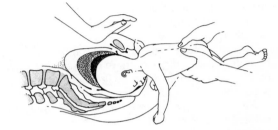

Birth of the Head

Descent: The head enters the pelvis when the shoulders are at the
outlet.

Flexion and internal rotation: The baby's head flexes so his chin rests
on his chest. When the head reaches the pelvic floor, it rotates so
that the face rests in the hollow of the mother's tailbone. The rest
of the baby's body also rotates, so that the baby's back is in the
same plane as the mother's belly.

Birth: The chin, face, brow and occiput pass over the taint, as the
nape of the neck pivots under the pubic bone.

Delivering the Breech Baby

There are three basic ways to deliver a breech.

1. *Spontaneous delivery*—The baby is pushed out by the mother
   with no assistance other than support of the baby's body.
2. *Assisted delivery*—The baby delivers up to the cord by himself,
   and you help with the rest.
3. *Breech extraction*—You help with delivery before the baby is
   crowned to his navel, as in a frank or a footling breech when you
   need to bring the feet down before the body is out to the navel.

Management of
Breech Labor and Delivery

First stage: The first stage proceeds as usual, although dilation of the cervix may take longer than the same woman would with a vertex birth. If the bottom is not engaged, the chance of a cord becoming prolapsed is increased; in this instance, keep the mother in bed in case her membranes rupture. *(With an unengaged bottom and rupture of membranes, a downward rush of amniotic fluid and gravity can wash the cord down before the bottom. Engagement of the baby's bottom will subsequently compress the prolapsed cord.)* Keep the membranes intact. If the membranes do rupture, listen to the fetal heart tones to rule out prolapse of the cord.

Breech babies often expel meconium during labor. As long as the baby's heart tones sound good, there is no cause for worry. Don't let the mother push, even though she may feel like it until you are certain that dilation is complete.

Second stage: In general the more upright the mother with a breech presentation, especially during the pushing stage, the less the chance for extension of the baby's arms or head.

Check the baby's heart rate frequently.

Delivery of the bottom:

1. Let the bottom come out and judge whether an episiotomy will be neccesary. This will depend on the size and stretchability of the mother and on the size of the baby. Support and oil the mother's taint with your hands as you would with a vertex delivery.
2. If you judge that an episiotomy is warranted, inject an anesthetic such as xylocaine into the mother's taint ("perineum") and make the cut when she is numb.
3. Do not pull on the baby or try to free the legs until the body is born to the navel.
4. Have your assistant keep manual pressure on the mother's belly in the direction of the baby's descent to help delivery and to keep the baby's head flexed.
5. Have the mother push only when her uterus contracts.
6. After delivery to the navel, pull down a loop of the cord so there is no strain on the baby's navel. The cord should have a strong pulse.

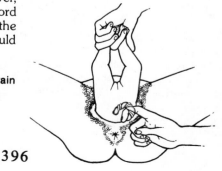

Fig. 93. Relieving Strain
on the Baby's Navel.

7. Once the baby is out this far, you want to be sure that you have a free airway to the baby's mouth within four to five minutes.

Delivery of the torso

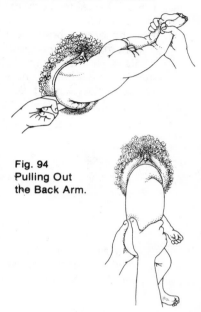

Fig. 94
Pulling Out
the Back Arm.

1. To deliver from the navel to the shoulder, cover the baby's body with a clean, warm towel and take the butt in your two hands with thumbs over the back of the sacrum, your index fingers on the front part of the hip bones, and the rest of your fingers spread evenly over the pelvis and thighs. This way you cannot injure the baby's internal organs.

Fig. 95. Delivery of
the Front Shoulder.

2. Have your assistant or the baby's father keep the pressure on the lower part of the mother's abdomen to keep the baby's head flexed.
3. Pull the baby downward and outward. Don't jerk or twist.
4. The baby's arms will usually be flexed across the chest. These can easily be brought down by slipping your index and middle fingers up the baby's back, over the shoulder, and down past the elbow to the forearm, catching the arm with your fingers and sweeping it across the baby's chest. Do the back shoulder first if it comes easier this way.
5. Lower the baby so you bring out the forward shoulder and arm. Again, hook your fingers over the shoulder and over the arm, and sweep it across the baby's chest.

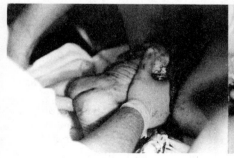
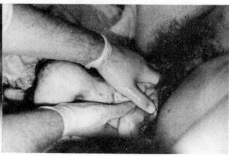

397

Delivery of the head:
1. The baby will almost always turn spontaneously so that his back is upward. Keep the baby in a belly-down position.
2. Lower the baby's body until you see the nape of the neck and the baby's hairline.
3. Put the baby's body over your forearm and put your first two fingers in the baby's mouth. Bring the baby's chin down so it rests on its neck, making the fullest flexion of the head. Put your other hand over the baby's shoulder, your first two fingers on either side of the neck. (See Fig. 97)

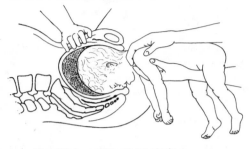

Fig. 96. Lowering the baby's body so that the occupit appears under the pubic bone.

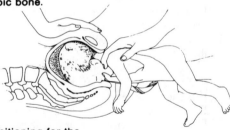

Fig. 97 . Hand positioning for the delivery of the head.

4. Have an assistant protect the mother's taint with her hand to prevent it tearing when the baby's head is pulled out. Have the mother push, and, pulling evenly with both hands, draw the head out. Lift the baby's body in an upward arc as you pull.
5. Have your assistant keep up the manual pressure on the mother's belly unless the head is moving rapidly.
6. An assistant should wipe the baby's nose and mouth as soon as they are exposed.
7. Deliver the rest of the head as slowly as possible. Use a strong, steady traction. Avoid suddenly popping the baby's head out of a tight place. Pressure on the mother's taint ("perineum") may be necessary to prevent the sudden expulsion of the head.

Stuck in Breech Position

Most breech babies will deliver spontaneously or with a minimal amount of help. If the breech delivery is to be safe, the diameter of the mother's pelvis must be wider than the diameters of the baby's head. You can be sure that the pelvis is wide enough if you attempt breech delivery only for mothers who can move the babies down pretty quickly in the second stage. Progress downward should be steady, and clearly visible with each push. The second stage should not last more than two hours or so. Sometimes, though, the baby may progress well, and then stop at some point on his way out; then you must be prepared to maneuver him out.

Stuck at the Shoulders

Bring the baby out until the bottoms of the shoulder blades are beginning to show. Rotate the body clockwise 90 degrees, while pulling. The baby's left shoulder and upper arm should appear beneath the pubic bone.

To bring out the arm, run your index and middle fingers up the baby's back, over its shoulder, down past its elbow to the forearm, and sweep it out. Turn the baby so its back is again upward. Then rotate the body counterclockwise 90 degrees so the right shoulder and arm emerge. Then you can bring out the right arm. You can rotate and counter-rotate the baby a few times if need be, as this will tend to bring the shoulders further and further out, and the arms will come down lower and lower until they can be brought out with your fingers.

Stuck at the Arms

Extended arms: Sometimes the baby's arms will be extended up alongside his head or, more rarely, one or both arms may be caught behind the head. In this case, you must free the arms in order to deliver the head.

1. Try to sweep the arms across the chest in the usual way.
2. If an arm is caught behind the head, you may need to rotate the baby's body to free the arm. Rotate the baby's body in the direction to which the hand is pointing until the arm is freed or loosened, possibly as much as 90 degrees. (Fig. 99). Be careful not to exert too much twist on the baby's neck, as this can cause injury and paralysis. The rotation should free the arm from behind the neck. Reach in and sweep down this arm, then rotate the baby back into face-down position so that you can deliver the head. If both arms are bent behind the head in this fashion, you'll need to rotate the baby in one direction to dislodge the first arm, sweep it out, and then rotate the baby in the opposite direction to dislodge the other arm, which you can then bring down. In order to find out which way the arms are hooked behind the head, you'll have to swivel the baby a little one way so you can know which one to free first. If it doesn't get you anywhere one way, try the other way, until you bring an arm down.

Your helper should be pushing on the baby's head from above all this while, keeping the head well-flexed in the best possible position for delivery.

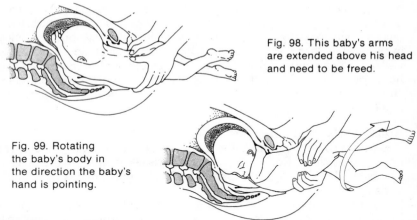

Fig. 98. This baby's arms are extended above his head and need to be freed.

Fig. 99. Rotating the baby's body in the direction the baby's hand is pointing.

Stuck at the Head

The baby's head can be held up at the pelvic rim, particularly if it is extended. If this is the case, it is best to have your assistant or the husband apply manual pressure to the mother's belly while you hold the baby straddled across your left arm (if you are right-handed) and reach the middle finger of your left hand into the baby's mouth, with your index and ring fingers on each of the baby's cheekbones. Pull downward on the head. With your right hand across the baby's shoulders, you can increase traction on the baby's head until it is born.

If you can't pull the baby's head all the way out, you should dry the baby's mouth and nose, and the birth canal adjacent, with a sterile towel; clear the airway with a suction bulb; and stimulate the baby in this position. The baby will be able to breathe even though it is still partially inside its mother. Then you can pull the baby the rest of the way out. Use a strong, steady traction. If the head cannot be delivered with a good amount of traction, forceps can be used to prevent injury to the neck or spinal cord.

Fig. 100. Delivering the head by traction and pressure on the mother's belly.

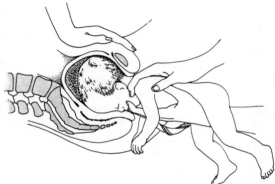

Tailbone Behind Position

This is the rarest and most difficult position in which to deliver a breech, as the head can become trapped, so prevent the baby's bottom from rotating so that his tailbone is towards the mother's back. Take hold of the baby's body with both hands and gently rotate it the way you want it to turn. You want to deliver the breech baby with the head facing downward—toward the mother's bottom.

If you do have a baby who rotates so that the back of his head rests in the hollow of his mother's tailbone, first try to turn him so his face is downward. If this fails, try to deliver his head by raising his body so that the occiput, vertex, and forehead can pass over the taint, in that order. Be careful not to overstrain the baby's neck. A large episiotomy will be necessary.

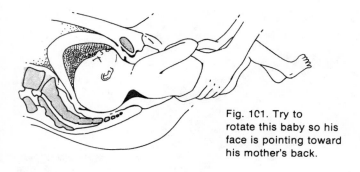

Fig. 101. Try to rotate this baby so his face is pointing toward his mother's back.

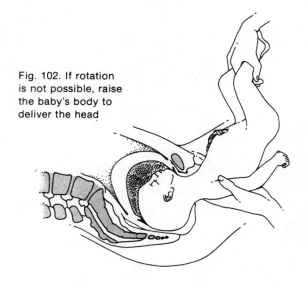

Fig. 102. If rotation is not possible, raise the baby's body to deliver the head.

401

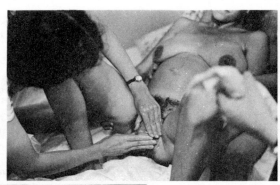

A first-time mother's breech delivery. Her son's bottom is starting to emerge.

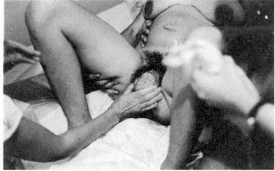

Pressure on the taint helps to prevent a tear.

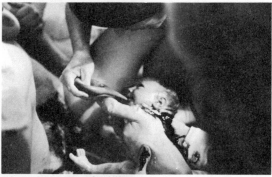

Five seconds old.

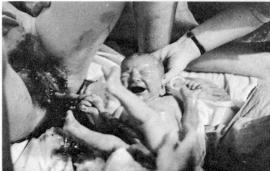

Ten seconds old. Baby's weight, 6 lbs. 9 oz.

11. Unusual Presentations and Positions

Persistent Occiput Posterior

The occiput posterior presentation, also called face up or sunnyside up, is when the baby's back is lying next to the mother's back. The baby's head presents with a slightly larger diameter than when the back of the baby's head lies toward the mother's front, so labor is usually longer and more difficult. The baby's head may be more molded than usual from passage down the birth canal.

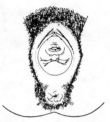

Fig. 103. Face Presentation from Below.

One obstetrics text states that occiput posterior position occurs in 15 to 30 percent of all births. Other midwifery and obstetrics texts estimate the number of persistent occiput posterior babies to be in the range of 6 to 10 percent. Our rate for 1723 births on The Farm has been under 2 percent. I can only guess about this comparatively low rate of such labors. It is certainly possible that the relative freedom of the mother to choose the position in which she felt most comfortable during the first phase of labor and to change positions frequently facilitates the rotation of the baby during the process of labor.

Face Presentation

The baby who presents face first is unusual, occuring once in about 500 deliveries. You may never see one. Face presentations occur more frequently in women whose abdominal muscles are very loose than in those with good muscle tone. A face presentation makes for a slower labor, but the baby usually can be born vaginally. The diameter of the head in this presentation is the same as that of the baby who is presenting occiput posterior. If the baby's head has not descended far into the birth canal, it may be possible to reach inside and tip the baby's head into a flexed position. Dilation of the cervix may be slower in a face presentation than in an ordinary vertex presentation; don't be surprised by this. Once the mother begins to push in an effective and coordinated way, you should see good downward progress.

Anencephalic babies are likely to present face first. In this case, delivery is not difficult, as the head will be small.

The normal face presentation baby's face will be swollen for a few hours after birth. Reassure the parents that this swelling will quickly subside. Almost always a face presenting baby will be born with the chin turned towards the mother's pubic bone. If the chin is turned towards her anus, a very unusual circumstance, delivery will be far more difficult; a cesarean will be necessary.

I have never seen a face presenting baby who suffered from breathing difficulties because of edema around the throat, but this can happen. Be prepared.

403

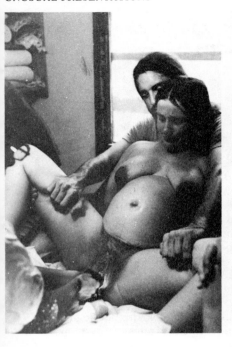
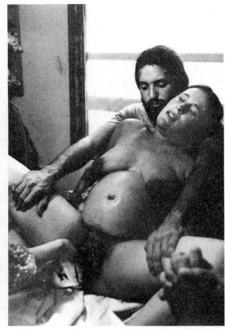
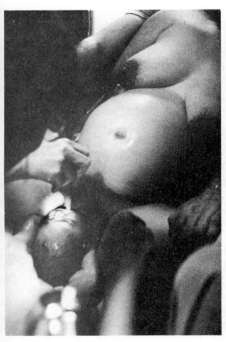
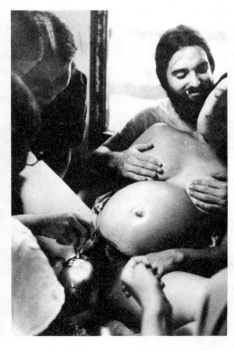

Brow Presentation

The brow presentation happens less frequently than face presentations—once in about 2,000 labors.

You can suspect a brow presentation if the head is very high and the presenting diameter unusually large. Back labor is likely, progress is likely to be slower than usual. Sometimes babies who present with their brows will have the umbilical cord wrapped several times around the neck. Some brow presentations will convert to an ordinary vertex presentation during the pushing stage.

Most texts state that vaginal brow births are possible only if the maternal pelvis is large or the baby small, or both. There is no question that a brow presentation makes for a more difficult birth than otherwise. But our series of births includes two vaginal brow births and one brow baby born by cesarean. One was a second twin, six and a half pounds, and born easily, and the second baby was a seven and a half pound baby, born in excellent condition.We helped this mother's efforts by having her stand during a few pushes. We were able to increase the size of her pelvic outlet by having an assistant stand on each side of her and push inward on the uppermost part of each of her hip bones. The effect of pushing the upper part of the hips together is to spread the hip bones slightly farther apart at the bottom.

I read about this technique, called the "pelvic press", in Nan Koehler's book, *Artemis Speaks,* and have used it in several situations in which the baby's head was slow to descend. I have seen it produce dramatic results.

Transverse Lie

Sometimes a baby will turn so he is lying sideways in the womb. Obviously the baby cannot be born while in this position. If the shoulder or arm does present, a cesarean is necessary as soon as possible.

There are several possible causes: placenta previa, multiple pregnancy, prematurity, polyhydramnios, contracted pelvis, febroid tumors, or very soft abdominal muscles.

If you discover a transverse lie in the last six weeks of pregnancy and can't turn it to a vertex or breech presentation, check with your doctor. It may not be hard to turn the transverse baby if the mother is not in labor or is in early labor, but if labor is advanced, a cesarean is likely to be necessary. (See External Version, p. 331.)

Sometimes a second twin will be transverse. If this is the case, the baby should be turned and the membranes ruptured so that the baby can be delivered quickly. (See p. 409 for diagrams of above presentations.)

12. Multiple Pregnancy and Birth

When there is more than one baby inside, it is called *multiple pregnancy*. Twins happen about once in every 90 births in the United States. Triplets occur only once in 9,000 births, and more babies at a time are much rarer.

There are two types of twins:

Identical, or monozygotic, twins result from the fertilization of one egg by one sperm. Very early in the fertilized egg's development, the cells that are starting to form the embryo divide, forming two identical embryos. Since the two babies have exactly the same genes, all their inherited characteristics will be exactly the same and they are always the same sex. These twins most often have one placenta and one chorion, but occasionally there are two of each of these. Almost always, each twin is enclosed in its own amniotic sac; monoamniotic (one sac) twins are rare.

Fraternal, or dizygotic, twins start from two eggs fertilized by two sperm. These babies may or may not be the same sex and don't necessarily look very much alike, as they have the same genetic relationship that any brother and sister do. They always have two water bags, two chorions, and two placentas, but the placentas may grow together (fuse) and look like one.

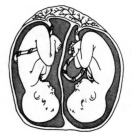 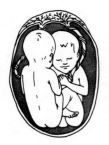 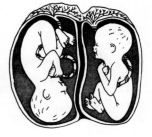

Fig. 104A.
Single Egg Twins.

Fig. 104B.
Monoamniotic
Single Egg Twins.

Fig. 104C.
Double Egg Twins.

In the United States, about 30% of twins are identical and the rest are fraternal. The incidence of fraternal twins varies greatly with various factors; the older the mother is and the more children she has had, the more likely she is to have fraternal twins. Black people have more fraternal twins than white, and Oriental people have fewer. There is evidence that fraternal twinning is influenced by heredity, probably through the mother. She would have to release two eggs at once in one cycle instead of the usual one. In contrast, all ages and all races of mothers, regardless of how many children they have had, have identical twins with the same frequency. There may be hereditary factors predisposing some people to have identical twins, but there is no strong evidence at this time to support this.

The use of fertility drugs sometimes causes the ovaries to release more than one egg at a time, so it has been responsible for more than a few sets of fraternal twins, triplets, quadruplets, and even more babies at a time in recent years.

Prenatal Care

It's good to keep alert to the possibility of twins in ladies in your care. They are common enough that it's likely you'll run into some. If you find out fairly early that a lady has twins and have her get plenty of rest, this may prevent her from going into labor prematurely, which could make it harder on the babies.

Some signs that might cause you to suspect twins are a very large belly, kicking everywhere, more pressure occurring earlier in pregnancy than usual, and an increase in weight without swelling or fat. Even more indicative would be if you could feel three or four large parts or hear two distinct fetal heart tones (though this is tricky to tell and you can't positively affirm or deny the presence of twins by hearing or not hearing two FHTs). Even with excellent prenatal care, and especially when they are premature, twins are often not diagnosed until after the birth of the first baby.

A pregnant lady with twins is more likely to become anemic than a lady with one baby. She is building blood supplies for two babies, and of course that takes more iron. Toxemia and polyhydramnios are more common than usual in twin pregnancies, so watch carefully. Weight gain of course can and should be more than usual.

The most common complication associated with twins is prematurity. Much before term the uterus gets as full as it would be at term with one baby, and this tends to bring labor on. This frequently is started by premature water bag rupture. Lots of rest in the last three months minimizes the chance of prematurity. Even with rest, they are likely to be two or three weeks early. If you are pretty sure of the length of gestation and they seem to be big enough, this is fine. After 30 weeks, twin babies are likely to be smaller than single babies of the same gestational age, but they tend to do as well.

Where To Deliver

When you know in advance that a lady is going to have twins, you can decide whether to deliver them yourself or do it in a hospital by how well set up you are and by how premature the babies are if labor starts early. There is a 50-50 chance of at least one of them being breech or (much less likely) transverse, so this is a strong consideration. In all probability everything will go very smoothly, but it is a fairly high-risk situation and you need to be well prepared. Because of all the possible complications, it would be advisable to at least have a doctor in attendance.

Presentation

It's helpful to know in advance the presentatations of the babies. You may or may not be able to determine this by touch. The most common combinations of presentations are the easiest ones to deliver. Both babies are head first in about half the deliveries. There are six possible combinations of presentations.

Fig. 105. Possible Twin Presentations in Order of Occurrence.

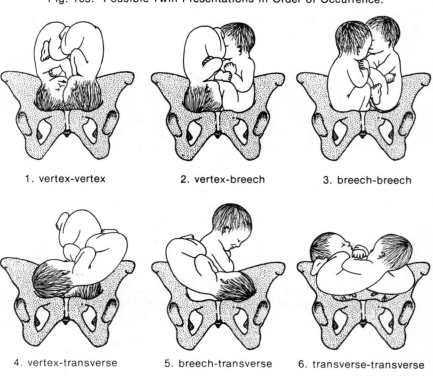

1. vertex-vertex   2. vertex-breech   3. breech-breech

4. vertex-transverse   5. breech-transverse   6. transverse-transverse

Management of Labor and Delivery

Labor is conducted the same as a single labor until after the delivery of the first baby. As soon as this baby is born, clamp the cord to prevent possible bleeding from the second twin through the umbilical cord.

It's best for the second twin to come out within 15 minutes or so after the first. Second twin babies tend to have more trouble in the perinatal period than first ones, and the likelihood of trouble for the second baby gets higher the longer time after this that he stays inside. If the babies share a single placenta, it may separate after the birth of the first one, and this would endanger the second twin. It is possible but rare for two healthy babies to be delivered hours and even days apart.

When the first twin is delivered, check inside the mother to find out what part of the second baby is presenting and how far it has descended. If the baby is in a transverse position, try to turn it into a breech or vertex externally. If the head or butt is down far enough so that the cord won't prolapse, you can break the water bag.

It will take less time to push out this baby, as the cervix is well dilated and the mother's bones are already stretched apart as far as they need to be. Check the FHT often. Keep track of how much time has passed, but go by how the energy feels. If the time lapsed is feeling like too much, you may need to pull the second twin out by "internal podalic version," which means taking hold of the baby's feet and turning the baby's body so that the feet come out first, pulling the baby slowly out, and delivering as for a breech. Wear a long sterile glove.

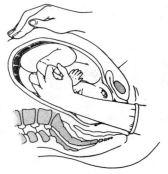

Fig. 106A. Grasp the Feet.

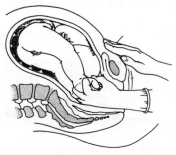

Fig. 106B. While pulling down on the baby's feet, push upward on his head.

This maneuver should not be done routinely; it should be used only if the spontaneous delivery of the second twin does not happen within 20 minutes or if there is fetal distress.

The placenta or placentas will deliver after both babies are born. Since it or they cover more of the inner surface of the uterus than a placenta of a single baby, there is more possibility of problems with its separation. (This also makes for a higher than usual incidence of placenta previa and low implantation in twin pregnancies.) Postpartum hemorrhage is also more common than usual in twin births, because of lack of tone in the uterus caused by its being stretched so much.

Some Possible Complications

Monoamniotic twins

This is when there is only one water bag, and it's rare. It happens only with identical twins, and can be hard on the babies. Fetal death because of cord accidents happens more often than usual, because the two babies and two cords can easily get tangled. If after the first baby is born there is no second water bag, you need to get the second baby out right away or he is fairly likely to asphyxiate.

Conjoined twins

These are always monozygotic and are the result of incomplete splitting of the embryo in two. They are very rare, and can be joined in several ways. They may cause protracted labor, and a cesarean is likely to be necessary.

Locked twins

These are another possible cause of non-progressing labor. There are several ways the babies can be jammed together so that neither of them can get out. All of them are very rare. It may be possible to reach in and push them apart with a finger or hand, or a c-section may be necessary

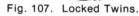

Fig. 107. Locked Twins.

After the Babies Are Born

A lady with twins needs lots of help. Part of your responsibility as a midwife may be to round up some help for her so that she doesn't become exhausted in the months following the births.

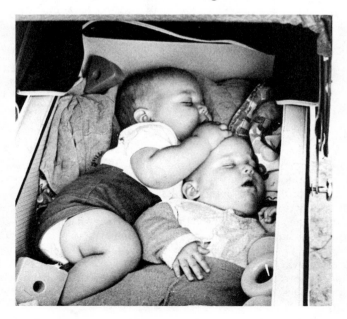

13. Complications of Pregnancy

Miscarriage or Spontaneous Abortion

These terms cover the non-induced expulsion of the contents of the uterus at any time before the twenty-eighth week of pregnancy, when the baby is considered to have some chance of making it. (A few babies born earlier do live.) Miscarriages are most common in the earliest part of pregnancy and are less likely as pregnancy progresses. In fact, it's not uncommon for a lady to miscarry so early that she never knew she was pregnant.

Some causes of miscarriage
- Defective egg or sperm
- Unfavorable implantation site
- Failure of the cells forming the embryo to divide and differentiate properly
- Failure of the corpus luteum to produce its hormones
- Failure of the placenta to function, either in nourishing the baby or producing its hormones
- Infections the mother may have—high blood pressure, hyper- or hypo-thyroidism, some vitamin deficiencies, malnutrition, diabetes, and others
- Uterine defects, such as a double uterus, scar tissue, or a tumor
- Incompetent cervix: This is a cervix that will not stay closed once the baby is putting a certain amount of pressure on it. It opens, usually in the second trimester, and the baby, who is often too immature to survive, is born. It can be a cause of repeated late miscarriages or premature deliveries. Incompetent cervix can be caused by trauma to the cervix from previous birthings or surgery, or it can (rarely) be congenital. A doctor can sew up the cervix of a lady who has this condition so she can keep the baby in. This is usually done between the fourteenth and eighteenth weeks of pregnancy. When it's time for the baby to be born he will undo it and the baby can be born.
- Exposure to toxic chemicals in the environment

Stages of miscarriage
Miscarriages are described in three stages: *threatened, inevitable,* and *complete.*

A *threatened* miscarriage is when any bloody discharge happens in the first twenty weeks of pregnancy. It may be accompanied by menstrual-like cramps or backache. Two out of every ten pregnant women will have some spotting or bleeding in the early months, but

411

only one of them will have a miscarriage. So if someone's spotting it doesn't mean she will lose the baby. We always consider any spotting or bleeding to be a threatened miscarriage, and have the mother take it easy and not make love until she's good and done with any spotting.

This miscarriage is *inevitable* when there is a fair amount of bleeding with clots, and cramps that may come and go rhythmically, and the cervix is dilating. It is *complete* when the baby and the placenta both come out, leaving the uterus empty.

The baby and placenta are usually passed together before ten or twelve weeks, and separately after that. Miscarriages that happen between the twelfth and twentieth weeks tend to be *incomplete,* which means there's some placenta or membrane still up inside. If bleeding or cramping is severe or if a fair amount of bleeding persists longer than a few days, especially after the twelfth week of pregnancy, the lady should see a doctor. She may need to have her uterus cleaned out with a D & C (dilatation and curettage). See p. 59, Mary's story.

A lady who has miscarried needs your continued care and support after the miscarriage in the same way that a lady who has just given birth does. The hormonal changes that her body is going through are much the same as if she had had a full-term pregnancy and lost the child, so she is likely to need help in making the transition to no longer being pregnant.

Missed abortion

When the baby is kept inside for two or more months after it has died, this is called a missed abortion. Sometimes the lady has bled or spotted and cramped and then stopped, but sometimes she hasn't had any signs of miscarriage. The uterus stops growing and may actually get smaller; changes in the breasts and other signs of pregnancy stop. There may be a brownish discharge, but there is still no period. Usually a missed abortion will end up with the baby coming out spontaneously. If a lady in your care seems to have one, consult with your doctor.

Habitual abortion

When a lady has three or more consecutive miscarriages, it is called habitual abortion. They can be caused by anything that can cause one miscarriage, especially when the cause is a chronic condition. It is not uncommon for a lady who has had several miscarriages for no apparent reason to finally carry a pregnancy to term.

A lady who has had a couple of miscarriages in a row should take it fairly easy when she gets pregnant again. If her miscarriages were in close succession, she should wait a while to get pregnant again, getting her general health back and getting her hematocrit back up, as she is likely to be anemic after starting and losing several pregnancies. She should have peace of mind and stability.

I knew a lady who had eight miscarriages before she gave birth to a full-term baby. She just kept trying. — Ina May

Ectopic Pregnancy

An ectopic pregnancy is a fertilized egg that is growing outside of the uterus; in the fallopian tubes (this is most common—90% of all cases), on the ovary, in the abdomen, or (very rarely) in the cervix. Ectopic pregnancy occurs about once in every 200-300 pregnancies.

It is often caused by some condition of the fallopian tube that prevents the egg from completing its trip to the uterus. This can be because of an unusually long and twisty tube, any condition (such as an inflammation) which changes the delicate chemical balance there, or by an obstruction such as scar tissue. The inflammation from a pelvic infection can result in scar tissue which may affect the tube; ectopic pregnancy may follow such an infection. In most cases the tube will rupture when the pregnancy grows too large for it, and this is when ectopic pregnancy is usually first suspected.

Be alert to the possibility of ectopic pregnancy with pain and vaginal bleeding usually starting by the eighth week of pregnancy. The symptoms are sharp lower abdominal pain, which may radiate into the neck and shoulder if there is bleeding into the abdomen, and vaginal bleeding, which is usually scanty and dark brown but can be profuse. The bleeding can be either continuous or intermittent. Rupture of the tubal pregnancy can cause dizziness, fainting, and shock. It can be confused with appendicitis, infection in the tubes, a miscarriage, or a ruptured or twisted ovarian cyst.

If a lady has some of these symptoms, you should be in touch with your doctor. A ruptured tubal pregnancy can be a life-threatening condition, and if you suspect that a lady has one, immediate medical care is necessary. Treatment is generally removal of the tube.

Abdominal pregnancy

Rarely, a fertilized egg which gets into the abdominal cavity will be able to survive and keep growing. Much more rarely, such an extrauterine pregnancy will result in a live baby which is mature enough to make it. In such a pregnancy, the mother would tend to have more discomfort than usual. The baby's movements are easily felt and can even be painful to her. If she has had other babies she is likely to say that this pregnancy feels different. On examination, the baby's outlines are easy to feel and the baby is often in a breech or transverse position. The FHT may be louder than usual. There are no Braxton-Hicks contractions. Since regular delivery is of course impossible (though false labor can happen), the baby must be delivered by abdominal surgery.

413

Hyperemesis Gravidarum, or Excessive Vomiting of Pregnancy

Hyperemesis gravidarum is excessive and hard-to-control vomiting in pregnancy, and is to be distinguished from the normal, mild and temporary vomiting of pregnancy, usually called morning sickness. The dangers in persistent vomiting are that the fluid and mineral balances in the mother's body can be messed up, and dehydration and even malnutrition can result. In the USA, one pregnancy in 2,000 requires hospitalization for vomiting, and this incidence is decreasing.

Loving help should be given the mother with any aspect of her life which makes her unhappy, whether it be her reluctance to have a child, her sex life, her fear of labor, or whatever. Encourage her to increase her activity, rather than laying around, and to do things that will get her attention outside of herself. If you can counsel a lady and give her *real* help, you can stop a condition which, left to itself, could require hospitalization.

Dehydration can occur after even a day or two of persistent vomiting, so you need to watch for this and notify your doctor in case he wants to hospitalize the lady. If a lady has become malnourished as a result of too much vomiting, the malnutrition needs to be corrected, and your friendly doctor should be consulted. Also, it is important to remember that there can be underlying physical causes for severe vomiting of pregnancy, and you must make certain not to assume that all of vomiting of pregnancy is psychically based.

Hydatidiform Mole

A hydatidiform mole is a kind of degeneration of the chorion. Exactly how it happens is uncertain. The villi enlarge into many little translucent cysts which contain a clear fluid. Their size varies from about 1 millimeter to 1 centimeter in diameter—the larger ones look something like grapes. As the mole grows, the embryo is absorbed in it. The moles grow at varying rates, and in many cases, the uterus grows more rapidly than in a normal pregnancy.

Hydatidiform mole is uncommon in the United States (about 1 in 2,000 pregnancies), and is known to be more common (1 in 150-500) in several Eastern countries and Mexico. It is also more common among older pregnant ladies, especially those over 45.

Signs and symptoms are vaginal bleeding, usually beginning by the twelfth week (occasionally a few of the little vesicles are also passed), nausea and vomiting more than with ordinary morning sickness, sometimes pain or discomfort, and the uterus being larger than expected. Toxemia is common and may start in the second trimester, earlier than with a normal pregnancy. There is of course absence of fetal movement and heartbeat. It must be distinguished from twins and polyhydramnios, either of which can make the fetal heartbeat hard to hear, and a tumor with or without the presence of a fetus.

With hydatidiform mole, chorionic gonadotrophin continues to be secreted as long as the mole is there, where in normal pregnancy the amount decreases after ten weeks. A test can be done for the presence of this hormone in the blood and the urine. Hydatidiform mole can also be diagnosed after 3 months by X-ray or ultrasound. However, it is not usually diagnosed until it is expelled spontaneously, which almost always happens by the seventh month. If the mole is diagnosed before it comes out, it is often because of threatened miscarriage, which is then allowed to proceed or can be helped along with pitocin in some cases. If the mole does not come out spontaneously, a doctor can remove it vaginally or if necessary, surgically. Both before and after the mole comes out, hemorrhage and infection are fairly common, so removal is done very cautiously.

A small percentage of. ladies develop tumors, some malignant, with or following hydatidiform mole, so very thorough follow-up care is necessary. The malignant tumors are virtually 100% curable with chemotherapy if they are found early.

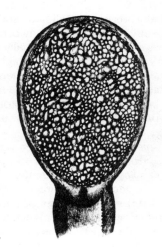

Fig. 108.
Hydatidiform Mole.

TOXEMIA

Toxemia, or pre-eclampsia, is the name given a group of symptoms that forms one of the most common and serious complications of pregnancy. Most doctors don't really know what causes it; there are many theories. Signs of toxemia include generalized swelling, protein in the urine, high blood pressure, hyper-sensitive reflexes and sudden and excessive weight gain. The results we have had with the 1723 pregnancies under our care tend to support Dr. Tom Brewer's contention that toxemia is a disease of malnutrition, especially when the mother's diet is very low in protein. Seven cases out of more than 1700 pregnancies is a very low rate of toxemia by anyone's estimation.

415

While Brewer advocates that pregnant women eat plenty of meat, fish, eggs and dairy products to prevent toxemia, it would appear from the very low rate of toxemia among the women of The Farm, all of whom were complete vegetarians during the period of their childbearing, that a diet heavily based in soy protein works just as well as one based in animal protein for the prevention of toxemia.* Only one woman among all The Farm residents who gave birth under our care had toxemic symptoms in her pregnancies (which numbered four), and she appeared to have some other factor affecting her pregnancies. The placenta of each of her pregnancies was about half the normal size, even when she was eating as much protein as she could, as well as a well-balanced diet in all other respects, and she led an otherwise healthy lifestyle. All her babies had low birth weights and quickly began to flourish once breastfeeding was established.

Toxemia is more common in first pregnancies, in adolescent mothers, multiple pregnancies, mothers with diabetes, polyhydramnios, and a history of high blood pressure. It usually starts in the last six weeks but can start as early as 24 weeks. It usually improves dramatically as soon as the baby is born, and all signs and symptoms clear up within a few days.

Toxemia is divided into two types:

Pre-eclampsia—This usually starts in a mild form and may progress. In its mild form it consists of high blood pressure with edema (swelling) and protein in the urine. Severe pre-eclampsia can cause symptoms related to the high blood pressure and to swelling of the brain, retina, and other tissues. These symptoms include severe persistent headache, nervous irritability, dizziness, visual disturbance, nausea, and pain in the upper abdomen.

It is very important to screen very carefully for toxemia throughout pregnancy. Routine check of blood pressure, weight, edema and urine will bring any cases to your attention. Nutritional counseling throughout pregnancy is your best means of prevention of toxemia.

Eclampsia—Pre-eclampsia may or may not develop into eclampsia. It rarely does and its incidence is decreasing. Eclampsia comes on suddenly, and consists of convulsions and coma. The mother may die from heart failure, edema in her lungs, or shock. Maternal mortality in eclampsia is about 10%. Eclampsia is almost wholly preventable through thorough prenatal care.

Toxemia affects the baby in that the placenta doesn't function as well as normal, which may cause a small-for-dates baby or fetal death. Since labor must be induced early in some cases, prematurity is another danger to the baby. There is a higher incidence of abruptio placenta than usual with toxemia, which is dangerous both to mother and baby.

---

* See "Pre-eclampsia and Reproductive Performance in a Community of Vegans." J.P. Carter, MD, Tami Furman, MS, & R. Hutcheson, MD, **Southern Medical Journal**, Vol. 80, No. 6, June 1987).

Third Trimester Bleeding

Third trimester bleeding can have a variety of causes, some placental and some nonplacental. Nonplacental bleeding can be caused by such things as blood disorders, cervical or vaginal infection, polyps, or cancer of the cervix. Placental bleeding is by far the most often seen, and is caused by two of the most common and most serious complications of late pregnancy, placenta previa (the placenta presenting) and abruptio placenta (premature separation of the placenta).

If a lady in your care is having any bleeding in the third trimester, check it with your doctor. In 90% of such cases, bleeding will quit at least temporarily with 24 hours of bed rest. But the bleeding may not stop, or it may start again later, and it's good to already have your doctor in on it. *Don't ever do a vaginal or rectal exam on a lady with third trimester bleeding, because if the placenta is presenting, the examination can cause a major hemorrhage.*

Placenta previa is a placenta that is set low in the uterus. A *complete* placenta previa completely covers the cervix, a *partial* one partially covers it, and a *marginal* placenta previa comes close to the cervix.

Placenta previa occurs once in about 200 deliveries. It is more common in ladies who are older and in ladies who have already had babies. Its only symptom is painless vaginal bleeding, which usually starts after the 28th week of pregnancy. This happens when the lower part of the uterus stretches and the placenta can't stretch with it, so it separates a little and bleeds. Bleeding may not start until labor starts; then the cervix dilates and opens but the placenta doesn't move. The bleeding is usually not excessive and may come in small gushes of dark blood and clots. It will usually stop, then start again later. The first time the bleeding starts, it is usually not serious, but it can be heavier when it recurs.

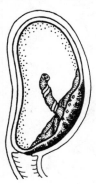

Complete placenta previa requires c-section. Partial or marginal placenta previa may not be discovered until labor. During labor the head may compress the placenta against the lower uterus and cervix enough to prevent all but a little bleeding. When this is the case, regular delivery is possible.

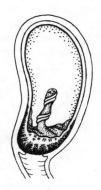

Fig. 109A. Partial Placenta Previa.

Fig. 109B. Complete Placenta Previa.

Placenta previa can be diagnosed by ultrasound. It can also be diagnosed by vaginal examination. However, putting a finger into the cervix of a lady with placenta previa can open up a major blood vessel and cause profuse bleeding. So this examination shouldn't be done except in an operating room with everything ready for blood transfusion and c-section. If the mother's condition permits, which it usually does, such examination should wait at least until the baby is mature enough to make it.

Abruptio placenta is separation of the placenta from the uterine wall before the baby is born. It is about as common as placenta previa. It usually happens after 28 weeks and is more common in ladies who have had several babies. It can be caused by toxemia, high blood pressure, a short cord, or injury to the mother, but usually no cause is apparent.

Wherever the placenta separates, it bleeds. The bleeding can be concealed, with all the blood contained inside the uterus and unable to escape; apparent, with all the blood escaping; or partially concealed. Concealed bleeding is painful because the blood creates pressure in the uterus. Abruptio placenta is characterized by varying amounts of pain which may be constant or severe, tenderness in the belly, a hard belly, and shock even without vaginal bleeding. Fetal distress may start, with the FHT first increasing, then dropping, and vigorous baby activity from hypoxia, as the placenta supplies the baby with less and less oxygen.

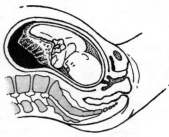

This is a dangerous complication for the mother because of blood loss, and it is particularly hard on the baby, who is in danger of death from asphyxia. So it is of greatest importance to recognize concealed bleeding early and get the mother to the hospital immediately. She may need a c-section to save the baby, and might lose enough blood to need a transfusion, and she might need treatment for a blood clotting defect which is an occasional complication of abruptio placenta.

Fig. 110A. Concealed Abruptio Placenta.

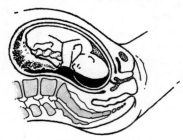

Fig. 110B. Partially Concealed Abruptio Placenta.

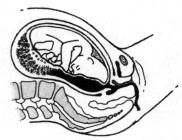

Fig. 110C. Apparent Abruptio Placenta.

418

Polyhydramnios

Polyhydramnios means too much amniotic fluid. There is usually about a liter (a little more than a quart) of amniotic fluid—over about two liters is considered polyhydramnios. Its cause is not known for sure, but it is often associated with twins, diabetes, toxemia, and other problems of either the mother or the baby. Over 20% of the cases are associated with congenital malformations of the baby, especially of the nervous system and the gastrointestinal tract. Normally, the baby swallows the amniotic fluid and this is thought to be one of the ways the amount of it is controlled. There is almost always polyhydramnios when the baby can't swallow it for some reason, such as intestinal obstruction. In babies with anencephalus and spina bifida, there are theories that it is caused by cerebrospinal fluid leaking from the exposed meninges into the amniotic sac.

You would probably recognize polyhydramnios on the basis of having seen a lot of bellies and felt a lot of babies. The uterus may seem larger and more tense than usual, which makes it harder to feel the fetal parts and hear the fetal heartbeat. You will need to check the lady's pee and blood pressure carefully, as this condition is more common with diabetes and toxemia. Minor degrees of polyhydramnios (up to 3 liters of fluid) are fairly common. If there is more fluid than that, or if the mother is having an unreasonable amount of discomfort, she should see a doctor. He may recommend X-rays or ultrasound to check for sure on what's happening in there.

During pregnancy, polyhydramnios can cause more edema of the legs and vulva, difficulty breathing and difficulty sleeping, indigestion, heartburn, and constipation. Polyhydramnios has several possible effects on labor. The cord is more likely to prolapse. Premature labor can happen because of the overstretched uterus. Difficult presentations are more common because the baby can float around more. Because of the uterine muscles being so stretched out, and because the amount of water can keep the baby's head "floating," instead of bearing down on the cervix, labor may be slower than usual. There may be postpartum hemorrhage because of the overstretched uterus.

Both the problems that cause polyhydramnios and the problems that result from it contribute to the relatively high perinatal mortality rate which is associated with it, and which gets higher as the amount of fluid increases. Because of this a lady with severe polyhydramnios should be considered a high risk pregnancy and should not be delivered at home.

Fetal Death

Sometimes the baby dies in the uterus. This can happen for a number of reasons, such as placental insufficiency or accidents with the cord. If this happens to a lady in your care, consult with your doctor to confirm your diagnosis and for advice on the delivery, as the mother runs a greater risk of infection, and labor sometimes is not so effective because of deterioration and softening of the baby. This mother needs your special love and attention. The best way to tell the parents is to be as simple and direct as you can. Hold on to the mother if that is all right with her. There's not much you can say to comfort parents who have just lost their baby, other than to let them know that time will eventually heal the rawness of the hurt. Feeling their grief with them is a non-conceptual way you can help share their load.

Diagnostic Tests

There are several diagnostic tests which have become nearly routine for prenatal care in the United States as provided by the medical profession. Amniocentesis, chorionic villi sampling and alphafetoprotein screening are considered part of the standard prenatal packet in many areas of the country. All three of these tests are appropriate only for women who could choose to abort a fetus at risk for Down's syndrome or other chromosomal abnormalities, anencephalic babies, and those with microcephaly, hydrocephaly, and spinal bifida. None of the above tests is 100 percent accurate, and the risks of chorionic villi sampling are not yet fully known. A significant drawback to alfafetoprotein screening is its 20 percent false positive rate. A normal maternal reading is no guarantee against having a baby with an open neural tube defect (as in anencephally, hydrocephaly, spinal bifida and microcephaly), as 10 percent of affected fetuses are missed.

Amniocentesis is a procedure in which a needle is passed through the abdominal wall into the uterus and amniotic cavity to pull out amniotic fluid for study. Amniocentesis is usually performed between fourteen and sixteen weeks of pregnancy. It is more accurate than alfafetoprotein testing, but it is considerably more expensive and risky to the fetus. In about one tenth of cases, the procedure needs to be repeated. Both minor and major complications have been reported. Uterine cramping, vaginal bleeding, leaking of amniotic fluid and pricking of the fetus occur in about one percent of the tests. Major complications include permanent injury to the fetus, maternal bleeding at birth, and miscarriage (in about a quarter of a percent of cases). There are emotional drawbacks to the procedure of amniocentesis, in my opinion. The waiting period for results of amniocentesis can be a very difficult time for couples; they often find they must deal with contradictory emotions when they don't know whether or not they will decide to continue the pregnancy. No one who received care at The Farm Midwifery Center opted to undergo prenatal diagnostic testing.

There are a few other nonroutine tests that may be done in pregnancy when there appears to be a particular risk. One in every thirty Jews of eastern European descent is a carrier of Tay-Sachs disease, so a random marriage of any two individuals from this ethnic group has a one in nine hundred chance of bringing together two carriers. If the parents are of Mediterranean descent, the fetus is at risk for thalassemia (or Cooley's anemia). One out of ten African-American parents carries the gene for sickle-cell anemia. Any of the parents in the above groups who have previously given birth to an affected infant will surely be concerned about possible recurrence and should be referred to genetic counseling.

14. Diseases That May Complicate Pregnancy

A pregnant woman has as much chance as anybody to get a number of diseases, some of which may have an effect on her pregnancy.

Infectious and Parasitic Diseases

AIDS and HIV Infection

AIDS, which is an acronym for acquired immunodeficiency syndrome, is a late manifestation of infection with human immunodeficiency virus (HIV). This disease came to the attention of the medical community in 1981, when small groups of individuals began showing up with a host of opportunistic infections that were severe and often fatal. These people died of different infections; what was common to them was the inability of their immune systems to fight the opportunistic infections. Medical researchers following these leads were able to isolate the human immunodeficiency virus.

Most people infected with the AIDS virus have no symptoms for long periods. It usually takes three months after infection for detectable antibodies to develop in the blood. A confirmed positive antibody test means that a person has the HIV infection and can transmit the virus to others. The time between infection with HIV and development of AIDS ranges from a few months to ten years.

AIDS is chiefly transmitted through intimate sexual contact or through the use of needles contaminated with the virus among intravenous drug users. The only way to prevent AIDS is to prevent the initial infection with HIV. When it comes to sexual transmission, there are only two ways to make sure that the virus is not passed; sexual abstinence or choosing only partners who are not infected with the virus. Since many HIV-infected people have no symptoms and are unaware they are infected, it is difficult to identify them without an antibody test. Because of this, knowledge of antibody status is desirable before a sexual relationship is initiated, and even this may be difficult to obtain. Even with antibody tests, it is important to know that these tests cannot detect infections that have occurred in the several weeks before the test. People need to be counseled that when they initiate a sexual relationship, they should use sexual practices that reduce the risk of HIV transmission. Women who have sex with an infected partner have more risk of acquiring the infection from anal intercourse than from vaginal intercourse. The relative risk of oral-genital contact is probably a little lower than the risk of transmission by vaginal intercourse. Other sexually transmitted diseases or trauma to the mucus lining of the vagina or mouth probably increase the risk of HIV transmission. The correct use of condoms further reduces the risk of HIV transmission.

Midwives, like other health care professionals who come into contact with bodily fluids in the course of their work, should take precautions to reduce the risk of acquiring HIV infection from an infected client. Thorough handwashing is still the most important method of preventing transmission of disease. Gloves must be worn during activities in which body fluids will be encountered, such as starting IV's, drawing blood from the umbilical cord or vein, vaginal exams, handling the placenta or cord, handling soiled linens, pads or dressings, changing diapers, specimen collection, and handling the baby prior to the first bath. Care should be taken to protect eyes, nose and mouth from splashing or spattering with blood or amniotic fluid. Protective eyewear and a mask are options here. Gowns or clothing splashed with body fluids should be changed immediately. Decontamination of surfaces and any devices or instruments that enter the vascular system or otherwise come into contact with body fluids can be done with soap and water, followed by household bleach solution (one part bleach to ten parts water).

Unfortunately, babies born to women with HIV infection may also be infected with HIV. The risk for this transmission is estimated at 30 to 40 percent. Sometimes a mother who has passed the infection on to her baby is still asymptomatic. Babies born with HIV infections are not usually recognized at birth, as they are still asymptomatic. The infection may not become evident until the child is between a year and a year and a half of age. All pregnant women with a history of sexually transmitted diseases or intravenous drug use should be steered toward HIV counseling and testing.

Gonorrhea

Gonorrhea can be treated effectively but it is often unsuspected or undiagnosed. The culture for gonococcus is a fairly simple lab test. You may want some or all of your pregnant women to have this test, depending upon the population you serve. Treatment of gonorrhea in the United States is influenced by the following factors: a) the spread of new antibiotic-resistant strains of the disease; b) the high frequency of chlamydial infections in women with gonorrhea; c) recognition of the serious complications of chlamydial infections and gonorrhea; and d) the absence of a fast, cheap, and accurate test for chlamydia. Nearly half of women infected with gonorrhea in some populations are now infected with chlamydia as well.

Pregnant women should be cultured for gonorrhea and tested for syphilis at the first prenatal visit. Those who are at high risk for sexually transmitted disease should have a second culture for gonorrhea, as well as a test for chlamydia and syphilis, last in the third trimester.

Untreated gonorrhea in the mother may result in infection in the baby's eyes. Topical antibiotics alone are insufficient to treat such an infection. A prophylactic agent is recommended to be put in the eyes of all newborn babies to prevent gonococcal infection of the eyes of the newborn. You may use erythromycin (0.5%) ophthalmic ointment once or silver nitrate (1%) aqueous once. We prefer the erythromycin ointment to the silver nitrate, because the latter frequently irritates the baby's eyes. This prophylaxis should be done within an hour after birth.

Chlamydia

Chlamydia is now the most prevalent sexually transmitted disease in the United States. Nearly five million new cases were estimated to have occurred in the United States in 1986. Chlamydia is particularly widespread among sexually active adolescent girls; the more sexual partners the woman has had, the higher the risk. The problem with the disease at the time of this writing

422

is that testing is not universally available, accurate or affordable. Babies born to infected women may develop pneumonia.

Cytomegalovirus

Cytomegalovirus (CMV) is a common infection that occurs in pregnant women. It is passed by close contact between humans, as in kissing or sexual intercourse. The virus can be found in urine, saliva, breast milk, semen, and cervical mucus. About half of all pregnant women in the United States have antibodies to CMV. An actively infected adult has very mild symptoms, or, often, none at all. From 0.5 to 2 percent of all babies of women infected with the virus are affected while still in the womb; most of these babies are only mildly affected. It does seem that the risk of severe congenital disease (deafness, visual problems and mental retardation) is highest when primary CMV infection is present. Between 5 and 10 percent of babies are infected with CMV during the weeks following birth. It is not known if these infections cause permanent damage. Recurrent CMV may also cause severe congenital infection. There is no accepted routine therapy for either maternal or neonatal infection.

We had dealt with one congenital CMV infection in a baby. Our infant was full-term but weighed only five and a half pounds. His mother noticed that he was not a very active baby during the pregnancy. He required two weeks of hospitalization and a few transfusions of platelets. I'm sure that his mother's determination to breastfeed him hastened his recovery.

Infectious Hepatitis

There are several types of infectious hepatitis to consider during pregnancy: hepatitis non-A and non-B, viral hepatitis A and viral hepatitis B. The first two types are diagnosed by excluding the second two. Viral hepatitis A is transmitted through contaminated feces. Viral hepatitis B is transmitted through blood, blood by-products, vaginal secretions, semen and saliva. Mothers infected with viral hepatitis B can transfer the virus to their babies at the time of delivery. Infectious viral hepatitis may be detected through history, physical examination and lab tests. Infected people often show lack of appetite, nausea, vomiting, fatigue, jaundice, a full feeling in the abdomen, and a sudden dislike for cigarettes and coffee. Infectious hepatitis may trigger premature labor. Infected women may need hospitalization for intravenous feeding.

Herpes

Genital herpes is a common venereal disease in the United States. No known cure exists, and the disease may be chronic and recurring. Treatment with the drug acyclovir may accelerate healing, but it does not wipe out the infection or affect the frequency, severity or risk of future attacks. Recurrences are usually brought on by physical or emotional stress. Painful sores develop on the cervix and inside the vagina; after the first attack, there may be sores on the thighs or butt. Sores may be active for several days, which then subside until a recurrence.

The risk of transmission of genital herpes to the baby is highest among women with their first herpes outbreak near the time of delivery. The risk is not so high among women with recurrent herpes. Babies who contract the herpes virus during birth may die or suffer central nervous system or eye damage.

Consistent emotional and physical support during pregnancy may prevent recurrent attacks in the mother. I have had good results with using echinacea drops applied directly to areas where lesions threaten to erupt.

A woman who has active lesions in her vagina at the time of labor should have her baby by cesarean. If the lesions are on the thighs, bottom or anal area, safe, vaginal delivery may be possible. Women with a history of herpes should have cultures of the birth canal each week from the 35th week of pregnancy. A vaginal exam, using a sterile speculum, should be done at the onset of labor or if the membranes rupture early, to rule out the presence of lesions.

Syphilis

Pregnant women should be screened early in pregnancy for syphilis. There are some populations and areas in the United States in which there has been a resurgence of syphilis in recent years. In some areas, screening should be repeated in the third trimester. Medical treatment is necessary to avoid spontaneous abortion, stillbirth, and damage to internal organs. Syphilis damages the baby mostly in the third trimester because it doesn't cross the placenta until then. Congenital syphilis in the newborn often has no visible symptoms at first; sometimes the baby develops a rash at the age of a month or so. It can be treated effectively if it is discovered, but if it is not treated by about a year of age, permanent bone damage can result.

Toxoplasmosis

Toxoplasmosis is an infection caused by a parasite. It causes severe congenital malformations and may result in the death of the fetus or in prematurity. The disease is contracted by eating infected meat that hasn't been cooked long enough, or by contact with cat droppings. Prevention involves cooking all meat well, and having someone else clean the cat box.

Rubella

Rubella, or German measles, in the pregnant woman is known to affect approximately 20 percent of babies involved. The risk is even higher during the first month of pregnancy. Common malformations from infection with this virus are heart defects, deafness, and cataracts. Many of the babies will have low birth weights, and some may be retarded.

Any woman of childbearing age who has never had rubella and is definitely not pregnant, and who will not be pregnant for a couple of months, can be immunized against rubella. Immunization will protect her future babies from any complication with congenital rubella. An antibody titre can establish present or past rubella.

Severe Anemia

A mild degree of anemia is common and even normal in pregnancy. This is discussed on p. 318. However, there are several different kinds of anemia, and you may find it necessary to find out what you are dealing with in a difficult case. This would be one where the mother's hematocrit is less than 32 or 33 and her health seems impaired.

Iron Deficiency Anemia

Iron deficiency anemia, which accounts for about 95% of the cases of anemia in pregnancy, may continue although the lady is taking iron pills. If she has difficulty absorbing the iron in that form, she can try time-release capsules, which are easier on the stomach, and try taking the pills along with vitamin C, which aids in the absorption of iron. If this doesn't help, your doctor may try injectable iron. If the anemia is still a problem, you should check further the possibility of another form of anemia.

Megaloblastic Anemia

This can cause tiredness, lack of appetite, nausea, and sometimes vomiting and diarrhea. It can be caused by deficiency of either vitamin B-12 or folic acid. Vitamin B-12 deficiency anemia takes a long time to develop and is rarely found in pregnant ladies. It can be caused by a vegetarian diet that does not supplement this vitamin. Folic acid deficiency anemia occasionally develops in pregnancy. It is usually caused by malnutrition, which can result from poor eating habits, alcoholism, or excessive vomiting. It is cured by taking extra folic acid. It's good to be sure the lady is getting enough vitamin B-12 also, because if she does have a B-12 deficiency, taking folic acid alone can mask the symptoms but the deficiency may cause nerve damage.

Anemia From Infection

Many kinds of infection, some so mild as to remain unrecognized, can cause anemia in the pregnant lady. This can result in a case of anemia that doesn't have any detectable cause and isn't helped by iron or folic acid.

Aplastic Anemia

Aplastic anemia is a rare and serious disease, and is extremely rare during pregnancy. It is sometimes caused by certain drugs or poisons, and can be treated to some extent with drugs and transfusion. It carries fairly high risks of premature labor and fetal or maternal death.

Hemolytic Anemia

This is a condition in which the body produced antibodies which destroy its own red blood cells. It may be a part of a progressive disease, in which case the drug therapy it is treated with can be continued through pregnancy, or it may be brought on by the use of certain drugs and other substances. There is a certain metabolic disorder found almost only in black people, in which the use of some substances which are harmless to most people will cause a hemolytic reaction. In this condition, keeping away from the substances that cause the anemia will prevent it, or cure it if it does develop.

Sickle Cell Anemia

Sickle cell anemia is a hereditary condition found mostly in black people. Pregnancy can be hard on ladies with sickle cell anemia. The anemia becomes more severe, infection is more common, and there are often other problems. There is a much higher than usual incidence of miscarriage, stillbirth, and neonatal death.

Management of Severe Anemia

These anemias can be found through lab tests. If a lady is found to have aplastic, hemolytic, sickle cell, or any other serious anemia, she should be under a doctor's close care. There are drugs which may help the various kinds of anemia, and transfusion of blood or packed red cells is necessary in some cases.

Diseases of the Gastro-Intestinal Tract

Acute Appendicitis

Appendicitis complicates about one in 2,000 pregnancies. The symptoms are similar to those in nonpregnant people but pregnancy may make it harder to recognize. Since the appendix is higher in the belly than usual, the pain is not in the usual place. When it occurs in the first trimester, it may be mistaken for ectopic pregnancy or infection in the tubes, both of which have similar symptoms. The treatment, as for anybody, is immedate removal of the appendix.

Miscarriage or premature labor can result from appendicitis. The main danger to the pregnant lady is widespread peritonitis (severe infection) if the appendix ruptures. As pregnancy progresses, the appendix moves higher into the abdomen, and this position makes it easier for the peritonitis to spread. So early recognition of appendicitis is important.

Gastroenteritis

Gastroenteritis is the inflammation of the digestive system causing stomach cramps, nausea, vomiting, and diarrhea. It can be caused by any kind of stomach bug. It may be serious enough to cause premature labor, so a lady who has this should take it easy and get treatment if necessary.

Peptic Ulcer

Ulcers rarely develop during pregnancy, and if a lady had one previously, it is likely to improve. However, very rarely pregnancy will aggravate an ulcer, possibly even resulting in hemorrhage.

Ulcerative Colitis

Pregnancy can improve this condition or aggravate it, and occasionally it will reactivate a case that has subsided. Treatment is the same as for anybody.

Inguinal Hernia

If this occurs during pregnancy, it is likely to disappear by the middle of pregnancy. Treatment is for the symptoms, and surgery is avoided if possible.

Diaphragmatic Hernia

A diaphragmatic or hiatus hernia is a piece of stomach or esophagus pushing through the diaphragm. It can result from pregnancy, because of the increased pressure under the diaphragm. These hernias may be present in more than 15% of pregnant ladies, but usually cause no symptoms and go undetected. Sometimes in the second half of pregnancy they are associated with heartburn, vomiting, abdominal pain and a sensation of pressure, especially while lying down. If a lady has these symptoms, you may want to check with your doctor. The lady usually makes an almost total recovery after delivery. The hernia generally disappears completely within several months after delivery.

Urinary Tract Problems

In pregnancy, the ureters—the tubes that carry the urine from the kidney to the bladder—get very dilated, especially the right one. This is due partly to the pressure of the enlarged uterus or ovarian veins on the ureters as they cross the pelvis, and partly to hormones that cause the smooth muscles to relax. Because of the loss of muscle tone, the urine doesn't move as well but tends to sit still, and if bacteria are present, infection is more likely to occur. These problems happen more often in the later part of pregnancy.

The condition of dilated and obstructed ureters may cause the urine to back up into the kidney. This condition is called hydronephrosis, and may cause pain on either or both sides of the lower back. These pains are often vague and intermittent. If a lady has this kind of pain, she'll have to have her pee checked for urinary tract infection. Check with your doctor.

Cystitis is an infection in the bladder only. It causes urgency and frequency of peeing, which is often accompanied by a burning sensation. If it is not treated, it will often go on to pyelonephritis.

Pyelonephritis is not uncommon in pregnancy. It is a general urinary tract infection including the kidney, and is what is commonly called a "kidney infection."

About 5-10% of pregnant women develop urinary tract infection, and it is also a risk after delivery. Symptoms may be gradual and slight, but they often come on fast and strong. There is usually a fever, sometimes 103° or more, with chills and shaking. There is pain in the back just below the ribs, on one or both sides—the right side is most often affected. Sometimes the pain is in the abdomen. There can be painful or frequent peeing, and general discomfort. Pyelonephritis can cause premature labor.

If you suspect a lady has a urinary tract infection, consult with your doctor about what to do.

Chronic Kidney Trouble—The kidneys keep the body cleaned out of waste products and keep its minerals and fluids in balance. A lady's body has to work a lot harder to grow a baby than it does normally, so the kidneys will have to work harder while she's pregnant. Kidney disease, including recurrent infections, complicates pregnancy because of the added strain on the kidneys. Chronic kidney trouble increases the chance of acute urinary tract infection during pregnancy. It also often causes high blood pressure, and

427

toxemia is more common in ladies with kidney trouble. Any lady who has chronic trouble with her kidneys should see a doctor at least once during her pregnancy.

Chronic Conditions

A lady with any chronic conditions should be checked by a doctor when she gets pregnant. These include things like rheumatic heart disease, diabetes, chronic high blood pressure, kidney problems, and hypothyroidism.

Heart

In pregnancy, the blood volume is increased by one-third, the heart enlarges, and the volume of blood pushed through on each beat is increased. By term, the heart also has to work harder to maintain circulation for an extra 20 or more pounds. Many ladies with heart conditions can go through pregnancy and labor without any problems. But some ladies may need to be watched closely, and sometimes a hospital delivery is necessary because of the extra strain that labor causes. If a lady has a heart murmur or any heart condition, be in touch with your doctor.

Chronic High Blood Pressure

About 10% of pregnant ladies have pre-existing high blood pressure, especially those who have had several babies and those over 35. If a lady has high blood pressure before the 20th week of pregnancy, she probably had it before she was pregnant. Uncomplicated high blood pressure usually has no effect on pregnancy, but these women are more prone than most to toxemia, so they must have careful prenatal care. There may be some protein in the urine (up to + 1), but if the protein is much over + 1 and if there is unusual weight gain or edema, it is likely that toxemia is developing.

Hypothyroidism

Mild hypothyroidism, or underactivity of the thyroid gland, is a fairly common condition. Pregnancy puts an additional workload on the thyroid gland, so in hypothyroidism it needs extra help. A doctor can determine how much, or how much more, thyroid supplement is necessary, and with use of this supplement, there should be no problems with the pregnancy.

In more severe cases or cases where inadequate treatment is given, hypothyroidism can result in miscarriage, premature labor, or abnormalities of the baby.

Diabetes

Pregnancy causes a strain on the carbohydrate metabolism even in healthy ladies. It can unmask a prediabetic state by adding extra stress. The body's sugar tolerance is changed, so the dosage of insulin needs to be regulated more carefully throughout pregnancy. Toxemia and polyhydramnios are more common than usual in diabetic ladies. The main risk with diabetic pregnant ladies is to the baby. There is a higher than usual incidence of intra-uterine deaths after 36 weeks, and a higher neonatal mortality rate. These babies tend to be unusually large and are prone to several problems that are common in premature babies but rarely affect other term babies. Because of these possible problems, we don't recommend home deliveries for diabetic mothers.

15. Complications of Labor

Complications Occurring Before Term

Premature Labor

When labor begins three weeks or more before term, it is considered premature. Over 10% of deliveries in the United States are premature. Prematurity, along with its resultant problems, is the most common cause of neonatal death, so you want to do everything possible to prevent it.

Premature labor can be caused by injury to the mother, by some diseases or conditions she may have, or by multiple pregnancy (because of the great enlargement of the uterus). Usually, though, no cause is apparent.

If a lady may be starting labor early, check her cervix once gently to determine dilation. Then don't check again unless her labor seems to be progressing—checking too often can stimulate labor.

If there has been no bloody show and there is no (or very little—1 cm.) dilation of the cervix, try getting the mother drunk. Alcohol is a depressant, and it suppresses the release of oxytocin from the pituitary gland. It works well for stopping labor in the third trimester. Alcohol should not be used in the first two trimesters to inhibit labor because of possible damage to the developing baby. The lady should stay in bed and everything should be as nice and quiet around her as possible. If she has no more rushes for 24 hours, she can be up and around the house a little bit, gradually increasing her time up as she goes through more days without any rushes. If a certain amount of activity (even just standing up) increases her rushes, she should not do it. Once in a while, complete bed rest for several weeks is the only way to keep the baby in. Making love tends to start rushes if a lady is on the edge of starting labor, so the couple should abstain a while in favor of "cooking" their baby a little longer.

Sometimes you may think you are dealing with a premature labor when you actually have a case of misfigured due date. Check the size of the baby, recheck the history of the last menstrual period and make your best judgment. Check with your doctor if the lady is in labor and you are not sure if the baby really is early.

If labor keeps progressing and the baby is premature, the baby should be delivered in a hospital, where all the equipment necessary to take care of him is available.

Premature Rupture of Membranes

Sometimes the membranes rupture before labor starts. If labor does not begin within six hours after rupture, you should consult with your doctor. He may want to induce labor, or he may, under some circumstances, put the mother on an antibiotic to prevent infection, monitor her temperature and the baby's heartbeat carefully, and wait for her to go into labor. Sometimes labor doesn't start for days after the water bag breaks, and this is okay if there's no infection present. But the water bag acts as a barrier to bacteria and once it has broken, there is nothing to stop bacteria from going on up inside the uterus and causing an infection. This would be dangerous to the baby and could happen even if the lady were on an antibiotic. If the water bag breaks several weeks or more before a lady's due date, the prematurity of the baby is another factor to consider. Occasionally, the water bag will break or leak, then reseal and stay sealed for weeks.

When the water bag ruptures prematurely, there is a possibility that the umbilical cord can be washed down through the cervix past the presenting part.

Check the mother's cervix and the baby's heartbeat just after the bag ruptures to rule out prolapse of the cord.

If you have any doubts about whether the water bag is leaking or has just broken, you can do the *nitrazine test* to find out. You can get nitrazine paper from a medical supply house or maybe from your druggist. It works like reagent strips for testing pee. To do the test, wash the ladys's puss and expose the cervix with a sterile speculum. Hold a piece of nitrazine paper in a sponge clamp and touch it to the cervical os. There is a chart with the paper that tells what pH each color indicates. Usual secretions from the puss are acid (4.5-5.5). Urine is acid (about 6). Amniotic fluid is alkaline (7.0-7.5). So it is likely that what is coming out is amniotic fluid if the pH is over 6.5 or so. Blood is alkaline, so if there is bloody show the result may be alkaline whether or not the membranes have ruptured.

Another way to test for amniotic fluid is to put some of the leaking fluid on a glass slide and examine it under a microscope. Amniotic fluid will show a fern pattern when dried.

Complications of the First and Second Stages

Prolapse of the Umbilical Cord

The cord is prolapsed when it drops through the cervix before the presenting part, after the membranes have ruptured.

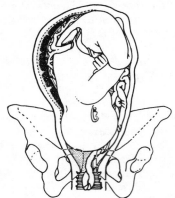 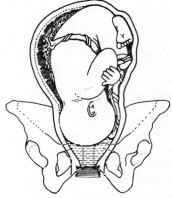

Fig. 111A. Complete Prolapsed Cord.   Fig. 111B. Hidden Prolapsed Cord.

It is presented when part of it lies below the presenting part of the baby while the membranes are still intact. The mortality rate for the babies is about 50% under these conditions. Fortunately it doesn't happen very often.

Usually, with prolapse of the cord, the presenting part is not well fitted into the bottom of the uterus. This sometimes happens with poly-hydramnios, prematurity, breech presentation, or a baby lying sideways in the uterus. Sometimes the cord is unusually long.

Always check for a prolapsed cord when the water bag breaks or if the baby's heartbeat is irregular. A loop of the cord may be long enough to be visible outside the mother's puss but a prolapse is usually discovered by vaginal examination

What To Do

If the cord is still pulsating, you can assume that the baby is in good condition. You want to keep the baby in good condition and deliver the mother as soon as possible.

1. Have the mother get into knee-chest position.

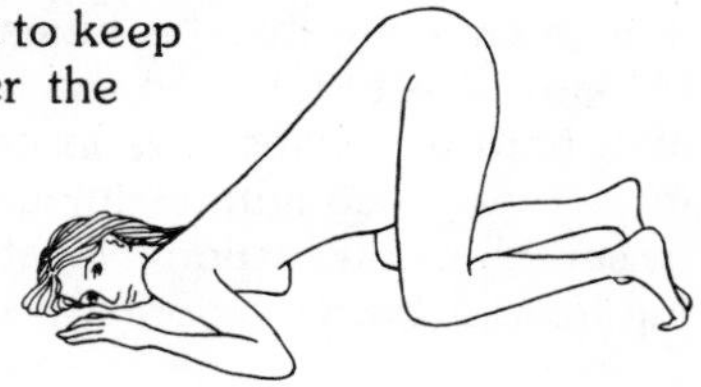

Fig. 112. Knee-Chest Position.

2. Put your hand, with a long sterile glove on, into the mother's birth canal and push up on the baby's head (or bottom) during the rushes. The idea is to keep the head far enough up to keep it from compressing the cord during the rushes.

3. If the cord is outside the mother's puss, keep it warm and protected with a warm, damp, sterile cloth so that the blood vessels don't go into a spasm.

4. Give the mother oxygen.

5. *Get her to a hospital as quickly as possible.*

If prolapse of the cord happens in the first stage, a cesarean section is necessary unless the doctor can quickly replace the cord. If prolapse happens in the second stage, the baby can be delivered quickly by forceps, or if the baby moves down right away, it can be delivered quickly with or without an episiotomy.

Fetal Distress

Fetal distress happens when the baby isn't getting enough oxygen and starts getting hypoxic. This can be caused by prolonged labor, trouble with the placenta or cord, or conditions such as toxemia or diabetes of the mother or a congenital defect of the baby.

If the baby lacks oxygen during labor, his anal sphincter tends to relax and meconium is passed into the amniotic fluid, turning it brown or green. Prolonged slowing of the baby's heart rate, prolonged speeding up of the baby's heart rate, meconium staining if the baby is not

431

in breech position, and abnormally vigorous movements of the baby are all considered signs of possible fetal distress. It is not at all uncommon for one of these signs to occur in a labor resulting in a live, perfectly healthy baby. You might even notice two indications of distress and have a fine, healthy baby, although statistically the chances of the baby being in trouble would be much greater.

If the heartbeat is low or high, you can try having the mother change her position. This will sometimes make the heartbeat return to normal. If the baby's heartbeat drops below 100 beats per minute for longer than a minute after a rush, you should get the baby out as soon as possible. If the mother is late in the second stage, give her oxygen, do an episiotomy if necessary and deliver quickly. If the mother is in the first stage, a cesarean may be necessary. Take the mother to a hospital. Give her oxygen on the way.

Meconium aspiration—When there is meconium in the fluid, the baby may suck some into his lungs (aspirate it) before or during delivery. Meconium is irritating to the lungs and may cause respiratory distress after birth and difficulties in eating and breathing for several days. If there was meconium staining of the amniotic fluid prior to the birth, be sure that you suction the baby's nose and mouth carefully as soon as the head is born—*before the baby attempts to breathe.*

Complications of the Third Stage

Post-Partum Hemorrhage

Be alert to the mother's condition and amount of blood loss after the baby is born. Sometimes the uterine muscles can lose their tension, not contracting enough to squeeze off the blood vessels of the placental site. By definition, post-partum hemorrhage is the loss of at least 500 ml. of blood during and after the birth of the baby. 500 ml. is about 2 cups. Remember that a little bit of blood can look like a lot. You can best tell how severe a hemorrhage is by its effect on the mother. Post-partum hemorrhage most often happens after the birth of the baby before the placenta comes out or directly after it comes out, but it can happen any time during the first day.

The risk of post-partum hemorrhage is increased in some ladies:

1. A lady who has had previous hemorrhages.
2. A lady who has had three or more children very close together. (This risk is less if the mother has exercised her body back into good condition between pregnancies.)
3. A lady with twins or polyhydramnios. An over-stretched uterus may have trouble keeping its tone.
4. A lady with anemia.
5. A lady who has suffered blood loss earlier in labor as with an abruptio placenta or placenta previa.
6. A lady who has had a prolonged labor.
7. A lady with a low-lying placenta.

If the uterus has anything extra in it, such as a partly retained placenta or a retained blood clot, it can't contract down as effectively as necessary to constrict the blood vessels of the placental site.

Treatment of Post-Partum Hemorrhage

While a post-partum hemorrhage is defined as the loss of 500 ml. of blood or more, you should not wait for that amount before you act. If there is a sudden gush of blood from the mother's puss, act immediately.

Lay the mother flat on her back.

Make the uterus contract by massaging it. The uterus has a wonderful ability to respond to the stimulus of touch. Massage as hard as necessary to make a contraction. You may have to squeeze and "tickle" it pretty vigorously.

At the same time have your assistant give an intramuscular injection of 10 units of pitocin or 0.2 mg. of methergine. Elevate the mother's feet.

Keep massaging the uterus as long as it has a tendency to lose its tone when left alone. If the mother has lost enough blood to be pale and weak, get her to a hospital. She very likely will need some blood or fluids intravenously. Give her oxygen and fluids by mouth, if she is alert enough to drink, on the way to the hospital.

In a more extreme case of hemorrhage following the birth of the baby and the expulsion of the placenta, you may need to compress the uterus between your hands, putting one sterile-gloved hand closed into a fist into the birth canal and the other on the abdominal wall. The second hand dips down behind the uterus, and pulls it toward the pubic bone. Press the two hands firmly together until the uterus contracts and stays hard.

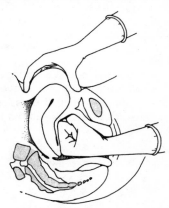

Fig. 113. Compression of the Uterus to Stop Excessive Bleeding.

Note: You shouldn't give more than one methergine shot to a lady for post-partum bleeding because it can cause the blood pressure to go too high. Never give it at all if the blood pressure before delivery is above 140/90. If you need to give more, use pitocin, while someone massages her uterus.

Retained Placenta

If the placenta does not come out within an hour after the birth of the baby, and the uterus remains firm (no extra bleeding), consult with your doctor about whether transport to the hospital is necessary.

If there is extra bleeding, transport the mother to the hospital. Sometimes you may need to remove the placenta manually to control bleeding. Use a long sterile glove.

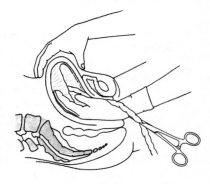

Fig. 114. Manual Removal of the Placenta.

Inversion of the Uterus

This complication of the third stage is fortunately very rare (one in 15,000 deliveries).

The inversion may be partial, or complete (the uterus will be visible outside of the puss). The mother may go into shock or may hemorrhage.

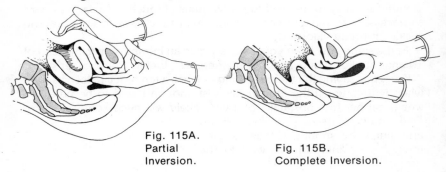

Fig. 115A.
Partial
Inversion.

Fig. 115B.
Complete Inversion.

Put on a long sterile glove. Immediately replace the uterus to its usual position, having your gloved hand inside the mother and the other on the abdominal wall pressing against the inside hand so that you can cause the replaced uterus to contract.

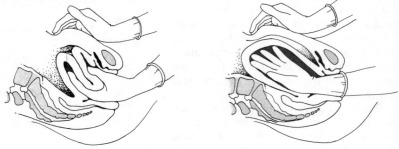

Fig. 116. Replacing the Inverted Uterus.

Shock

Shock can result from hemorrhage, dehydration, anemia or fear. Symptoms of shock are:

1. A pulse rate of more than 90.
2. Low blood pressure—a systolic pressure of less than 100 mmHg.
3. Paleness of the skin, with cold sweat.
4. Low body temperature.

Transport the mother to the hospital. Give her fluids by mouth on the way if she is able to drink. Raise the foot of her bed so that her blood will gravitate towards her heart and vital organs, and give her oxygen. Keep her warm enough that she doesn't shake, but don't raise her skin temperature until she is flushed, as she needs all her available blood near her vital organs.

16. Birth Injuries

Birth injuries are unlikely to occur in deliveries without the use of oxytocics or forceps, but you should know about some injuries.

Swellings of the Head

Caput succedaneum is the swelling of the head that can happen during labor because of the pressure of the head against the dilating ring of the cervix. The pressure hampers circulation of the scalp, resulting in congestion and edema in the loose scalp tissues. The swelling can vary a great deal in size according to the amount of pressure and the length of time the scalp is under pressure. The swelling pits with pressure and may be bruised as well. This swelling is harmless; it's present at birth and subsides within a day or so. Be sure the parents know that this swelling is harmless.

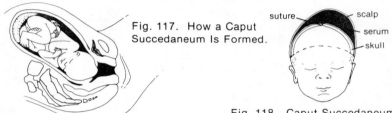

Fig. 117. How a Caput Succedaneum Is Formed.

Fig. 118. Caput Succedaneum.

A **cephalohematoma** is a swelling of the head that happens because of the escape of blood between the skull and the membranes that cover the skull (the periosteum). Small blood vessels can rupture because of strong pressure on the head during labor. This type of swelling is usually located over a parietal bone, but can never cross a suture because the periosteum under which the blood collects covers each bone separately. Sometimes there may be two swellings.

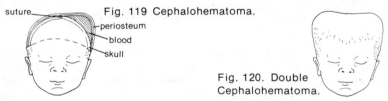

Fig. 119 Cephalohematoma.

Fig. 120. Double Cephalohematoma.

A cephalohematoma usually doesn't appear until a few hours after the birth, and it may increase in size for a day or so. There is no discoloration, and it does not pit with pressure. No treatment is necessary. The swelling will subside over a period of several weeks. Reassure the parents that it will eventually go away.

Fractures

Sometimes an arm or collarbone can be fractured in getting a large baby out of a small hole. If this happens, you will probably hear the fracture when it occurs and the injury will be obvious to touch. Check with your doctor: A fracture in a new baby will mend very quickly.

17. Congenital Abnormalities

There are some congenital abnormalities that can occur in babies, which the midwife should be able to recognize so that she can refer the baby to a doctor for treatment. All of the abnormalities are rare. Only the treatable abnormalities are mentioned.

Abnormalities of the Central Nervous System

Spina Bifida

This is an abnormality in the formation of the spinal cord. The bones which normally enclose it fail to close all the way, leaving the cord exposed and sometimes protruding. A mild case may have no symptoms, other than a slight dimple in the baby's back, and present no problems. A more severe case may involve a protrusion of the meninges (the tough membranes covering the spinal cord), called a meningocele, or the protrusion of the spinal cord, a meningomyelocele. Sometimes the skin is stretched over the bulging meninges, and sometimes they are completely uncovered. The child has a good chance of survival. The midwife must take care to cover the meningocele with a sterile dressing to prevent infection (meningitis is possible), and let the doctor know, and transport the child to the hospital. Spina bifida is often accompanied by hydrocephalus, but either condition can occur by itself.

Hydrocephalus

The hydrocephalic baby's head is unusually large because there is an increased amount of cerebrospinal fluid. This condition can cause obstructed labor—because the head can be too large to get through—unless it is diagnosed early. A cesarean may be necessary. In milder cases, the child lives and may be treated.

Abnormalities of the Digestive System

Pyloric Stenosis

Pyloric stenosis is a narrowing or abnormal thickness of the pyloric sphincter (the lower opening of the stomach, leading to the intestine). This condition causes projectile vomiting and should be suspected if the mother tells you that the baby has had projectile vomiting during the second or third week after birth. Projectile vomiting is the kind in which the contents of the stomach are thrown out of the mouth with some force, rather than dribbled out. Sometimes the baby can be treated with relaxing medications, and sometimes surgery is done to correct this condition. It most often occurs in first-born boys.

Closed Duodenum

Very rarely the upper part of the small intestine (the duodenum) will be closed off. This condition is called duodenal atresia. The baby will have vomiting soon after birth and the abdomen may be distended. This can be corrected surgically.

Closed Esophagus

This is a very rare formation, called esophageal atresia, in which the upper end of the food tube (the esophagus) ends in a pouch instead of leading to the stomach. The lower end is usually connected with the breathing tube (the trachea) by a small tube called a tracheo-esophageal fistula. You should suspect this condition if the baby keeps dribbling mucus from his mouth (more than the usual dribbling of partially swallowed fluids) immediately after birth. Taking any fluids makes the baby cough and turn blue. Polyhydramnios often accompanies this condition. Do not feed the baby, as the fluid most likely would go into the baby's trachea and lungs. An immediate operation is necessary.

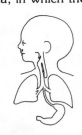

Fig. 121. Closed Esophagus with Tracheo-Esophageal Fistula.

Other Abnormalities

The other ends of the baby's tube may be closed off too—both the pee tube (the urethra) or the baby's butt-hole (anus). Rarely, a baby boy's foreskin may be so tight that he can't pee. All of these conditions are surgically correctable, but they must be recognized early in order to avoid danger to the baby; watch for them if the baby does not pee within the first 12 hours after birth or if he does not shit during the first day.

Abnormalities of the Heart and Blood Vessels

Congenital heart disease (CHD) includes many developmental abnormalities of the heart and the major vessels near it. There can be obstruction of the major vessels or of the openings between the heart's chambers and there can be extra openings. They can make it so the blood that is sent out by the heart isn't carrying as much oxygen as is needed, or so that good oxygenated blood gets recirculated through the lungs and heart instead of going out into the body. The symptoms may be similar to those of other disorders which interfere with breathing.

Signs and symptoms of CHD are:
- pulse rate of under 100 or over 160 at rest
- breathing difficulties
  * shallow and fast respirations—over 45 for a term baby and over 60 in a preemie. Respiration will be faster while feeding and with any increase of activity
  * retractions (above, below or between the ribs)
  * grunting
  * wheezing
  * coughing
  * moist crackling breath sounds heard with a stethoscope
- cyanosis, either all the time or only with feeding and increased activity

437

*signs of fluid overload: distended scalp or neck veins, enlarged liver, swelling of the skin, excessive weight gain
*sweating
*cool extremities
*heart murmurs

Some kinds of CHD will cause no symptoms and may never even be noticed, and some kinds can be controlled with medication. Some kinds will require surgery, either immediately or later. If you suspect CHD, take the baby to the hospital right away. Rarely, a baby can make it as long as his circulation hasn't completely switched over from the fetal kind but he'll die within a few minutes when it does. (It usually switches between a few hours and a few days after birth.)

While you are taking a baby who has suspected CHD to the hospital, give him oxygen if he needs it, and have him sitting up or semi-sitting. He can breathe most easily in this position.

Abnormalities of the Limbs

Club Feet

This condition is caused by the contraction of muscles or tendons on the inner side of the baby's legs. It can be corrected by exercise, massage, and splinting while the baby is still very young.

Extra Fingers and Toes

Extra fingers and toes usually have no bone and are connected to the hand or foot by a thin thread of skin. If there is a very narrow base and no bone, you can just tie them off with a silk suture—very tight—and they will fall off in a few days. If the extra digit has a broad base, see your doctor.

Congenital Dislocation of the Hip

In this condition, one or both hips are abnormally formed. Suspect it if you aren't able to flex the baby's hip to 90° or if the creases below the baby's buns, viewed from behind, look asymmetrical. This condition is more common in girls and can be treated if diagnosed early. It should be found right after birth by the routine test described on p. 373.

Abnormalities of the Skin

Birthmarks

Strawberry marks are not too unusual after birth—small, red, raised marks. They often grow larger for a while, then spontaneously disappear. They are harmless.

Purple, stain-like marks do not disappear, but they, too, are harmless.

Other Abnormalities

Phenylketonuria [PKU]

This is an abnormality of the metabolism in which the baby is not able to process the essential amino acid phenylalanine because of an enzyme missing in his liver. It is a very rare condition, occurring about once in 10,000 babies. If a baby has this condition, his diet can be managed so there is no damage to any of his systems (mental retardation occurs if the baby's diet is not properly managed)

These babies appear normal at birth. A PKU test is a simple blood test to determine if a baby has this disorder. All babies should have this test by the time they are ten days old; in some states this test is required by law.

Craniosynostosis

Craniosynostosis is the premature fusing of the sutures of the skull. It results in there being no bone growth perpendicular to the suture that is fused. The skull needs to allow for the growing brain, so it grows parallel to the fused suture, which results in an oddly-shaped head. You should check for a lack of soft spot in the newborn physical exam. It can cause increased pressure in the head, and eye trouble. The treatment is surgery.

Undescended Testicles

The testes usually descend into the scrotum during the last trimester If they aren't there at birth, they will probably descend during the first year. The mother should keep in touch with the doctor about this

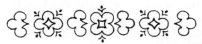

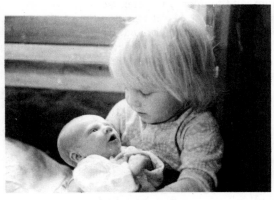

Rabbi Mordecai of Neskizh said to his son, the rabbi of Kovel: "My son, my son! He who does not feel the pains of a woman giving birth within a circuit of fifty miles, who does not suffer with her, and pray that her suffering may be assuaged, is not worthy to be called a zaddik."

His younger son, Yitzhak, who later succeeded him in his work, was ten years old at the time. He was present when this was said. When he was old he told the story and added, "I listened well. But it was very long before I understood why he had said it in my presence."

18. Tidbits on Energy and Attitude

A husband and wife form a single energy unit.

Some couples exchange energy by loving, and some do their main energy exchange by fighting. One couple I know got together in an interesting way. They noticed that whenever they got near each other, they usually ended up in an argument. After this had happened a few times, they figured it out that they must be pretty attracted to each other. They seemed to like to exchange energy with each other, even if it was by hassling. They soon noticed that their arguments were of no consequence, so they decided they would try exchanging energy in a friendlier way and see what that was like. They eventually decided to get married.

In some relationships, one partner will be in the habit of short-changing the other in energy transactions.

At one birthing, the mother's first, the husband was a big help to her. During a rush he would squeeze her back, trying to rub in exactly the right place for her and keeping his full attention on her to the very end of the rush. After a rush, he would smooch her, give her a lot of love and encouragement, and she wouldn't acknowledge that he had said anything to her. It was uncomfortable because the way she was being with him left the energy unbalanced. He had been giving her his best, and she hadn't acted like it was good enough to be noticed. He was so obviously feeling her labor with her and trying to share her load in any way that he could that she needed to give some energy back to make it feel right. I thought at the time that it must look to him like maybe she regretted having got familiar enough with him to have gotten pregnant. When I mentioned this (I tried to do it humorously), she laughed, and then she let him know that I hadn't been far off in my guess, and then she let him know that she loved him and that it was okay. From then on, they did fine. He helped her a lot, she accepted his help, and they had a nice baby girl not long afterward.

At another birthing, just before the birth of the baby, the lady would tell her husband that she loved him, feeling the energy of the baby very strong and wanting some graceful way to channel it, and he would just nod—wouldn't tell her that he loved her too and give her back as much as she had just given him. The midwives told him that it wasn't fair to be stingy about the energy that way, that this was the same energy that was trying to get his child born. They told him that he was really lucky to have such a nice lady, and encouraged him to have a good time at this birthing since it was one of the highest experiences that he would ever have. He loosened up and their baby was soon born.

Inhibition can block birthing energy.

If I suspect that inhibition is slowing down the progress of labor, I pay attention to the situation for a while, and observe the couple go through a few rushes. I look to see if this couple really loves each other. At the same time I am watching them, I am trying not to impose my own presence on them so much that they don't have any room to be together. Sometimes I will see that the husband is afraid to touch his wife's tits because of the midwives' presence, so I touch them, get in there and squeeze them, talk about how nice they are, and make him welcome. That way he can be uninhibited and loving at the same time. One of the strongest things a man can do to help his lady during their birthing is to let her know he loves her in all the ways that he can.
A marriage should be reliable, fun, and uninhibited.

Stephen taught us in the beginning that stimulation of the ladies' breasts had a powerful connection with bringing about contractions of the uterus. Our group of midwives had known this and used it as a tool for two or three years before we heard that the medical community, in doing experiments, had discovered that there is a powerful endocrine hormone called oxytocin that is produced by the pituitary gland, which can be prompted to do this by stimulation of the breasts. We had been using this in starting labor in the woman, or, where labor had begun, in speeding it up. We prefer to do this by pleasanter means than an IV drip.

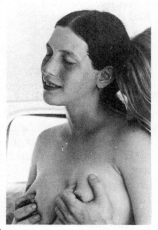

One time I was delivering a single lady whose cervix was fully dilated, but she wasn't able to move the baby. Her pelvic measurements were ample, but she couldn't get herself gathered together so that all her energy was working the same way. Usually it is possible to teach a mother how to push if she is pretty free of subconscious. She can usually learn in a few tries how to get all that energy focused into pushing. But sometimes, no matter how many times you go through it with a lady and demonstrate and do it with her, she always seems to move her leg or something at just the time when the energy is building. She moves that way, or forgets and lets out her breath or does something that you know she could be doing better. When I have a case like this, I usually begin to suspect there is some kind of subconscious that is tying up the energy. I have noticed that it is often sexual subconscious if the energy is blocked once the cervix is already dilated.

So in this case I started talking about it and since she was a single lady, I asked her about what the baby's father was like and what her relationship with him had been. It turned out that she didn't like him too much—she thought he was good-looking, but she didn't really like him too much. As she talked about it, and everybody in the room heard what she had to say about him, it seemed to free up a lot of energy that she had tied up in hostile feelings about him, and she could feel better about her baby being half that guy's genetic makeup. He wasn't going to have anything to do with the raising of the child, but she needed to feel okay about the part of the baby that was him.

I remember a similar situation with a married lady who had already had one baby with her husband. All through their relationship they questioned whether they ought to be together. Then they got pregnant again. They split up and got back together several times during the pregnancy and finally they just agreed not to do it together. During her labor, she had to come to peace about having his baby. The baby didn't want to come out until she felt okay about the regrets over what had gone on so far.

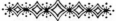

When someone says, "I love you" and means it, it opens up his throat—it literally does it. And when the throat opens up so does the cervix. I've been checking a lady's dilation at the same time she'd say that, and I could feel a distinct difference in her tissue, in how stretchy she was, that was exactly synchronous with her saying, *"I love you."* It made me really understand that words are vibrations and that some combinations of words have greater power than others. "I love you" is very strong.

One thing to remember is not to babble away all your energy by talking about insignificant or irrelevant things while the birthing is happening.

Sometimes laboring mothers get amazingly beautiful during a rush; you can see the prettiest one of that lady that you ever saw. These are very important moments to look for. Just to appreciate the way somebody is being tends to manifest it; nothing needs to be said.

"The flow of energy through a system tends to organize that system."
—Harold Morowitz

One of our single mothers who came to the Farm to have her baby was very unsatisfied with how she looked. At the time she came to us, she had a large patch of pimples on each cheek, and she would spend quite a bit of time looking critically at herself in the mirror, which didn't tend to help her complexion any. (What you pay attention to, you get more of.) I was present during part of her labor, when she was approaching transition. She was being very brave, and as I looked into her eyes during a rush, I would see that her pimples tended to fade whenever she could stay on top of the energy during a rush. If she would start to lose control a little bit and tighten up her face, the redness would come on again and the pimples would look exaggerated. By the time her son was born, she had managed the energy well enough that her pimples were about half as red as they had been at the onset of labor, and when I saw her again a few days later, her face was completely healed. Instead of looking in a mirror and not liking what she saw, she had been looking in her son's eyes. He wasn't critical a bit. He had that pure vision that newborns have, and he just loved her.

I remember an interesting birthing. The mother was a single lady who was about six feet tall and not really comfortable about being that big. She had this prim, proper, nicey-nice way about her that was a hang-up to the energy when she started having her first child. I arrived at the birthing when she was about four or five centimeters dilated. She was handling her rushes pretty well in that she wasn't complaining, but I noticed right away that her skin was not very fine-textured as is usually the case when a lady is running this much energy. Usually the facial skin looks very subtle and delicate; and you can see an amazing subtlety of expression. But her skin was more red and coarse-looking, and the level of expression was not too delicate—her face moved in bigger chunks at a time. Then, when she got to where she was almost fully dilated, she got very nauseous all at once. She turned green and had to throw up right away and had a hard time doing it. (It is interesting to notice how easily and gracefully somebody pukes, as this can tell you something about their very most basic attitudes. If a person has a hard time throwing up, to where it takes a very strong rush of nausea before she can do it and she gets a very revolted look on her face, not doing it as naturally as a dog or a new baby does it—it is because of conditioning, and it's best if you can point out the direction of this conditioning and help free her of it.) So this lady barfed a long time and went through all the colors of green that she could. There were a lot of secretions that day. After she was done throwing up and got to feeling all right about it, she started having a sense of humor and said, "This was not exactly what I had in mind that I would be doing at my birthing. I thought I was going to be having this fine spiritual experience." Here she was on her hands and knees throwing up all over the place on a hot summer day, etc. While all this was going on, I was noticing some very distinct changes in her appearance. She began looking rosy, and amused, and her face looked a lot more subtle and real. Her mouth looked very pretty, and I thought she was having her spiritual experience, even if it didn't fit her preconceptions.

Throwing up dilated her cervix the rest of the way, and she had a beautiful boy after a very short second stage. All that barfing freed her up so that she was ready for anything, and that's the attitude that a birthing mother needs to have.

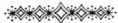

I saw a videotape once of a baby giraffe being born. The mother giraffe delivered standing up—while walking even. (Giraffes can't afford to lay down and do it—they would be too vulnerable to lions.) So the baby giraffe fell out of its mother six or seven feet to the ground. Its landing caused a small dust cloud. The baby breathed right away— (no wonder) and immediately began struggling to its feet with the help of mother. It figured out how to walk in the next minute or two, and mother and baby caught up again with the rest of the herd. Nature does not always arrange that birth be gentle. In the case of the giraffe, the chances for survival of the species seem to indicate that a rough landing on the planet is the best way.

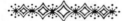

When I was going to college, my neighbor, whose pregnancy I had been following with great interest, had her baby in an unexpected way. She had started having some cramps, so she called her doctor. He told her to come by his office for a check-up. She went there and while on the examination table, went into full-scale labor and had the baby a few minutes later—didn't even have time to take her socks off. Her doctor let her rest for an hour or so, and then drove her home. I liked it that he didn't make her go to the hospital. And what an impressive way to have a baby! To just animal out on them so fast that they had to make the most practical decisions about what to do.

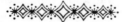

One Farm baby was born with a polycystic kidney. The way that we figured out that he needed special attention was that his mother noticed that he was not quite like her other two had been at that age, though it was a very subtle difference. But he did spit up easier than her others had, and it bugged her enough that she called us in the middle of the night. We took him right to the hospital where they diagnosed him and operated on him immediately. It turned out that one kidney was full of cysts and had to be removed, and the other was perfect. (He's currently doing well on just one kidney, which is all you need.) The miraculous thing about a new baby that needs surgery is that they are growing so fast and have so much life force energy at the time of birth that they heal very quickly. He did amazingly well in surgery and recovered much faster than a grownup would.

One time I was delivering a first baby for a lady, whose labor was coming on really fast. From the time I first checked her, every time she had a rush, her cervix dilated half a centimeter or so. The vibrations were very strong, and because she was physically very strong herself (she was quite a lot bigger than I), I didn't get very far in smoothing out her energy by rubbing her out. She weighed about 190 pounds at term, and was not at all fat. I felt like I was delivering this gorgeous giant lady. Instead of me getting her to relax, touching her tended to make me shake. This was the first birthing that I ever had Paul attend (he had been present for the hospital births of two of his kids), and I noticed that he was in the same condition that I was. I looked at him to see how he was doing, and he just waggled his eyebrows at me a little. (The lady was a lot bigger than he was too.) The rushes kept coming on stronger and more intense, so I knew that I had to get the energy feeling mellower so that my hands wouldn't be shaking when the baby came. I told the lady that I was really going to need her cooperation so that my hands could be steady and sure. She knew it was true as she had already observed the effect that her vibrations were having on Paul and me. I felt like I had her deep agreement then, and showed her how to breathe slow and deep no matter what else was happening. After it had got calmer, I had her and her man smooch through the rest of the opening-up rushes. They felt really good, and the energy was flowing very smooth and steady. A ten and a half pound girl was born without a tear after a total of four hours of labor.

Conscientious Objector

I shall die, but that is all that I shall do for Death.
I hear him leading his horse out of the stall; I hear the clatter
   on the barn-floor.
He is in haste; he has business in Cuba, business in the Balkans,
   many calls to make this morning.
But I will not hold the bridle while he cinches the girth.
And he may mount by himself; I will not give him a leg up.
Though he flick my shoulders with his whip, I will not tell him
   which way the fox ran.
With his hoof on my breast, I will not tell him where the black boy
   hides in the swamp.
I shall die, but that is all that I shall do for Death; I am not on his pay-roll.
I will not tell him the whereabouts of my friends
   nor of my enemies either.
Though he promise me much, I will not map him the route
   to any man's door.
Am I a spy in the land of the living, that I should deliver men to Death?
Brother, the password and the plans of our city are safe with me;
   never through me
Shall you be overcome.

—Edna Saint Vincent Millay

In 1972 The Farm Midwives made public an offer to mothers who desired to continue their pregnancies even though they were unsure about keeping their babies. They were invited to come to The Farm for prenatal and maternity care. They were provided room and board and all medical care free of charge during their stay. The expectant mothers, most of whom were single, were put under no pressure to give up their babies. After the time of birth, if a mother did not feel ready to assume responsibility for caring for her baby, the baby was placed with a foster family. The agreement was that if the biological mother ever changed her mind and wanted to reclaim her child, the foster family would return the baby to her. The foster families entered into this agreement freely, taking the risk of loving and caring for children who might not always be with them.

By early 1984, 269 women had taken advantage of the midwives offer. Remarkably, only 12 of them left their babies with foster families, and of these, half were later reclaimed by biological mothers or other relatives. The midwives observed that most of the mothers they served seemed to have developed such stong bonds with their babies — possibly from having given birth naturally — that they no longer were ambiguous about their ability to mother.

Hundreds of women besides those who gave birth at The Farm either telephoned or wrote to the midwives, applying for care or counselling by the midwives. A large percentage of these women later contacted the midwives, to let them know of the births of their babies and to say that the existence of the program had been the major factor in their decisions to continue their pregnancies. These mothers were able to find satisfactory care without travelling to Tennessee.

The program has helped mothers from all over the United States and Canada, as well as from Germany, Australia, England and Wales.

The cost of the program up to April, 1983, was totally borne by the members of The Farm, by then a community of 300 adults and their children. By late 1983, the community could no longer afford to fund the program because of the increasing cost of the occasional hospitalization that was sometimes necessary. Since that time, the help we give mothers in desperate straits has depended upon tax-deductible donations made to *Rocinante*, a non-profit foundation supporting the work of Stephen and Ina May Gaskin; 41, The Farm; Summertown, Tennessee 38483

APPENDICES

A. Further Reading

Taber's Cyclopedic Medical Dictionary, Clarence U. Taber. Philadelphia, Pennsylvania: F.A. Davis Co. Or any good medical dictionary.

Human Labor and Birth, Oxorn and Foote. New York: Appleton- Century-Crofts.

Handbook of Obstetrics and Gynecology, Ralph C. Benson. Los Altos, California: Lange Medical Publications.

A Text-Book of Midwifery, Johnstone and Kellar. London: A. and C. Black, Ltd.

Becoming A Midwife, Carolyn Steiger. Portland, Oregon: Hoogan House.

Heart & Hands: A Midwife's Guide To Pregnancy & Birth, Elizabeth Davis. Berkeley, California: Celestial Arts.

Sensitive Midwifery, Caroline Flint. London: Heinemann Midwifery.

Mayes' Midwifery, Rosemary E. Bailey. London: Bailliere Tindall.

Textbook for Midwives, Margaret Myles. Edinburgh, London and New York: Churchill Livingstone.

Where There is No Doctor, David Werner. Palo Alto, California: Hesperian Foundation. An excellent book on primary health care. Also available in Spanish.

Maternal-Infant Bonding: The Impact of Early Separation or Loss on Family Development, Klaus and Kennell. St. Louis, Missouri: C.V. Mosby Co.

Care of the High-Risk Neonate, Klaus and Fanaroff. Philadelphia, Pennsylvania: W.B. Saunders Co.

Artemis Speaks: V.B.A.C Stories & Natural Childbirth Information, Nan Koehler. Occidental, California: Jerald R. Brown, Inc.

The Human Body—Its Structure and Operation, Issac Asimov. New York: The New American Library of World Literature, Inc.

A Child Is Born, Nilsson, Ingelman-Sundberg and Wirsen. New York: Dell Publishing Co.

The Complete Book of Pregnancy and Childbirth, Sheila Kitzinger. New York: Alfred A. Knopf.

What Every Pregnant Woman Should Know: The Truth About Diets and Drugs in Pregnancy, Gail Sforza Brewer, with Tom Brewer, M. D. New York: Random House.

Home Birth: A Practitioner's Guide to Birth Outside the Hospital, Sagov, Feinbloom, Spindel, Brodsky. Rockbridge, Maryland: Aspen.

Babies, Breastfeeding and Bonding, Ina May Gaskin. Amherst, Massachusetts: Greenwood Press

B. RESOURCES
Periodicals

The Birth Gazette
(a quarterly magazine
published by Ina May Gaskin)
42, The Farm
Summertown, Tennessee 38483
$25/year

Midwifery Today
Box 2672-4
Eugene, Oregon 97402

Mothering
P.O. Box 8410
Santa Fe, New Mexico 87504

NAPSAC News
P.O. Box 429
Marble Hill, Missouri 63764

The Clarion
Cesarean Prevention Magazine
P.O. Box 152
Syracuse, New York 13210

Texas Midwifery
The Association
   of Texas Midwives
Suite 1A-202
603 West 13th Street
Austin, Texas 78701

Birth
Three Cambridge Center
Suite 208
Cambridge, Mass. 02142

Journal Of Nurse-Midwifery
Elsevier Scientific
   Publishing Co.
52 Vanderbilt Avenue
New York, New York, 10017

The Compleat Mother
RR 2
Orangeville
Ontario L9N 2Y9
Canada

MANA News
P.O. Box 1121
Bristol, Virginia 24203-1121

Check with the Midwives Alliance of North America (MANA) to find out the address of state and provincial midwifery organizations.

Birth Supplies

Moonflower Birthing Supply
P.O. Box 128
Louisville, Colorado 80027

Cascade Birthing Supplies
P.O. Box 12203
Salem, Oregon 97309

Naturpath Medical
   and Birthing Supplies
RR 1, Box 99C
Hawthorne, Florida 32640

B. Especially for Doctors

In my first writings on spiritual midwifery, I made the statement that sometimes I thought doctors became so uncompassionate that they behaved like mad scientists. Some people have thought this was a harsh thing to have said, so I have decided to include a couple of stories of birthings which will explain why I have felt this way at times.

The first story was sent to me by Mary, whose fourth baby died in her womb. Mary's previous birthings had all taken less than two hours, so she had a reputation as an excellent baby-haver. She is the same Mary whose description of her rushes of a previous birthing is on page 53.

Christina's Birth and Burial

One afternoon when I had about seven weeks left of my pregnancy, I suddenly realized that my baby hadn't moved all day. I had a job at the time that kept me very busy and I hadn't been paying that much attention to my pregnancy except that I had an exceptionally active baby—she seemed to wiggle all the time. So when I didn't feel her move for a whole day, I got a sort of sick, scared feeling in my stomach. I called Mary Louise who said to come on over to the clinic. She heard a heartbeat but it was some slow. She said we'd keep a close check. I went to see her every day. The baby still didn't move and I felt that something was really wrong.

In a few more days the midwives sent me to see Dr. Williams in town. He didn't hear anything inside me but said he'd seen cases before where you couldn't get a heartbeat for a while but would still have a live baby. Everyone encouraged me not to give up hope so I tried to think that way, but it felt really heavy to me. I managed to keep it together somehow that day until I got to Michael. We went off alone and I cried and cried. I felt an anguish and pain I'd never felt before. Michael was very strong and brave and solid. I was so grateful to have him.

I still tried to keep up hope that the baby was alive. A few days later I went to the clinic when Ina May was there. As soon as I walked in I felt a beautiful, clear aura of Truth in the room. Ina May listened and felt and then we looked at each other long and strong. We both knew my baby had died. She gave me so much love and strength in those moments that I knew I could handle whatever had to come next.

Michael stayed really available so I could get to him whenever I needed him, which was often. I wanted to have the baby on the Farm if at all possible and everyone agreed that we would try to do that. Dr. Williams said it would be safe to just wait and see if I would go into labor on my own. So I continued to work and tried to stay really busy. A few times Dr. Williams tried to break my water bag

449

to see if that would start me up but without success. We waited for five weeks but nothing happened. My emotions were getting very hard to control and I'd go through places where I thought I might just blow or something. Then I'd run to Michael and he'd keep me going by loving me and being strong and sane. I couldn't make love because every time we'd get that close and intimate there would be the three of us and I would feel so sad I just couldn't go on. Michael was very understanding.

Finally Dr. Williams said we could use pitocin to induce labor and he would come help us do it on the Farm. I felt very relieved and was looking forward to the day. On the appointed day Michael and I came home early to be together and get ready. While we were hanging out, we got a phone call that Dr. Williams had changed his mind—there were too many risks involved in inducing labor on the Farm for him to feel comfortable about it. When I heard that I felt a huge wave of despair sweep over me; I decided I just couldn't handle it anymore and felt my head sort of float off into some big empty space. Then I heard a far-off distant voice calling my name. I slowly realized it was Michael calling me and that if I checked out, I was going to leave him all alone with this problem—I loved him and certainly didn't want to do that. So I got it back together and we just lay there and loved each other for a long time. I'd never seen before what a freewill decision it is to be crazy.

Everyone knew that I just needed to get the baby out now, so we agreed to go to the hospital. Within a couple of days, the arrangements were made to go to a hospital and Michael could be with me. Michael, Cara and I drove to the hospital and were met by a really kind head nurse named Carol. She obviously had some sort of prestige around there and fixed us up very smoothly. She helped us through all the red-tape of admittance and let me skip all the "prep" stuff like getting shaved and hooked up to machines and all. She said Cara and Michael could be with me throughout the whole trip and that if anyone objected we should get her right away.

I got an X-ray and we saw that the baby was in breech position. Then they took me to the labor room and hooked me up to the pitocin. I looked around at the setup they have for having babies—it was awful. The rooms were very bare and sterile with no chairs for folks to be with you and there was a big clock right in front of you. The lady in the next bed was all gray and wasted-looking. She said she'd been in labor for 18 hours. Her body was numb from the waist down and she looked bored. A machine next to her told her when she was having a contraction, but she didn't seem very interested. Her husband sat in the only chair in the room and read a cheap novel. Cara suggested maybe he could rub her legs or something because they obviously needed to get some kind of energy going, but the lady said never mind, she couldn't feel it anyway. Cara managed to pump them up a little, but it sure did look different from the way I was used to having babies. Four ladies had babies while we were there and no one noticed at all that it was a beautiful, Holy event. The ladies screamed things like, "I can't stand it," and, "Help," and the nurses told them to shut up and be brave. Then just after the commotion died down, we'd hear the baby's first cry. It was so pure and beautiful and Holy. We three would hold hands and rush together.

My labor was progressing mechanically. It really felt different from doing it myself. It felt like I was plugged into a machine that was doing my labor instead of my own body. At one point a short, fat male doctor came in to check my dilation. His vibes were so uppity and uncompassionate that it took everything I had for me to hold it together and let him touch me. After he left, Michael rubbed me a lot to smooth it back out.

After a couple of hours of labor, the shift changed and our guardian angel Carol went home. She told us if we had any trouble to call her at home and left us her number. When she had gone, we met our doctor, a young lady intern who had obviously never had a baby herself. She was cold and distant and didn't want to talk. The new nurse who came on looked like a growling bulldog who hated her job or people or both. She wouldn't look at us and refused to talk. The three of us looked at each other and knew we were alone, but we felt strong and competent and knew we'd do okay.

My rushes were building up stronger and it was good for me to see what a longer labor could be like—my others had all been so smooth and fast. In a couple more hours I got fully dilated and got to where I could push. At that point I could feel my body take over and now I could help out. I enjoyed pushing and putting out big surges of energy. This was more like it. Michael and Cara encouraged me a lot and told me how beautiful I looked and how good it sounded. Then someone came in and pushed my bed to the delivery room. When we got there, I had to get up off my bed and get on the delivery table. I couldn't believe they were making me do this absurd moving around while I was trying to have this baby, but I got through it and grabbed my knees and got into it again. Then the bulldog nurse grabbed my legs and pulled them down into those stirrup things that immediately put intense cramps into all my leg muscles and, worst of all, I couldn't push anymore. I wiggled and tried to get away and Cara said, "That really isn't necessary," but they would hear none of it. It was quite different getting out a dead baby because there wasn't any energy from the baby. I'd never realized before how much the baby puts out to get born, but now it was noticeably lacking. The baby came out quickly in a big rush of relief. We saw that the cord was wrapped very tightly around her neck four times. The doctor staggered back and said, "Oh, it stinks!" We just let that pass. The three of us rushed and felt good. I felt the same exhilarating rush and wave of gratitude that I'd felt just after delivering my live babies. I was really sorry I'd lost this one, but I was glad to bring the karma to rest.

I felt totally open, and I was lying there rushing when suddenly I felt a heavy stabbing pain in my abdomen. I screamed and we looked to see what was happening. With her fingers straight and stiff, the doctor was stabbing me repeatedly just below my belly button as hard as she could. We realized she was trying to deliver the placenta. Cara hollered, "Don't! It isn't necessary. Please stop!" Michael turned pale and looked like he was going to throw up, and I just hollered. They didn't pay any attention to us at all. Finally the placenta came out and I got pushed back to the labor room. We were all three shaking from having been involved in such a barbaric, cruel act. I had never been treated so violently before in my life and I was amazed. I don't think that doctor was particularly intentionally cruel—she'd just been taught like that—but it was hard to believe that anyone could be so gross and uncompassionate.

When we were safely back in our room, our first reaction was to get out of there as fast as we could, but Cara hadn't brought her birthing kit with methergine in it and we definitely didn't want me to hemorrhage on the way home. My body felt all fine and strong except for the bruises all across my abdomen, but we didn't want to take any chances, and decided to let me sleep for a while. In a couple of hours the lady doctor came in and said she'd heard we were thinking of leaving. She said I should certainly stay for three days or so because hemorrhaging would be very likely on the ride home. We didn't believe it but called Ina May to be sure. She said to come on home. Then we found out they wouldn't let us take the baby, so we called home again. Our lawyer assured us we could get the baby—we'd send someone to get her later—so we left amid lots of groans and head-shakings at leaving without the doctor's permission. We were very grateful to get out of there.

I was really appalled to see the setup they had for having babies—you could hardly make it any more uncomfortable or difficult if you tried. It was a shame to see what a rotten experience childbirth was for so many ladies under such conditions when it's really so beautiful, gratifying, and Holy. I realized like I never had before how *very* important our medical revolution is. The people really need us—most of them don't even know how bad they're getting ripped off. I was so grateful to drive back through the gate of the Farm—I am so very grateful every day.

Michael and I rested while someone brought our baby back home. Michael had made a little redwood coffin for her, so that evening he went to the clinic, cleaned her up, and put her in the coffin. When he got home, he said he felt he knew her well enough that she should have a name. We wanted a religious, pure-sounding name and decided on Christina.

The next morning Cara came over and told us Stephen and Ina May would be there soon to go with us to the funeral. Cara helped me get some clothes on. Stephen, Ina May, Michael and I drove to the

452

cemetery while Leslie and Cara came in another truck. Leslie had already prepared a place and Stephen gently laid our baby to rest. When I heard the first shovelful of dirt hit the coffin I felt such a wave of sorrow that I thought I might fall, but Michael was holding me on one side and Ina May had my hand on the other and I got strength from them. After a while Michael took the shovel and Stephen came to stand by me. He rubbed my belly gently and lovingly—I could feel him blessing me and healing me. I felt very grateful for his strength and love. As soon as Christina was buried, we all held hands in a circle around the grave. I had my eyes closed and saw a vision of a beautiful shaft of white light reaching from the circle that was made by our joined hands. I felt the purity of Christina's soul and what a blessing it was to have had her if only for such a short time. Then I opened my eyes and the same vision was there before me in reality. It was a truly beautiful moment and I felt calm and peaceful. As we walked back to the truck, I saw the tears running down Michael's cheeks—it was the first time I'd seen him cry. He had been so brave and strong through the whole thing—I was so grateful and I love him very much. On the way home Michael told Stephen how grateful he was to have the Teachings to carry him through such a heavy place. Stephen said yes, he knew; that's what he lived by too.

Michael and I picked up our three kids and spent the day being with them and loving them and being grateful for our fine family.

Four weeks after writing her story, Mary gave birth to a healthy baby girl in her home after a 30-minute labor.

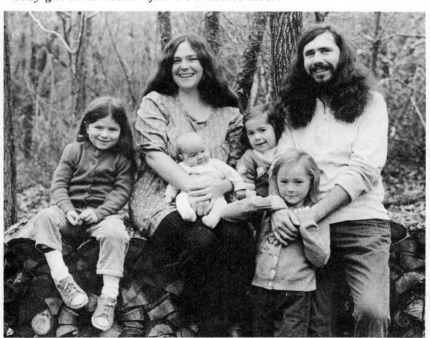

One of the most insensitive things I ever saw a doctor do was during a cesarean section, after the delivery of the baby, during the sewing up of the incision. The section had been necessary because the mother had developed a painful urinary tract infection while in labor, which had the effect of slowing down her labor considerably. But she had been incredibly brave throughout, especially ever since she had arrived at the hospital, and I found myself remembering that in Norse tradition, laboring women as well as courageous, fallen warriors were given a place in Valhalla, the life-after-death reward for valor. While going in after the baby, the doctor had cut too deep and had made an incision in the mother's bladder, which made the operation last about half an hour longer than it would have, and created the possibility of spreading the infection that was already in there. The mother had fallen asleep while her incision was being closed, and while her belly was still open about an inch deep, the doctor put his hands on either side of the incision and, moving the wound as if it were a puppet mouth, said, "Hi, Steve," to the young intern across the operating table from him. The remark was intended to be funny but wasn't, because the doctor was ignoring so totally the human dignity, not even to mention the bravery, of the lady whose life was in his hands.

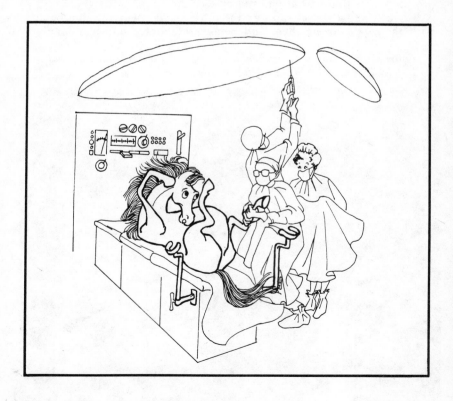

454

I want to tell you about the birth of Ira because it is a lesson in compassion.

Ira's Story

One warm June night I got a call to go out to a birthing. It was a relief to hear that this mother had finally begun her labor, as she and I had been expecting the same week. My baby had been born three weeks early and was now six weeks old.

When I got to the bus where the birthing was happening, I could see that the mother felt the same way I did. Her eyes were bright and dilated. Although this was her first baby, she did not fight the energy of her rushes, and before long, her cervix was nearly all the way open. I decided that it was time to check her dilation and did so, discovering then that the baby's face was presenting instead of the top of his head. When the head began to move down the birth canal, we began to see the baby's mouth, all beautiful and rosy and delicious-looking. During a rush I would put my finger to his lips and he'd suck it. I felt that I had a special kind of relationship with this little one, to get to communicate with him so strongly even before his birth.

When his head came out, I couldn't integrate what I was seeing at first. His body followed quickly, broad-shouldered, lean and long-limbed—proportioned more like a full-grown man than a brand new baby. I pulled myself together then and looked at his head. What I was seeing was his brain, for no skull had formed over it. I remembered then having seen pictures of babies like this in a couple of obstetrics textbooks, with the caption "anencephalic monster" underneath. The question arose in my mind whether it was right to help him start breathing. I knew right away that I had to help him. He wanted to live. That was obvious. I couldn't withdraw my love from him because he didn't look like the rest of us. Then after the initial shock had begun to wear off, we began to see that he did resemble two of us: his parents. His mouth, for instance, was an exact miniature of his mother's.

I decided that I should take him to the hospital. His parents agreed. I knew he wouldn't live long as he was, but thought perhaps they could help us out, make him some kind of plastic skull cap or something. He was so strong he almost kicked himself off my lap when I was taking him in—he had a kind of power that newborn babies don't usually have. I gave him to a nurse who felt kind about him, and went home.

When I'd get up to feed my baby in the night, I'd find myself thinking about Ira. (His mother decided to name him because it seemed like he ought to have a name.) About five days later, the doctors were amazed that he was still alive, and I found out why they were amazed. His parents found out by chance that the hospital as a matter of policy had not given him anything to eat or drink from the time they'd gotten him. This is common practice in hospitals in this country and these babies usually die within a few hours. When we heard that they weren't feeding him it came as a shock to us because we had assumed that they were at least feeding him. His mother felt very strongly that she wanted to care for him herself—that he was still her baby.

I called the pediatrician and said that we wanted to bring the baby home. She said that she didn't think it was a good idea, but she signed the papers and we went in and got him. There were nurses in the nursery who were unhappy about not feeding him because they wanted to help him too, but they would have been countering doctor's orders, so they didn't do it. Some of the people at the hospital treated us like we were weird hippies come to claim our weird kid, and others of them were very glad and felt that that was the right thing to do.

When the nurse handed him to me, he was as light as a feather because he hadn't eaten or drunk anything in five days. We felt that it was a miracle that he was still alive, and it was with gratitude and relief and love that we brought him home. He and his parents stayed at our house, and we fed him with an eye dropper because he was too weak to nurse. Both of his parents spent all their time with him as they knew he didn't have too long to live. His mother made him little hats and they sunned him on the porch. He never cried, but now and then, he called us. Both mine and Margaret's babies (both six weeks old) picked up that same call and used it for a few days after Ira had died. He lived for five more days. He was no longer a baby; he was like a wise old teacher. We felt very privileged to have a Holy thing being like that in our house.

It was a teaching to Dr. Williams too. When he talked about these babies he would use the medical term, "anencephalic monster," and we'd say, "No, a baby, not a monster, a *baby,*" and that you should treat them like babies, and I said, "Anyway, back in San Francisco when a lot of us were taking psychedelics, I saw a lot of my friends look weirder than that." He understood.

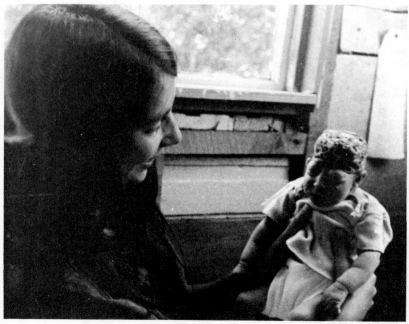

Margaret and Ira

C. Equipment and Supplies

The following is a list of instruments and supplies that we use in our sterile packs and midwife kits. You can modify it according to your needs and preferences.

Sterile Packs

We make up five separate sterile packs, each wrapped in heavy paper, tied with string and baked for 1 hour in a 250°F. oven. Each pack is marked with the date of expiration (7 days after sterilizing).

(1) 3 sheets
   2 midwife gowns

(2) 2 sheets
   2 hand towels
   20 gauze pads (4" x 4") separate package
   4 sanitary napkins, wrapped separately

(3) 3 towels
   20 washcloths

(4) For the baby:
   4 receiving blankets
   4 small cloths (soft flannel)
   1 kimono
   1 diaper
   1 cover sheet (a 2' x 3' or pillow case will do fine)
   2 pieces of 12" heavy cotton string (unless you use plastic or metal cord clamps)

(5) Extra:
   2 receiving blankets
   20 more gauze pads

The Midwife Kit

The following is a list of instruments and supplies that we carry in our kits.

Instruments

2 curved hemostats with long ends (Kelly hemostats)
2 blunt/sharp surgical scissors
1 toothed tweezers
1 straight needle holder
1 or more sterile sponge clamps (ring forceps)
1 speculum
1 emesis basin for holding sterilized instruments

These instruments should be kept sterile by one of the methods on p. 459
1 infant suction set (DeLee catheter)
24 sterile exam gloves

3 pair surgical gloves, size 6½-7½
2 test tubes for cord blood
2 thermometers (oral and rectal)
3 cord clamps
1 sterile baby bottle
2 sterile ear syringes
  plastic sheet
  blood pressure cuff
  stethoscope
  fetoscope
  lubricating jelly
  enema bag
  nail brush
2 bottles Betadine scrub
.1 quart sterile water
1 bottle baby oil
  lots of alcohol
  benzalkonium chloride for soaking instruments
  Betadine solution
  Argyrol eye drops
  triple dye for baby's cord

Supplies for Injections and Stitching

This is more syringes than you're likely to need at one birthing, but it's good to be amply supplied in case you attend two or three birthings close together.

10 3cc. syringes for injecting methergine and obtaining cord blood
5 10 cc. syringes for injecting xylocaine
3 tuberculin syringes for giving caffeine—these syringes are long and skinny, for accurately measuring a small amount
6 000 chromic sutures
5 23 gauge 1" needles
5 23 gauge 5/8" needles
5-10 sterile 4" x 4" gauze pads

Injectables

2 ampules caffeine
4 ampules methergine
4 ampules pitocin
1 bottle lidocaine
12-24 methergine or ergotrate pills

Papers

  birthing records
  new mother's instructions
  midwife check list
  post-partum exercises
  measuring tape
  cord blood tube envelopes

Keeping Your Supplies Sterilized

"Sterile" means "free from any living micro-organisms." Some of your equipment, such as syringes and gloves, will already be sterile when purchased and will come sealed in paper. These will stay sterile as long as they don't get wet (being wet makes it possible for bacteria to grow). Store wrapped, sterilized supplies in a clean, dry place.

You will need to routinely sterilize some of your equipment, such as instruments, linens, and ear syringes for suctioning the baby. There are several ways of doing this.

1. Carefully wash and dry the instruments and wrap them in paper or cloth (except for scissors, which need to be sterilized by either of the other two methods because repeated heating will dull them). Bake at 250°F. for one hour. Watch the temperature carefully. Put a pan of water in the bottom of the oven to help prevent scorching. The sterile linen packs (see p. 457) are also sterilized in a 250°F. oven for one hour.

2. A large pressure cooker can also be used for sterilizing and has the advantage of not scorching the material. Place the clean, wrapped instrument packs on a rack above water level (two quarts of water). Make sure the top is on tight and bring it up to 15 lbs. pressure for 20-30 minutes. Let the packs dry in a clean warm place, as they may be moist.

3. Soak the cleaned instruments in benzalkonium chloride solution (Zephiran) for thirty minutes.

•Rubber ear syringes need to be boiled in water for 45 minutes just prior to using unless you are sterilizing with a pressure cooker or an autoclave. If you are, wrap the syringe in gauze and then in a clean cloth before sterilizing. Rubber syringes can't be baked because they will melt, and they shouldn't be soaked in benzalkonium chloride solution, as some of the solution might remain inside the syringe.

•Supplies wrapped in paper and sterilized will need to be re-sterilized every week until used. If they are wrapped in a double thickness of tightly-woven cotton cloth before sterilizing, they will keep for 2 or 3 weeks. Write the expiration date on the wrapping before sterilizing.

•You need sterile water at a birthing. You can sterilize some by canning it up in canning jars beforehand, or by boiling it in a pan on the stove for 15 minutes, and letting it cool.

•When something is sterile, you have to be really careful not to touch it to something that is not sterile, or it will be contaminated. This requires developing a whole set of conscious habits about keeping sterile things sterile.

Portable Oxygen Kit

At all birthings on the Farm, we have a portable oxygen kit on hand in case the mother or baby needs oxygen. Our kits contain:
(1) a "D" size medical oxygen cylinder,
(2) a set of medical oxygen pressure regulator and gauges,

(3) a cylinder wrench,

(4) adult and infant oxygen masks and

(5) an infant bag mask resuscitator (with 100% oxygen adapter).

All of this equipment can be bought at a medical supply company. It's a good idea to compare prices of oxygen cylinders and regulators at an industrial gas supply company. A "D" size medical oxygen cylinder costs about $45 plus $5 for the contents. Regulators come in different types and prices. All of ours have a pressure gauge to let us know how much oxygen is in the cylinder, and a liter-flow gauge to know how much you are delivering. A new regulator commonly costs $50.

We've built kits that are divided into two parts: an open compartment for the masks and bag mask, and a circular slot for the cylinder. The kit is made of plywood and covered with vinyl, making it waterproof and strong enough to protect the equipment.

Use of the equipment

Begin by taking the cylinder wrench and slowly opening the valve at the top of the cylinder, allowing a short blast of oxygen to come out. Then close it back up. This clears the valve of any dust that could be blown into the regulator.

Next, install the regulator onto the cylinder. Make sure the plastic washer is inserted between the regulator and the cylinder. Tighten the regulator exactly and securely to avoid accidents, leakage, or damage to the equipment.

Now open the valve at the top of the cylinder. The pressure gauge should read 2200 pounds on a full tank. Make sure there are no leaks. You can now turn on the flow meter to the desired liter flow (4-8 liters per minute for anyone except emphysema patients).

The adult oxygen mask is used when the mother needs oxygen. The infant oxygen mask is used when the baby is born, is breathing, but does not have good color. The infant bag mask resuscitator is used when the baby is born but is not breathing on his own. The 100% oxygen adapter for the bag mask should be used on any newborn who is not breathing on his own and who does not have a good color after 1 or 2 minutes. Some bag masks have an adjustable pressure cut-off to insure safety of the newborn's lungs. Bag masks that don't have a pressure cut-off can be outfitted with a manometer (an airway pressure gauge) which will show how much pressure is being delivered (15-20 cm. of water is safe). After bag-masking a newborn with 100% oxygen, his color will hopefully get better. When that happens, take the 100% adapter off and use the mixture. One hundred percent oxygen should only be given as long as it is needed to keep the baby pink, because it is known to be damaging to the newborn's eyes—especially the premature newborn—if it is used for prolonged periods. Infant bag masks are an expensive but useful tool. They retail for about $75.

Always handle your oxygen equipment with care. Be sure it is well secured before you move it. To clean the masks and bag mask, use acetone and not alcohol because alcohol will dry and crack the plastic.

Remember: *Oxygen is not flammable and will not explode, but it will support combustion.* Sparks or a burning cigarette may become a problem in an oxygen-enriched atmosphere.

This oxygen kit can be an invaluable tool if these directions and precautions are used.

Use of the DeLee Infant Suction Set

The DeLee infant suction set is a portable suction device that works like a water pipe. It's a small plastic bottle with two tubes coming out of the top. It is used when an ear syringe doesn't reach deeply enough into the airway to clear out all the mucus. To use it, place one tube in your mouth and put the other tube through the baby's mouth into his trachea. Slide it down carefully about 4 or 5 inches (depending on the size of the baby) until you meet a little resistance. This will be the bottom of the trachea, where it divides into the bronchi. As you slide it in, suck in on the tube in your mouth. Then pull the tube slowly out of the airway, continuing to suck on the other tube. This will draw out mucus and any fluids from the baby's airway and trap them in the bottle. *Keep the tube that touches the baby sterile.*

D. Necessary Nursing Skills

Blood Pressure

Blood pressure is the term that refers to the (liquid) pressure exerted by the blood on the walls of the vessels at a given point in the circulatory system. The beating of the heart forces the blood through the arteries, maintaining the pressure of the blood within them. The arteries are made up of elastic tissue, so they expand a little bit as the blood pulses through them.

The blood pressure is greatest in the arteries nearest the heart. It becomes less as the blood is forced into the arterioles, then the capillaries, and finally reaches the veins on its way back to the heart.

When you measure blood pressure, you are interested in two kinds of pressure:

Systolic pressure is the pressure in the arteries when the heart is contracted and is pushing the blood at the peak of its force.

Diastolic pressure is the pressure in the arteries when the heart is relaxed between beats.

To measure blood pressure, you use a blood pressure cuff, or *sphygmomanometer.* The usual method for measuring blood pressure in an adult is to measure the pressure at the brachial artery, on the inside of the arm, just above the elbow. The pressure is recorded in millimeters of mercury.

How to Measure Blood Pressure

The size of the cuff you use can affect the accuracy of your readings. If too large, the reading will be lower than accurate; if too small, the

461

reading will be higher than it should be. If you are dealing with a woman who is quite overweight, you may need to obtain a special cuff in order to obtain an accurate reading. Generally speaking, the width of the cuff should be about 20% wider than the diameter of the woman's arm.

Use the same routine when you take blood pressures: ask the woman to take the same position for each reading and take it on the same arm every time, as the blood pressure can vary between arms. The first blood pressure you take on the woman is important, since this will be the reference point for all future readings. Make sure she is well relaxed before you start.

Ask the woman to sit down with her forearm resting, palm upwards, on a flat surface. The cuff should be wrapped snugly around her arm at the same level as her heart, and her arm should be relaxed. Put the earpieces of the stethoscope in your ears (curved ends pointing forward). Locate the brachial artery by feeling its pulse beneath your fingers. Place the stethoscope on the artery. (You won't hear anything meaningful through the stethoscope until you have pumped up the pressure bag, putting pressure on the artery.) Tighten the valve screw on the rubber bulb, and inflate the pressure bag by squeezing the rubber bulb. Continue inflating the bag until the mercury column reaches about 150 mmHg. Then slowly release the valve screw so that the air is gradually released and the column of mercury begins to fall at a steady rate. If it starts to fall too fast, tighten the screw till you have adjusted the rate so you can easily tell what's going on. Note the pressure reading of the column of mercury when you first hear a faint beat of the pulse through the stethoscope. This is the systolic reading, the measure of the greatest pressure that the arterial system has to bear. Normal systolic pressure ranges from 100 to 125 mmHg, with some variation. The systolic pressure varies a fair amount according to exertion and emotional condition.

After noticing the point where the pulse is first heard (the systolic pressure), continue letting the air slowly escape from the bag. The diastolic pressure will usually be between 60 and 80 mmHg. The pulse will grow louder and more distinct for a while, then will change to a softer swishing sound, which indicates that the brachial artery is no longer under pressure. The diastolic pressure is recorded at the point where the sound changed from loud and distinct to soft and swishing.

When you record blood pressure, you write the systolic pressure first, followed by the diastolic. For instance: 115/70, or 105/60l.

462

Giving Injections

To inject a local anesthetic such as xylocaine or lidocaine to numb the area of a laceration or episiotomy before stitching:

Materials:
• a 25-gauge needle 5/8 inch long, with a 5 cc. syringe
• bottle of local anesthetic
• cotton balls
• alcohol

To draw the anesthetic up into the syringe, wet a cotton ball with alcohol and wipe it once across the rubber seal of the bottle of anesthetic. Remove the wrapping from the sterile syringe. Remove the plastic cap from the needle and make sure the needle is well-fixed to the barrel of the syringe. *Remember to keep the needle sterile at all times until you are finished with it.* Pull back the plunger so that you fill the barrel with air to the same amount as the amount of anesthetic you want to draw up. Stick the needle through the middle of the rubber seal, push the plunger down, pushing the air into the bottle. Invert the bottle, making sure that the tip of the needle is immersed in the liquid, and pull back the plunger to the amount of anesthetic you want. When the barrel of the syringe is as full as you want it, pull the needle out of the bottle. Holding the syringe with the needle up, flick your finger on the side of the barrel a few times to bring any air bubbles to the surface. Then push the plunger in a little bit to push out any air bubbles that may have collected.

Anesthetic should be injected just below the surface of the skin of each of the cut edges of the taint. Push in a small amount when the tip of the needle is 1/8 inch into the tissue, then, gently, push the needle up just inside the cut edge, pushing the plunger as you go. The anesthetic infiltrating into the tissue will plump the tissue out a little at the same time that it numbs. Be careful not to inject so much anesthetic that the tissue becomes over-swollen. Check what will be your stitching line for numbness by poking there gently with the needle. Usually no anesthetic is needed for repairing the deep muscle layers or the lining of the birth canal.

Fig. 122. Breaking the Ampule.

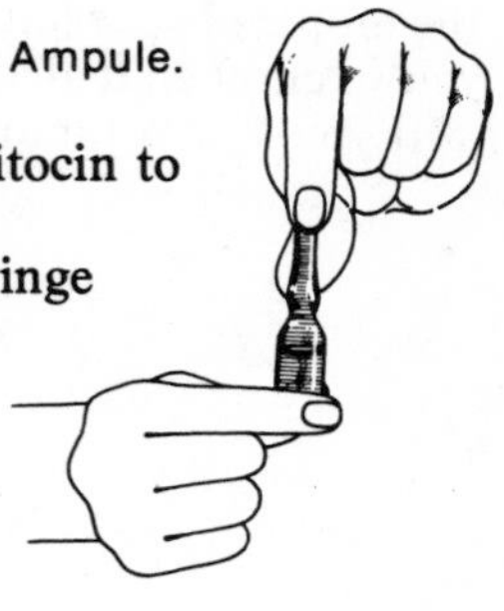

Injecting an oxytocic
To inject an oxytocic such as methergine or pitocin to control bleeding in the third stage, you'll need:
• a 21-gauge needle 1 inch long, with 3 cc. syringe
• ampule of oxytocic (methergine or pitocin)
• cotton balls
• alcohol
Break the glass ampule so that any glass slivers will fly away from you.

Remove the wrapping from the sterile syringe. Stick the needle into the slightly tilted ampule and pull the plunger back to the amount of oxytocic you want to inject. Locate the site on the mother's thigh for the injection and swab it with an alcohol-soaked cotton ball.

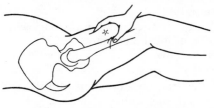

Fig. 123.
Site for Intra-
Muscular Injection.

Hold the needle perpendicular to the skin and make a quick insertion to as deep as the needle will reach. If the lady has a lot of fat there, use a longer needle. Use some wrist action in making the puncture, as if easily throwing a dart. Pull back the plunger slightly and if no blood enters the barrel, slowly inject the oxytocic and rapidly withdraw the needle, keeping it perpendicular to the skin. Place a dry, sterile cotton ball over the injection site and massage it for a few seconds.

E. Breast Self-Exam

Breast Self-Examination
Most lumps you find in your breasts are harmless, or *benign*. A lot of the breast tissue is fat, so they naturally feel a little lumpy. Feel them and get to know what they normally feel like. You should check them once a month, one week after you start your period. The reason for this is that they're less tender and they tend to get a little lumpier right before and during your period.
Stand in front of a mirror, and raise your arms. This tightens the skin so you can see any abnormalities easier. Look for any slight dents, since cancerous tissue sometimes causes this. Look and see that your nipples look normal. Then lie down, and put your left hand behind your head. With your right hand with the fingers flat, start at the nipple of your left breast, and move in a spiral motion outward until you've checked it all out. Do the other side. Then sit up and repeat it.
If you find a lump, see your doctor.

F. Keeping Records

These are some of the forms we use for prenatal clinic and birthings.

Prenatal Record

Name_____ Estimated Due Date_____ Parent's Address: ____

Address_____ Age _____ _____

_____ Birthdate _____ _____

Father's Name_____ Farm   Other Farm   Off the Farm   Hospital Bill Agreemeı.

PATIENTS HISTORY: (circle)

asthma, TB, respiratory disease, rheumatic fever, heart trouble, high blood pressure, low blood pressure, cancer, German measles, diabetes, thyroid problems, epilepsy, bladder infections, kidney disease or infections, phlebitis, ill effects from medicine, varicose veins, ulcers, hepatitis, pelvic infection.

Details: _____

Allergies (type): _____

List any injuries, surgery, or hospitalization with dates: _____

_____

_____

Blood transfusions?_____Give details _____

Gonorrhea: Yes _____ No_____Year _____Details of treatment _____

Syphilis: Yes_____ No _____Year _____Details of treatment _____

Herpes II: Yes_____ No_____Year _____Details of treatment _____

Birth control pills: Yes_____ No_____Type _____ Length of time taken _____

　　　　Age when began taking _____ complications or side effects _____

Intra-uterine devices: Yes_____ No_____ Still in place?_____

　　　　complications or side effects _____

Other methods of birth control: _____ How long used?_____

　　　　complications or side effects _____

Difficulty in conceiving: Yes_____ No_____ reason if known _____

On any medications now? (name)_____

Date of last Pap smear _____ Results _____

Diet: Vegetarian _____(complete veg., lacto-veg., fruitarian, macrobiotic) How long? _____

　　　　Non-vegetarian _____

Menstrual history: Age at onset _____ Length of cycle _____ days   Flow_____ days

　　　　Scant _____ Average _____ Heavy _____ Regular_____ Irregular _____

PREVIOUS PREGNANCIES:

Number_____

Live births_____

Stillbirths_____

Miscarriages_____

Abortions _____

Pregnancies ending in miscarriage or induced abortion:

Year	Length of Gestation	Miscarriage or Abortion?	Complications/Comments

PROBLEMS DURING PREVIOUS PREGNANCIES:

	Number of pregnancy	Which trimester	Details	Drugs or treatment (list all drugs taken)
Weight gain over 25 lbs.				
Morning sickness (1st trimester)				
Continued nausea (2nd or 3rd trimester)				
Water retention				
Bladder infection				
Varicose veins				
Kidney problems				
Protein in urine				
Glucose in urine				
Pre-eclampsia				
Eclampsia				
High blood pressure				
Anemia				
Spotting or bleeding				
Early onset of labor				
Vaginal infections				
Other				

PAST BIRTHS: Number_____; Number premature_____; Multiple Births_____; Now alive_____

	year	home, hosp., or other	sex	weeks gestation	hours labor	anesthesia	type of delivery*	presentation**	living now	Comments/Complications
1.										
2.										
3.										
4.										
5.										
6.										
7.										
8.										Mother: prolonged 2nd or 3rd stage, hemorrhage, polyhydramnios, postpartum depression, prolonged rupture of membranes Baby: birth injuries, cong. abnormality, jaundice, nursing problems, failure to thrive

* I=Induced, C= C-section, V= Vaginal   ** V=Vertex, B=Breech, F=Face, B=Brow, T=Transverse

History since last menstrual period: LMP_____

sure?   yes____ no____   normal?   yes____ no____

bleeding since?   yes____ no____   X-rays?   yes____ no____

rashes, virus infections yes____ no____   vaginal discharge   yes____ no____

Medications_____

Comments_____

FAMILY HISTORY:

	Patient's Father	Patient's Mother	Patient's Siblings	Paternal Relatives	Maternal Relatives	Outcome and Details
Allergies						
Cancer						
Congenital abnormality						
Diabetes (age discovered)						
Epilepsy						
High blood pressure						
Heart disease						
Kidney disease						
TB						
Twins						
Other						

PATIENT'S MOTHER'S OBSTETRICAL HISTORY:

Number of pregnancies_____ number of births_____

Number of hospital births_____ number of home births_____other_____

Number of cesarean sections_____ number of breech deliveries_____

Complications of pregnancy_____

Complications of labor or delivery (prolonged labor, hemorrhage, etc.)_____

Number of babies breast-fed three months or more_____difficulties_____

Attitude towards childbirth (positive, negative, so-so)_____ details_____

Hormones taken during any of pregnancies (estrogen, progesterone, diethylstilbestrol, others): Yes_____ No_____Don't know_____

Did she take diethylstilbestrol during pregnancy leading to birth of patient? Yes_____ No_____ Don't know_____

PHYSICAL EXAMINATION:

Height_____ Pre-pregnancy weight_____T.P.R. _____

General appearance_____

HEENT_____

Nodes_____

Neck and thyroid_____

Chest and lungs_____

Breasts and nipples_____

Heart_____

Abdomen and height of fundus_____

Joints and extremities (varicosities and edema)_____

Neuro_____

Skin_____

PELVIC EXAMINATION:

Puss_____ D.C._____ S/S notch_____

Cervix_____ Shape/sacrum_____ Spines_____

Uterus (size)_____ Coccyx_____ Bi-ischial dia._____

Ovaries and tubes_____ Arch_____ Largest baby delivered_____

Rectum_____ Evaluation_____

Examined by_____

NAME _____ DUE DATE _____

4

LABORATORY RESULTS:

Blood type_____ Rh factor_____ Blood type of father_____

Hematocrit			Antibodies			Urinalysis	Date	Results
	Date	Results		Date	Results	Urinalysis		
3 mo.			5 mo.			VDRL (Syphilis)		
7 mo.			6 mo.			Rubella titer		
			7 mo.			Gonorrhea culture		
			8 mo.			Hemoglobin		
						Pap smear		
						Other		

Roll over test (28-32 weeks): Negative_____Positive_____   (Blood pressure: Side_____ Back_____)

PRENATAL EXAMINATIONS:

date	weeks gestation	weight	fundus (cm.)	presentation	BP	urine		FHT	examiner	REMARKS (Headaches, dizziness, nausea, vomiting, bleeding, fever, edema, nutrition, urinary complaints, quickening, effacement, station)
						alb.	glu.			

NOTES:

DATE	

Birthing Record

Parents' Names_____

Baby's Name_____ Date_____ Time_____

Male_____ Female_____ Multiple birth_____ Midwife_____ Assistant_____

Others who attended_____

Live birth_____ Stillbirth_____ Father Present_____ Phase of the Moon_____

No. of Pregnancy_____   No. of previous births_____   No. of miscarriages or abortions_____

<table>
<tr><td>

BABY

Apgar: 1 min._____ 5 min_____

Wt._____Wks. gestation_____

Length_____Head circum._____

Presentation:_____

  Cephalic-vertex_____face____brow_____

  Breech: frank_____footling____complete__

  Other_____

Position: Occiput forward_____

  Occiput behind_____

  Other_____

Amniotic fluid (amount):_____

  Meconium staining____Time noted_____

Resp. problems_____

FHT: range_____

    decelerations_____

Birth injuries_____

Congenital malformation_____

Cord vessels_____

Medications·_____

</td><td>

MOTHER

Complications of pregnancy - polyhydramnios,

toxemia, other_____

Significant lab results: Hct, UA, VDRL,

rubella, other_____

Epis____Tear_____ 1°__2°__3°__Stitches_____

Length of labor (total):_____

  1st stage_____2nd stage_____3rd stage_____

  Precipitous labor_____

Rupture of Membranes:

  Date and time_____

  Premature_____1st stage_____2nd stage_____

  Ruptured artificially_____ Spontaneously___

Placenta normal_____

Cervical lacerations_____

Post-partum hemorrhage_____

Intake_____Output_____

Medications: Pitocin-1 amp IM_____

  Pitocin-1 amp I.V. drip_____

  Methergine-1 amp IM_____

  Methergine-1q_h X_____

</td></tr>
</table>

NOTES ON LABOR AND DELIVERY

Date/Hr.	FHT	BP or pulse	Dilation	Station	Comments

POST PARTUM: Infection_____Hemorrhage_____RhoGam_____

6 wks. check: General appearance☐

Perineum ☐

Cervix ☐

Uterus, tubes, ovaries☐

Pap smear_____ Hct_____ UA_____

Baby☐

Breast-feeding Yes ☐   No ☐

NOTES:_____

_____

_____

_____

_____

Birthing record, side 2, bottom. Top is lined for notes.

Newborn physical record, side 1, top.

Newborn Physical

Name _____ Birthdate/hour _____

Parents _____ Midwife _____

General Appearance

Skin

Head

Eyes

ENT

Mouth

Neck

Chest & Lungs

Heart

Abdomen

Joints & Extremities

Neuro

Genito-Urinary

Head Circ.

Length

Weight

G. Tables and Charts

This is usually called the EDC—estimated date of confinement—but since we don't believe in confining ladies in labor, we're calling it the EDD—estimated due date.

The first line of each set of two is the date of the first day of the last menstrual period; the second line is the EDD.

January	1	2	3	4	5	6	7	8	9	10	11	12	13	14	15	16	17	18	19	20	21	22	23	24	25	26	27	28	29	30	31	January
October	8	9	10	11	12	13	14	15	16	17	18	19	20	21	22	23	24	25	26	27	28	29	30	31	1	2	3	4	5	6	7	November
February	1	2	3	4	5	6	7	8	9	10	11	12	13	14	15	16	17	18	19	20	21	22	23	24	25	26	27	28				February
November	8	9	10	11	12	13	14	15	16	17	18	19	20	21	22	23	24	25	26	27	28	29	30	1	2	3	4	5				December
March	1	2	3	4	5	6	7	8	9	10	11	12	13	14	15	16	17	18	19	20	21	22	23	24	25	26	27	28	29	30	31	March
December	6	7	8	9	10	11	12	13	14	15	16	17	18	19	20	21	22	23	24	25	26	27	28	29	30	31	1	2	3	4	5	January
April	1	2	3	4	5	6	7	8	9	10	11	12	13	14	15	16	17	18	19	20	21	22	23	24	25	26	27	28	29	30		April
January	6	7	8	9	10	11	12	13	14	15	16	17	18	19	20	21	22	23	24	25	26	27	28	29	30	31	1	2	3	4		February
May	1	2	3	4	5	6	7	8	9	10	11	12	13	14	15	16	17	18	19	20	21	22	23	24	25	26	27	28	29	30	31	May
February	5	6	7	8	9	10	11	12	13	14	15	16	17	18	19	20	21	22	23	24	25	26	27	28	1	2	3	4	5	6	7	March
June	1	2	3	4	5	6	7	8	9	10	11	12	13	14	15	16	17	18	19	20	21	22	23	24	25	26	27	28	29	30		June
March	8	9	10	11	12	13	14	15	16	17	18	19	20	21	22	23	24	25	26	27	28	29	30	31	1	2	3	4	5	6		April
July	1	2	3	4	5	6	7	8	9	10	11	12	13	14	15	16	17	18	19	20	21	22	23	24	25	26	27	28	29	30	31	July
April	7	8	9	10	11	12	13	14	15	16	17	18	19	20	21	22	23	24	25	26	27	28	29	30	1	2	3	4	5	6	7	May
August	1	2	3	4	5	6	7	8	9	10	11	12	13	14	15	16	17	18	19	20	21	22	23	24	25	26	27	28	29	30	31	August
May	8	9	10	11	12	13	14	15	16	17	18	19	20	21	22	23	24	25	26	27	28	29	30	31	1	2	3	4	5	6	7	June
September	1	2	3	4	5	6	7	8	9	10	11	12	13	14	15	16	17	18	19	20	21	22	23	24	25	26	27	28	29	30		September
June	8	9	10	11	12	13	14	15	16	17	18	19	20	21	22	23	24	25	26	27	28	29	30	1	2	3	4	5	6	7		July
October	1	2	3	4	5	6	7	8	9	10	11	12	13	14	15	16	17	18	19	20	21	22	23	24	25	26	27	28	29	30	31	October
July	8	9	10	11	12	13	14	15	16	17	18	19	20	21	22	23	24	25	26	27	28	29	30	31	1	2	3	4	5	6	7	August
November	1	2	3	4	5	6	7	8	9	10	11	12	13	14	15	16	17	18	19	20	21	22	23	24	25	26	27	28	29	30		November
August	8	9	10	11	12	13	14	15	16	17	18	19	20	21	22	23	24	25	26	27	28	29	30	31	1	2	3	4	5	6	7	September
December	1	2	3	4	5	6	7	8	9	10	11	12	13	14	15	16	17	18	19	20	21	22	23	24	25	26	27	28	29	30	31	December
September	7	8	9	10	11	12	13	14	15	16	17	18	19	20	21	22	23	24	25	26	27	28	29	30	1	2	3	4	5	6	7	October

Pound/Ounce--Gram Conversion Table

1 oz. = 28 gm.   1 lb. = 454 gm.

oz.	lbs. 3	4	5	6	7	8	9	10
0	1361	1814	2268	2722	3175	3629	4082	4536
1	1389	1843	2296	2750	3203	3657	4111	4564
2	1417	1871	2325	2778	3232	3685	4139	4593
3	1446	1899	2353	2807	3260	3714	4167	4621
4	1474	1928	2381	2835	3289	3742	4196	4649
5	1503	1956	2410	2863	3317	3770	4224	4678
6	1531	1984	2438	2892	3345	3799	4252	4706
7	1559	2013	2466	2920	3374	3827	4281	4734
8	1588	2041	2495	2948	3402	3856	4309	4763
9	1616	2070	2523	2977	3430	3884	4338	4791
10	1644	2098	2551	3005	3459	3912	4366	4819
11	1673	2126	2580	3033	3487	3941	4394	4848
12	1701	2155	2608	3062	3515	3969	4423	4876
13	1729	2183	2637	3090	3544	3997	4451	4904
14	1758	2211	2665	3118	3572	4026	4479	4933
15	1786	2240	2693	3147	3600	4054	4508	4961

Centigrade--Fahrenheit Conversion

C°	F°
35.5 =	95.9
36 =	96.8
36.5 =	97.7
37 =	98.6
37.5 =	99.5
38 =	100.4
38.5 =	101.3
39 =	102.2
39.5 =	103.1
40 =	104

$$F = 9/5\,C + 32$$
$$C = 5/9\,(F - 32)$$

CLINICAL ESTIMATION OF GESTATIONAL AGE

Examination First Hours

PHYSICAL FINDINGS		WEEKS GESTATION 20-48
VERNIX		APPEARS (20–24) · COVERS BODY, THICK LAYER (25–37) · ON BACK, SCALP, IN CREASES (38–39) · SCANT, IN CREASES (40–41) · NO VERNIX (42–48)
BREAST TISSUE AND AREOLA		AREOLA & NIPPLE BARELY VISIBLE, NO PALPABLE BREAST TISSUE (20–33) · AREOLA RAISED (34–35) · 1–2 MM NODULE (36) · 3–5 MM (37) · 5–6 MM (38–39) · 7–10 MM (40–43) · >12 MM (44–48)
EAR	FORM	FLAT, SHAPELESS (20–33) · BEGINNING INCURVING SUPERIOR (34–35) · INCURVING UPPER 2/3 PINNAE (36–37) · WELL-DEFINED INCURVING TO LOBE (38–48)
	CARTILAGE	PINNA SOFT, STAYS FOLDED (20–33) · CARTILAGE SCANT RETURNS SLOWLY FROM FOLDING (34–36) · THIN CARTILAGE SPRINGS BACK FROM FOLDING (37) · PINNA FIRM, REMAINS ERECT FROM HEAD (38–48)
SOLE CREASES		SMOOTH SOLES C CREASES (20–33) · 1–2 ANTERIOR CREASES (34–35) · 2–3 ANTERIOR CREASES (36) · CREASES ANTERIOR 2/3 SOLE (37) · CREASES INVOLVING HEEL (38–39) · DEEPER CREASES OVER ENTIRE SOLE (40–48)
SKIN	THICKNESS & APPEARANCE	THIN, TRANSLUCENT SKIN, PLETHORIC, VENULES OVER ABDOMEN, EDEMA (20–33) · SMOOTH THICKER, NO EDEMA (34–36) · PINK (37) · FEW VESSELS (38–39) · SOME DESQUAMATION PALE PINK (40–41) · THICK, PALE, DESQUAMATION OVER ENTIRE BODY (42–48)
	NAIL PLATES	AP-PEAR (20–23) · NAILS TO FINGER TIPS (34–38) · NAILS EXTEND WELL BEYOND FINGER TIPS (42–48)
HAIR		APPEARS ON HEAD (21–23) · EYE BROWS & LASHES (24–26) · FINE, WOOLLY, BUNCHES OUT FROM HEAD (27–35) · SILKY, SINGLE STRANDS LAYS FLAT (36–39) · RECEDING HAIRLINE OR LOSS OF BABY HAIR SHORT, FINE UNDERNEATH (40–48)
LANUGO		AP-PEARS (20–22) · COVERS ENTIRE BODY (23–33) · VANISHES FROM FACE (34–36) · PRESENT ON SHOULDERS (37–39) · NO LANUGO (40–48)
GENITALIA	TESTES	TESTES PALPABLE IN INGUINAL CANAL (34–35) · IN UPPER SCROTUM (36–38) · IN LOWER SCROTUM (40–48)
	SCROTUM	FEW RUGAE (34–36) · RUGAE, ANTERIOR PORTION (37–38) · RUGAE COVER (39–41) · PENDULOUS (42–48)
	LABIA & CLITORIS	PROMINENT CLITORIS LABIA MAJORA SMALL WIDELY SEPARATED (34–36) · LABIA MAJORA LARGER NEARLY COVERED CLITORIS (37–39) · LABIA MINORA & CLITORIS COVERED (40–48)
SKULL FIRMNESS		BONES ARE SOFT (20–33) · SOFT TO 1" FROM ANTERIOR FONTANELLE (34–36) · SPONGY AT EDGES OF FONTANELLE CENTER FIRM (37–38) · BONES HARD SUTURES EASILY DISPLACED (39) · BONES HARD, CANNOT BE DISPLACED (40–48)
POSTURE	RESTING	HYPOTONIC LATERAL DECUBITUS (20–27) · HYPOTONIC (28–30) · BEGINNING FLEXION THIGH (31) · STRONGER HIP FLEXION (32–33) · FROG-LIKE (34–35) · FLEXION ALL LIMBS (36–37) · HYPERTONIC (38–41) · VERY HYPERTONIC (42–48)
	RECOIL - LEG	NO RECOIL (20–30) · PARTIAL RECOIL (34–37) · PROMPT RECOIL (40–48)
	ARM	NO RECOIL (20–33) · BEGIN FLEXION NO RECOIL (34–35) · PROMPT RECOIL MAY BE INHIBITED (36–37) · PROMPT RECOIL AFTER 30" INHIBITION (38–48)

Confirmatory Neurologic Examination to be Done After 24 Hours

PHYSICAL FINDINGS		WEEKS GESTATION 20-48
TONE	HEEL TO EAR	NO RESISTANCE (26–29) · SOME RESISTANCE (32–33) · IMPOSSIBLE (34–35) (38–39)
	SCARF SIGN	NO RESISTANCE (24–29) · ELBOW PASSES MIDLINE (32–33) · ELBOW AT MIDLINE (34–37) · ELBOW DOES NOT REACH MIDLINE (40–48)
	NECK FLEXORS (HEAD LAG)	ABSENT (28–33) · HEAD IN PLANE OF BODY (38–39) · HOLDS HEAD (42–43)
	NECK EXTENSORS	HEAD BEGINS TO RIGHT ITSELF FROM FLEXED POSITION (32–33) · GOOD RIGHTING CANNOT HOLD IT (34–35) · HOLDS HEAD FEW SECONDS (36–37) · KEEPS HEAD IN LINE C TRUNK>40° (40–41) · TURNS HEAD FROM SIDE TO SIDE (44–45)
	BODY EXTENSORS	STRAIGHTENING OF LEGS (32–33) · STRAIGHTENING OF TRUNK (36–37) · STRAIGHTENING OF HEAD & TRUNK TOGETHER (40–41)
	VERTICAL POSITIONS	WHEN HELD UNDER ARMS, BODY SLIPS THROUGH HANDS (30–33) · ARMS HOLD BABY LEGS EXTENDED (34–35) · GOOD SUPPORT C ARMS (38–39)
	HORIZONTAL POSITIONS	HYPOTONIC ARMS & LEGS STRAIGHT (30–33) · ARMS AND LEGS FLEXED (36–37) · HEAD & BACK EVEN FLEXED EXTREMITIES (38–39) · HEAD ABOVE BACK (40–41)
FLEXION ANGLES	POPLITEAL	NO RESISTANCE (20–28) · 150° (30–31) · 110° (32–33) · 100° (34) · 90° (36–37) · 80° (38–39)
	ANKLE	45° (32–33) · 20° (34–35) · 0 (38–39) · A PRE-TERM WHO HAS REACHED 40 WEEKS STILL HAS A 40° ANGLE (44–48)
	WRIST (SQUARE WINDOW)	90° (28) · 60° (32) · 45° (34) · 30° (36) · 0 (38)
REFLEXES	SUCKING	WEAK NOT SYNCHRONIZED C SWALLOWING (28–33) · STRONGER SYNCHRONIZED (34–35) · PERFECT (36–37) · PERFECT HAND TO MOUTH (38–39) · PERFECT (42–48)
	ROOTING	LONG LATENCY PERIOD SLOW, IMPERFECT (28–30) · HAND TO MOUTH (31) · BRISK, COMPLETE, DURABLE (34–37) · COMPLETE (40–48)
	GRASP	FINGER GRASP IS GOOD STRENGTH IS POOR (28–33) · STRONGER (34–37) · CAN LIFT BABY OFF BED INVOLVES ARMS (38–41) · HANDS OPEN (46–48)
	MORO	BARELY APPARENT (24–27) · WEAK NOT ELICITED EVERY TIME (28–33) · STRONGER (34) · COMPLETE C ARM EXTENSION OPEN FINGERS, CRY (35) · ARM ADDUCTION ADDED (38–39) · ?BEGINS TO LOSE MORO (46–48)
	CROSSED EXTENSION	FLEXION & EXTENSION IN A RANDOM, PURPOSELESS PATTERN (28–33) · EXTENSION BUT NO ADDUCTION (34) · STILL INCOMPLETE (36–37) · EXTENSION ADDUCTION FANNING OF TOES (38–39) · COMPLETE (42–45)
	AUTOMATIC WALK	MINIMAL (31) · BEGINS TIPTOEING GOOD SUPPORT ON SOLE (34) · FAST TIPTOEING (36) · HEEL-TOE PROGRESSION WHOLE SOLE OF FOOT (38–41) · A PRE-TERM WHO HAS REACHED 40 WEEKS WALKS ON TOES (44–45) · ?BEGINS TO LOSE AUTOMATIC WALK (46–48)
	PUPILLARY REFLEX	ABSENT (26–28) · APPEARS (30–31) · PRESENT (38–48)
	GLABELLAR TAP	ABSENT (28–31) · APPEARS (32–34) · PRESENT (39–48)
	TONIC NECK REFLEX	ABSENT (28–30) · APPEARS (32–36) · PRESENT (40–48)
	NECK-RIGHTING	ABSENT (30–33) · APPEARS (34–36) · PRESENT AFTER 37 WEEKS (37–48)

Reproduced with permission from Kempe CH Silver HK O Brien D (editors): Current Pediatric Diagnosis & Treatment 4th ed. Lange 1976.

H. STATISTICS FOR 1723 BIRTHS MANAGED BY THE FARM MIDWIVES
from October 8, 1970 to December 31, 1989

Total Births	1723	
First time mothers	746	43%
Residents of The Farm (complete vegetarians)	797	46.4%
Amish mothers	92	5.3%
Others	835	48.5%
Home Births	1650	95.8%
Hospital Births	73	4.2%
Cesarean sections	25	1.4%
Births with anesthesia	26	1.5%
Vaginal births with forceps	8	.46%
Vaginal births by vacuum extraction	0	0
Vertex births	1670	96.9%
Breech births	52	3%
Frank breech	41	
Footling breech	10	
Complete breech	1	
Face presentations	6	0.3%
(All vaginal births)		
Brow presentation	3	0.17%
(One cesarean, two vaginal)		
Transverse lie	1	
Occiput posterior births	29	1.7%
Twins (including one fetal death in utero; no cesareans)	8 sets	
Meconium staining	140	8.1%
(6 of these babies had respiratory distress syndrome; mortality 0)		
Maternal mortality	0	
Neonatal mortality*	10	(5 per 1000)
Three of these babies had lethal abnormalities		
Perinatal mortality**	18	(10.4 per 1000)
Three of these babies had lethal abnormalities. Six were hospitalized.		

Intact perineums	1220	70.8%
First degree tears & episiotomies	228	13.2%
Second degree tears & episiotomies	271	15.7%
Third degree tears & episiotomies	4	0.2%

Premature rupture of membranes	33
(2 cases of respiratory distress syndrome, 1 neonatal infection; no mortality)	

Congenital abnormalities	18	1%

Apgar scores for 1310 births
(75% of births resulted in Apgars of 8/10 or better)

10/10	583	44.5%
9/10	287	22%
8/90	122	9.3%

Pregnancy complications

death in utero	3
hypertension	11
pre-eclampsia	7
just 1 mother of the vegan (complete vegetarian) group	
blood incompatibility	2
placenta previa	3
urinary tract infection	1
pendulous abdomen	2
small gestation age baby/placental insufficiency (same mother)	4
incompetent cervix	4
prematurity	16

*Neonatal mortality is defined in North America as "death of a live born infant up to 28 days of age."

**Perinatal mortality is defined in North America as "fetal deaths of 28 or more weeks' gestation plus infant deaths under 7 days of age. Mortality figures include births which took place in the hospital.

Total perinatal mortality in the United States in 1980 was just under 18 per 1,000, according to the U.S. definition of "perinatal mortality".*** This figure does not include deaths in utero, which I have included in our perinatal mortality figure, which corresponds to that used by most European countries and included the intrauterine deaths from 20 weeks of gestation on.

****Obstetrics and Gynecology: The Clinical Core*, Fourth Edition, Ralph M. Wynn, Lea & Febinger, 1988.

Index

Terms that might be looked for in emergencies are set in **bold type**.
Page listings for illustrations are set in italics—for example, *437*.

477

EDITORS: Rachel Sythe   Matthew McClure   Kathryn McClure
Margaret Nofziger   Dr. Jeffrey Hergenrather, *Medical Consultant*
Paul Meltzer, *Medical Consultant* Eleanor Martin Sarah Hergenrather
Eleanor Dale Evans   Cynthia Holzapfel

ART: Mark Schlichting, *Art Director*   Peter Hoyt   Nancy Presley
Edith Lucas   Drury Grigsby   Bonnie Kaufman   Richard Martin
James Hartman

PHOTOGRAPHY: Daniel Luna   Clifford Chappell   Edine Frohman
David Frohman   Valerie Epstein   Catherine Hartman   Anne Queeney
Vance Glavis   Brian Hansen   Steve Owens

Order these fine books directly from Book
Publishing Company:

Please send $1 per book for postage and handling.

Mail your order to:
    Book Publishing Company
    PO Box 99
    Summertown, TN 38483